The Guide to Good Health

for Teens & Adults with Down Syndrome

The Guide to Good Health

for Teens & Adults with Down Syndrome

Brian Chicoine, M.D. & Dennis McGuire, Ph.D.

Woodbine House ◆ 2010

Publisher's note: The information contained in this book is not intended as a substitute for consultation with your child's health care providers. Although the authors, editor, and publisher made every attempt to ensure that the information in this book was up to date and accurate at the time of publication, recommended treatments and drug therapies may change as new medical or scientific information becomes available. Additionally, the authors, editor, and publisher are not responsible for errors or omissions or for consequences from application of this book. Any practice described in this book should be applied by the reader in close consultation with a qualified physician.

Library of Congress Cataloging-in-Publication Data

Chicoine, Brian.
  The guide to good health for teens & adults with Down syndrome / by Brian
Chicoine and Dennis McGuire.
      p. cm.
  Includes bibliographical references and index.
  ISBN 978-1-890627-89-8
  1. Down syndrome--Patients--Health and hygiene--Popular works. 2. Down
syndrome--Complications--Popular works. I. McGuire, Dennis Eugene. II. Title.
  RC571.C43 2010
  618.92'858842--dc22

                                                                    2010018783

Printed in the United States of America

First edition
10 9 8 7 6 5 4 3 2 1
                        JAN 2011

Table of Contents

Acknowledgements

We want to thank our patients of the Adult Down Syndrome Center and their families who welcome us into their lives and share their stories with us. We have the privilege of becoming repositories of the information we have learned from them. This book is an opportunity to compile that information and share it with them and others.

We also have the benefit of working with a fine group of colleagues and staff at the Center. Their outstanding and compassionate care for people with Down syndrome is exemplary. These individuals include Erin Dominiak, MD, Physician; Janet Bilodeau, CNP, Nurse Practitioner; Laura Iatropoulos, CMA, Office Coordinator and Certified Medical Assistant; Sharon Giannone, MOA, Medical Office Assistant; Carol Machiela, LPN, nurse; Jenny Howard, Outreach Coordinator; Nancy Wilson, Advocate; Shirley Lange, Patient Representative; Carol Jacobsen, Transcriptionist; and Eileen Walsh, RD, Nutritionist. We also thank dedicated volunteers Catherine Chicoine, Pat Brand, and Pat Lasch.

In addition, we want to recognize Advocate Health Care and the division that manages the Center, Advocate Medical Group. The Adult Down Syndrome Center is part of the mission of this faith-based health care system, and the support of many individuals needs to be recognized, including James Skogsbergh, President and CEO, Advocate Health Care; James Dan, MD, President Physician and Ambulatory Services; Tony Armada, President Advocate Lutheran General Hospital; Kevin McCune, MD, Chief Medical Officer Advocate Medical Group; Cynthia Job, Vice President, Practice Operations; Nancy Christie, Director Physician Practice Management; and Carol Rizzie, Advocate Foundation.

We are extremely fortunate for our patients to receive additional care, when needed, from other physicians in Advocate Medical Group and through Advocate Lutheran

General Hospital. There are many fine physicians who treat our patients with respect and dignity while providing quality care. These physicians include our fellow Family Medicine faculty: Judith Gravdal, MD, Chairman Department of Family Medicine and Director Family Medicine Residency, Stuart Goldman, MD, Greg Kirschner, MD, Bruce Perlow, MD, Tamar Perlow, MD, Bill Briner, MD, Mayank Shah, MD, Robin O'Meara, MD, Pat Piper, MD, Inna Gutman, MD, Kara Vormittag, MD, and Deb Haley, PhD.

We also benefit from working with the National Association for Down Syndrome. Their Executive Director, Diane Urhausen and their former Executive Director, Sheila Hebein, have been instrumental in the development of and support of the Center.

We also want to thank Susan Stokes, our editor at Woodbine House. With her guidance, this book has become more than we could have hoped.

Brian's Personal Acknowledgements

I would also like to thank the many people in my life who have supported and guided me, including:

- ◆ Louis Isert
- ◆ My parents
- ◆ My siblings, Mary Jo, David, Mark, Beth Ann, Mike, and Julie
- ◆ My daughters, Emily, Caitlin, and Laura
- ◆ And especially, my wife, Kathy.

Dennis's Personal Acknowledgements

I am so fortunate to have the support and encouragement of my wife, my son, my siblings, my parents—who were my first teachers—and all the people with Down syndrome, their families, and caregivers who continue to teach me.

Introduction

Is there really a need for a book on health care just about adults with Down syndrome? Couldn't you just read a general medical text and get the necessary information?

In fact, most of the information in a general medical text is just as important to the care of adults with Down syndrome as it is to the care of other adults. This book is not intended to replace a general medical text. What this book will do, however, is highlight differences in promoting

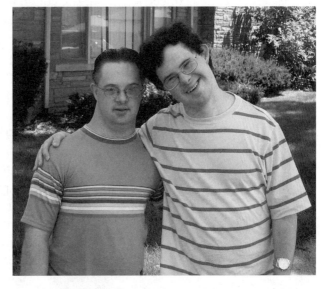

the health of adults with Down syndrome, address the health problems that are more common and those that are less common, and focus on how health problems sometimes present uniquely in adults with Down syndrome.

This book is written as a practical guide to health care for adults and adolescents with Down syndrome, and therefore does not cover medical problems that are concerns for people with Down syndrome of all ages. Other books in print already address health care concerns that can begin in childhood. This book is filled with case examples (in fact, each chapter starts with a case example). It is intended not only to help families and other caregivers promote health at home, but also to educate professionals about special treatment considerations for adults with Down syndrome in a health care setting. It is not meant to take the place of your health care providers' assessments or treatments. Instead, it is a supplement to that care; to assist in improving the understanding of health promotion and health care for people with Down syndrome.

Before we address these issues, it is important for you to understand how this book came to be written, understand the authors' approach to health, and define some ideas that are basic to this approach.

The authors have based the information in this book on their experiences in delivering health care to adults and adolescents with Down syndrome at the Adult Down Syndrome Center of Advocate Lutheran General Hospital in Park Ridge, Illinois. The Center was developed by the hospital and Advocate Medical Group at the request of the National Association for Down Syndrome, the parent group that serves the Chicago metropolitan area. These parents believed that their sons and daughters had received fine health care when they were children but were not receiving the same level of care as they reached adulthood.

The NADS members were concerned that their children's health problems were frequently dismissed as "just the Down syndrome." For example, shortly after the Center opened, the mother of a young man with Down syndrome (DS), a new patient of the Center, called concerned about the cough he had had for three weeks. He had recently been examined twice by his physician, and his mother had been told each time that the cough was "just the Down syndrome." We then examined him and

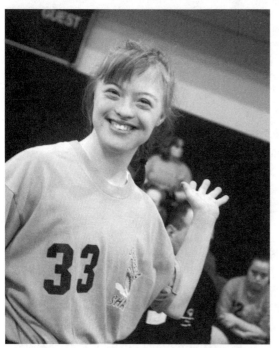

diagnosed pneumonia. The patient responded well to antibiotics and his cough disappeared.

With these types of concerns in mind, the Executive Director of the National Association for Down Syndrome, Sheila Hebein, approached the president of the hospital and asked that a clinic for adults with Down syndrome be established. The Center opened in 1992 and has served about 4500 adults and adolescents with Down syndrome as of this writing. This book is based on the knowledge we have accumulated in serving these patients and their families.

When the Center was being developed, families often asked the staff two questions. The first was, "Do you have a son or daughter with Down syndrome?" The underlying question seemed to be, "Can we trust you with the care of our son or daughter?" While neither of the authors has a child with Down syndrome, hopefully over the course of time, we have demonstrated our trustworthiness. (Interestingly, since the Center opened, the first author has discovered that he had a great uncle with Down syndrome who died in 1948 at the age of 40.) We believe that the trustworthiness comes not only from a desire to serve people with Down syndrome, but also to a willingness to listen to people with Down syndrome, their families, and their caregivers. One of the keys is being aware of, and willing to look for, health concerns that might be causing a problem rather than just blaming it on "the Down syndrome."

The other frequently asked question was about our training in caring for adults with Down syndrome. There was little education about adults with Down syndrome in the first author's medical school training or the second author's Ph.D. training in social work. In fact, the first author jokes that he had "five minutes of training in medical school about adults with Down syndrome and that is probably a five-minute exaggeration." While this lack of education would seem to be a huge detriment at the outset, it has actually been used to our advantage. Each of us approached our patients with an open mind (and a clean slate). This has allowed us to learn a great deal about our patients and to avoid getting stuck on some of the inaccurate information that was in print about adults with Down syndrome.

We did bring some of our own ideas to the development of the Center. The first was the definition of health. We use this definition:

> *Health is more than the absence of disease; it involves physical, mental, and spiritual wellbeing.*

This definition guides the type of care that we seek to provide.

One of the other preconceived notions that we had, based on our discussions with members of the parent group, was that behavioral and mental health issues would be an important part of the Center's services. In addition, we perceived that it would be essential to develop an understanding of how physical health problems could contribute to mental health issues, and to evaluate patients for these connections. Therefore, we developed a multidisciplinary center with this mission statement:

> **To enhance the well-being of adults with Down syndrome by providing comprehensive, holistic, community-based health care services by a multi-disciplinary team.**

We definitely believe in this mission statement and think it aptly describes what the Center does. However, the first author believes that our efforts could be summed up in more down-to-earth terms by this observation that Atticus Finch makes in *To Kill a Mockingbird*: "You never really know a man until you stand in his shoes and walk around in them."

We will never completely know what it is like to be a person with Down syndrome. However, we repeatedly find that if we try to understand our patients' perspective, it improves our care. Sometimes the most enlightening question we can ask ourselves is, "How would I feel in that situation?"

Patient Care at the Adult Down Syndrome Center

We see people with DS age 12 and older at the Adult Down Syndrome Center. Some patients use the Center for their primary care as well as to address issues more specifically associated with Down syndrome. They are seen for an annual evaluation but also when they develop medical problems such as a cough, sore throat, etc. Other individuals, particularly those who live further away, have a primary physician at home but visit the Center annually for an evaluation. A third group has a primary physician at home, comes annually for an evaluation, and also regularly receives care at the Center for specific issues—most commonly psychosocial issues.

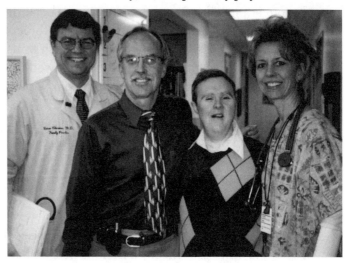

The annual evaluation at the Center includes a complete history and physical exam by a medical practitioner. A complete psychosocial assessment is also done by the psychosocial team. This evaluation includes questions about expressive language, activities of daily living, social support, social skills, and other related information. We diagnose and treat medical conditions as well as mental health conditions.

The Medical Home

In addition to treating medical and mental health conditions, the staff of the Center provides advocacy and coordination services. These services include providing educational materials, directing patients and families to additional resources, and assisting them through bureaucratic systems. We also help coordinate care with other specialists who are involved in the care of the individual.

In the pediatric arena, providing comprehensive primary care to the individual while also coordinating care with specialists is an approach referred to as the "medical home." The medical home is not a place. It is a family-professional relationship. It is based on mutual respect, involves coordination of care, and relies on good communication between the family and the professionals.

We think people with Down syndrome of all ages benefit from having a medical home. However, as the person with Down syndrome reaches adolescence and adulthood, we think it is necessary to "remodel the medical home." It is necessary to expand the relationship to three parties: the person (with Down syndrome), the family, and the professional. No one would expect an infant or young child with Down syndrome to participate in decision-making about his health care. But as that individual matures, it is important for the adult with Down syndrome to participate in his own health care (to the extent possible). This includes asking the person to provide his own history, listening to his concerns, and providing information that helps him make treatment decisions.

"Two Syndromes"

Through our work at the Center, we have learned a great deal from our patients and their families and caregivers. Sometimes, however, in discussing what we think we know about adults with DS with the family of a younger person with Down syndrome, family members will question our findings. They express a concern that "that is not our experience." These types of comments have helped us learn a great deal about younger adults with Down syndrome and the respects in which they may differ from those in their forties, fifties, and older.

We have called this phenomenon "two syndromes." The genetic basis for Down syndrome is the same for the older generations as for the younger generations. However, there are several issues that are different: expectations, life expectancy, opportunities, and goals.

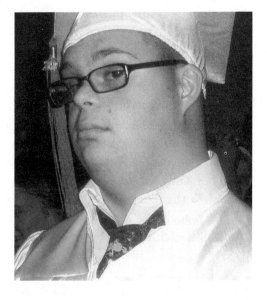

In the past, families were often told at the birth of their child with Down syndrome that he would never walk, talk, attend school, or "have any meaningful development even with therapy or working with him." This information had a very significant impact on many families, who then did not expect their child to develop these skills.

This lack of expectations was coupled with the lack of opportunity for therapies, school, work programs, recreational activities, and other supports that are now available (although not always adequately available). Therefore, many adults with Down syndrome who were born in the 1970s or earlier received very little of the assistance that benefits so many now. (On the other hand, many families developed their own work programs, schools, and recreational programs.)

Another difference between the older and young generations that strongly influenced families was the predicted life expectancy of a person with Down syndrome. In 1900, the life expectancy of a person with Down syndrome was nine years. When our older patients (now in their sixties and seventies) were born, the life expectancy was still only in the twenties. These families did not expect their child to live into adulthood

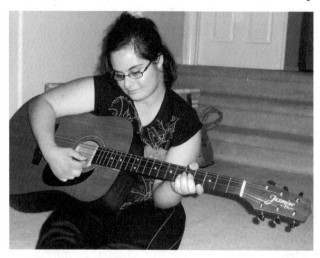

(or at least, older adulthood). Therefore, there was no reason to prepare for adulthood. And there was no reason to prepare for the person with Down syndrome outliving his parents.

Because of the lower life expectancy, the medical professionals' predictions of limited development, and the lack of opportunities, the families of many of our older patients set significantly different goals than the families of our younger patients. They didn't plan for adulthood because they didn't anticipate their son or daughter would live that long. They didn't pursue opportunities for their son or daughter because there were so few available, and, even if there were, they were told their efforts were pointless—the person with DS would never develop skills. (Of course, some families of our older patients "bucked the system" and made goals that were closer to the goals of the families of people with Down syndrome who are children now.) Just as we know from early intervention efforts today, these adults often function better in many regards than those whose parents had lower expectations and had less opportunity to grow and develop.

The difference in goals can have a very significant impact on the life of the person with Down syndrome and may be a big factor when families tell us, "That is not our experience." Only time will tell us to what extent our theoretical "two syndromes" will be evident. With a longer life expectancy, greater opportunities, changing expectations, and expanded goals, the jury is out on what impact these will have on people with Down syndrome. It is exciting to have the opportunity to observe and participate in these changes.

HELPING A TEEN OR ADULT WITH DOWN SYNDROME BE HEALTHY

♦ ♦ ♦ ♦ ♦ ♦ ♦ ♦ ♦ ♦ ♦ ♦ ♦ ♦ ♦ ♦ ♦ ♦

The rest of this book will describe our observations and participation in helping teens and adults with Down syndrome be healthy. We will discuss common issues, health promotion, health issues, the interaction between physical and mental health, and medical intervention.

Our hope and expectation is that this book will be used by people with Down syndrome, their families, and caregivers, as well as professionals. As has been true with

Choosing a Physician

Down syndrome groups or families from cities outside of Chicago often ask us how they can start their own clinic or how they can choose a physician. In particular, they often ask us about finding "an expert" in providing health care for adults with Down syndrome. As indicated above, physicians generally receive little training in caring for adults with Down syndrome in medical school. Our experience suggests, however, that despite lack of training, a physician can be successful in providing care for adults with Down syndrome. Still, there are certain qualities that often make one medical professional a better choice than others looking for a physician for a teen or adult with Down syndrome.

Although we don't think this is an all-inclusive list, we believe it is helpful to look for medical professionals who have:

- ◆ a belief that all people with Down syndrome deserve the same respect and care provided to any patient;
- ◆ a willingness to listen to and learn from the patients, the families, and the care providers;
- ◆ a willingness to learn from other people providing care for people with Down syndrome (a succinct guide to some of this information is available as the Health Care Guidelines developed by the Down Syndrome Medical Interest Group; see Dr. Len Leshin's web page at www.ds-health.com);
- ◆ a willingness to consider that problems that occur in a person with Down syndrome are not necessarily part of the syndrome and may have another cause that requires specific treatment;
- ◆ an understanding of human development—especially childhood development—and a willingness to assess an adult with Down syndrome in that light;
- ◆ an interest in the psychosocial aspects of health as well as the physical.

Although there are a few practitioners who are providing care for a large number of adults with Down syndrome, most practitioners have limited experience. In our experience, being willing and open to caring for and learning to care for adults with Down syndrome is more important than having received the limited training available to most physicians. It is also helpful if the family and care provider are willing to share general information (such as the Health Care Guidelines) with one another.

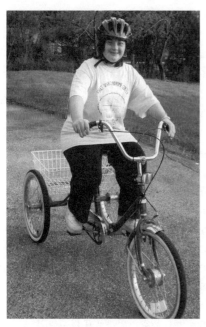

other publications (such as the Down Syndrome Medical Interest Group's *Health Care Guidelines*), we anticipate that families will share this information with their physicians and other professionals as they develop their own medical home.

While this book focuses on physical health issues, it also addresses some mental health issues. As noted above, physical and mental (as well as spiritual) wellness are part of the definition of health. We believe they are linked and have an impact on each other. (For a fuller discussion of mental health, see our previous book, *Mental Wellness in Adults with Down Syndrome: A Guide to Emotional and Behavioral Strengths and Challenges*.)

As you read this book, we ask you to remember "Joe." Joe is not a real person, but a compilation of people and ideas first introduced in our book on mental wellness. He reflects what we believe are key points in keeping a person with Down syndrome healthy. Joe is 29 years old and healthy. We believe that there are some important contributing factors to his health:

- ◆ He is accepted as an individual.
- ◆ He is (and always has been) given choices.
- ◆ He has expectations placed on him that are neither too low nor too high.
- ◆ He gets regular exercise.
- ◆ His need for routine is supported.
- ◆ He is encouraged to develop some flexibility.
- ◆ He has opportunities to do for others (people who are always "done for" need an opportunity to "do for").
- ◆ He gets annual health evaluations.
- ◆ He has been encouraged and supported to develop and improve his communication skills.
- ◆ He received vocational training as part of his schooling.
- ◆ He is part of a community.
- ◆ He has opportunities to integrate (into the general community).
- ◆ He also has opportunities to congregate (with other people with disabilities).
- ◆ He is heard. (When Joe has a concern, people listen. They don't always say "yes" to his requests, but his concerns are addressed.)

We recommend ensuring that all adolescents and adults with Down syndrome be provided with the same opportunities and supports as a foundation to optimal physical and mental wellness.

Chapter 1

Understanding
Common Issues That
Affect Health Care

Jim, a 21-year-old man with Down syndrome, had been refusing to go to work for a week. He lived in an apartment with three other men with intellectual disabilities. Each man worked in the community and the routine was that a van picked them up each morning and took each of them to their place of employment.

The supporting staff reported that Jim was refusing to walk out to the van, and that he became upset when they encouraged him to go to work. Upon further questioning, we discovered that Jim had also been declining to participate in other activities and that he was sometimes seen limping (although he had not limped into the office).

The physical exam revealed a red, swollen joint on Jim's great toe. Jim stated that he had not reported his pain because in the past, when his hand had been red and swollen, he had been diagnosed with an infection and hospitalized for five days. This time he really wanted to go on the special recreation trip to St. Louis next week and didn't want to take a chance that he would be in the hospital and miss the trip. We diagnosed gout, treated Jim with an anti-inflammatory medication, and he enjoyed the trip to St. Louis.

As discussed in the Introduction, it is important to avoid attributing every change in a person with Down syndrome to "just the Down syndrome." People with Down syndrome (DS) can get a number of health problems that are not unique to people with DS and that often have a specific treatment. However, it is also necessary to understand some of the common characteristics of adolescents and adults with DS to better understand the health problems that may be present. This chapter briefly reviews these characteristics to help readers improve their ability to understand and care for individuals with DS.

The Interaction between Physical Health and Mental Health

There is an interaction between physical and mental health. This statement is neither a new concept nor uniquely true of people with DS. Physical health problems can have a psychological impact on all people. We may respond to an illness with fear, anger, depressed mood, anxiety, and other emotions. In addition, when we don't feel well, we may not function as well physically or mentally. This is also true for people with DS. However, the relationship between physical and mental health can at times be more complicated and more difficult to assess in adults with DS. This is discussed further in Chapter 5.

Communication Issues

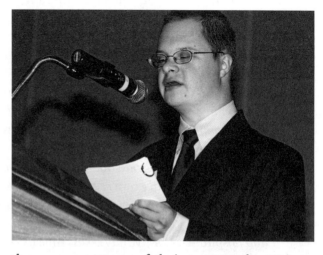

One reason it can be more difficult to assess the relationship between physical and mental health in adults with DS is because communication challenges are common. Many people with DS have difficulties with expressive language. They may readily express their feelings nonverbally through a look of sadness, anger or anxiety, or through expressions of joy and exhilaration. However, it may be very difficult for them to verbally communicate the cause or source of their expressed emotions, particularly negative feelings. Caregivers are usually good observers and will often know that something is wrong, but they may not know what or why. Often the only means that an adult with DS has to communicate the presence of a problem is through a change in mood or behavior. This may be especially true if a major problem or stress is involved, such as the loss of an important supervisor at a job, or the presence of a physical problem, with pain or discomfort.

When looking at behavior as a communication issue, it may be helpful to consider how "loud" the person's nonverbal or behavioral communication needs to be for others to "hear" it. Some professionals in the mental health field have discussed what they call the level of "selective deafness" that occurs in one's social environment (Minuchin and Fishman, 1981). For example, if there is a slight change in someone's mood or behavior, others may ignore it. If the problem persists, then the person's behavior may amplify until others "hear" that something is wrong. Not surprisingly, as someone experiences more pain or discomfort (whether physical, mental/emotional, etc.), his behavior may change (such as by becoming more agitated or restless) and become more obvious to others.

Once a problem is "heard" by significant others, the next step is to find the cause or source of this problem. This usually requires digging and detective work on the part of parents, caregivers, and any professionals who have been engaged to help solve the problem. At the Adult Down Syndrome Center, we look high and low for any clues to help explain the source of a change in behavior. We look for physical problems by conducting a thorough physical exam. We also ask about stress in the person's life. We seek out and talk to as many people, in as many settings, as we can to help explain a problem. This may include teachers in schools, staff in residential settings, supervisors at a worksite, etc. In short, we try to gather information from any source to help us find what the person is trying to communicate through a change in their behavior.

Due to the frequency of communication problems, we view any and all behavioral change in adolescents and adults with DS as a possible communication tool. Particularly if the person is nonverbal or has limited verbal skills, a behavioral change can be his means of communicating discomfort or a feeling of illness. Even some of our patients with excellent communication skills do not communicate their discomfort via spoken words or writing. The physical illness affects them mentally, and they communicate it through a change in behavior.

In cases like these, we like to think that it is not that our patients are not communicating well; it is just that we are not listening correctly. In short, we urge others to look very carefully at any behavior as a form of communication.

Why is this so important? People who may be unable to communicate the presence of a problem, whether or not they have good verbal skills, may be at greater risk for mental health problems. Their inability to communicate a problem may contribute to a condition described by a psychologist as "learned helplessness" (Seligman, 1975). Learned helplessness occurs when people do not get enough experience solving problems they encounter in their daily lives, and, as a result, tend to give up rather than try to meet the challenge. In other words, they have literally "learned to be helpless." This, in turn, often leads to a state of hopelessness and depression.

Ensuring that people with DS have a means to communicate the need for help, whether through verbal or nonverbal communication, may go a long way to help to prevent or reduce learned helplessness. Once people learn that they have a responsive environment and that they can communicate successfully when there are problems, this greatly increases the chance that they will use this strategy when faced with future challenges. Taking these differences into account can improve our ability to diagnose health problems and also develop treatment plans.

PAIN

◆ ◆ ◆ ◆ ◆ ◆ ◆ ◆ ◆ ◆ ◆ ◆ ◆ ◆ ◆ ◆ ◆ ◆

It is important to understand how pain affects people with DS when diagnosing and treating illnesses and injuries. For years we have heard family members say that their son, daughter, or sibling with DS does not feel pain in the same way as they do. They appear to have an increased pain tolerance. Although no studies of people with DS have proven this to be true, one study has demonstrated an increased pain tolerance in mice with trisomy 16 (Martinez-Cue et al., 1999). (Mice with trisomy 16 have many of the physical and medical characteristics of people with DS and are referred to as "a mouse model for Down syndrome.") When these mice were subjected to painful stimuli, they had less of a response than the mice without the extra chromosome. This study demonstrated in the mice what families had been saying about people with DS for years.

It is also important to consider how a person's difficulties with communication might contribute to an apparent increased pain tolerance. In other words, sometimes when an individual with DS is not expressing that he is in pain, the problem may be that he is not able to effectively communicate his pain to others, not that he does not perceive the pain.

Another issue that we have seen involves denial. It is usually in the form of refusing to acknowledge pain to avoid evaluation or treatment. A number of our patients, like Jim in the case example at the beginning of the chapter, have not told us of pain because "the last time I told you, you did (this test or that procedure)."

So, what is the best way to avoid missing painful episodes that need treatment? We recommend:

◆ Watch for subtle signs that something is wrong (facial expressions, holding an extremity differently, a change in appetite, etc.).
◆ Watch for behavioral changes, including changes in appetite, changes in mood, and changes in activity level.
◆ Consider the possibility that the person has a reduced ability to perceive pain.
◆ Consider communication issues, since symptoms may be misinterpreted if the person has difficulties in communicating. (Consider using pictorial representations of pain, a number scale, or something similar if you suspect communication issues.)

SELF-TALK AND IMAGINARY FRIENDS

We have repeatedly heard at the Center that our patients with DS talk out loud to themselves, and many also have imaginary friends. Although this behavior concerns some parents and professionals, we urge caution when evaluating it. Too often the behavior is viewed as pathology when it is quite normal in most cases.

Many children in the general population talk to themselves at some time in their childhood and many have imaginary friends. For these children, the self-talk and imaginary friends usually continues up to the age when they are able to internalize their thoughts. Many people with DS continue to talk out loud to themselves and to have imaginary friends throughout their lives. This should not be considered odd or abnormal in teens or adults with DS, given that many of them continue to have intellectual functioning that is similar to a child's, at least in some respects.

Usually when an adult with DS continues self-talk or imaginary friends into adulthood, we view the behaviors as a social skill issue. Talking out loud in public settings can be upsetting to others and draw attention unnecessarily. We recommend that the adult be taught to use self-talk only in a private space, such as the bedroom or bathroom at home. (Be sure to note that stalls in a bathroom at work are *not* a "private space.")

If the adult can learn to use self-talk in a private space, there are many benefits (which we have described in detail in *Mental Wellness in Adults with Down Syndrome*). Briefly, the adult can use self-talk to direct his own actions, particularly with a new task—that is, to talk himself through the steps. Self-talk can also allow someone to review previous events and to plan for future events. It may help the person solve problems or express his feelings and frustrations and calm himself down. Some people use self-talk to help themselves learn new skills or to entertain themselves. For example, many people enact scenes from their workplace or school to practice needed skills or because they enjoy activities from these settings.

In addition, self-talk may actually play an important role in communicating the presence of a problem. The key is for others to be sensitive to this medium of expression. People with DS may be able to say things in or through their self-talk that they are not able to say directly to others, including parents or other caregivers. This might be because the person does not want to offend or disappoint others by directly telling them what is really on his mind, or because he does not feel comfortable confronting others or making direct comments.

Whether or not parents or other caregivers can understand the words expressed in the self-talk, they may still hear a change in tone or see a change in expression that provides a clue as to what the problem is. If the adult is angry or self-critical in his self-talk, this may be a clear message that something is amiss in his life. Angry self-talk may not be a concern if it only occurs occasionally as a means to vent frustration, and most of the self-talk is more positive. On the other hand, if more and more of the self-talk is negative, it is worth investigating to see if something is wrong. The person may be experiencing something in his day-to-day life that is disturbing or upsetting. For example, there may be a conflict or problem at work or in the person's residence. Or the self-talk could be an indication of some type of physical pain or discomfort.

Again, self-talk is just one means for letting others know there may be a problem. We just need to be alert and open to this means of communication. See Chapter 8 of *Mental Wellness in Adults with Down Syndrome* for a more detailed discussion of self-talk.

THE GROOVE

One of the more interesting and consistent findings at the Center is that people with DS have a need for sameness, repetition, and order in their lives. We call

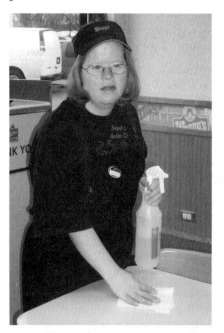

this a tendency for "grooves," because people's behavior tends to follow set patterns or grooves in their thoughts and actions. Like all patterns of human behavior, these grooves can be either productive and adaptive or unproductive and maladaptive. For example, people with DS can get stuck in "ruts" involving unhealthy eating habits and a sedentary lifestyle or they may get into the groove of having healthy eating habits and an active lifestyle.

The good news about people with DS is that because they tend to maintain set patterns or grooves, once a healthy pattern is established, they are often incredibly conscientious and reliable with maintaining these patterns. Time and time again, we have seen adults with DS stay with a pattern of healthy eating and physical activity, lose weight, and develop a sense of pride and self-esteem that comes from a healthy lifestyle. It also helps if they repeatedly hear from others how good they look. People with DS are often especially aware of, and sensitive to, praise and support from others.

One important thing for caregivers to consider is that people with DS may not be able to set up a healthy pattern of behavior on their own. However, once a program is established, they will often keep the schedule going, "come hell or high water." Parents and other caregivers will attest to the tenacity of people with maintaining a healthy (as well as an unhealthy) routine.

In short, we have all repeatedly heard that people with DS are "stubborn and set in their ways." If there is some truth to this, then why not use the tendency as a strength to develop and maintain routines and grooves that actually help people with DS feel better and live longer?

MEMORY

Researchers have consistently found that people with DS have difficulty remembering and acting on what they hear or what is told to them. On the other hand, we have found that people with DS tend to have exceptional visual memories and are very good visual learners. Consequently, they are far more likely to remember and

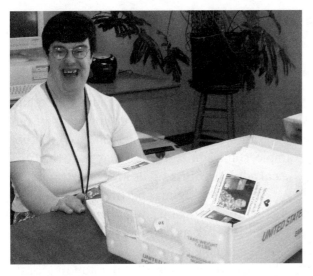

respond to a request from others if shown rather than told what to do. Examples of the use of visual cues will be given in many of the case vignettes discussed throughout this book.

We have also learned at the Center that visual cues can be combined with a person's need for sameness and grooves to develop very effective problem solving strategies or to promote independence and adaptive behavior. For example, many people with DS are very reliable and conscientious about following a list of healthy foods, which they then check off at every meal. It may be even more reinforcing if they also use a calendar to mark their food choices at the end of the day and record their success with the plan. A calendar can be a very effective incentive in and of itself.

GRIEF

Grief is another issue to consider when trying to get to the bottom of a change in mental or physical health. We commonly see a delayed response to grief in adolescents and adults with DS. For a period of time (often about six months), many of our patients seem to be little affected by a death in the family or other loss. Only later does the person seem to grieve. It is not exactly clear why this delay occurs, but it may be that some people with DS take longer to really understand the magnitude or the permanence of the loss.

Interestingly, some of our patients have not initially appeared to grieve after a significant loss such as the death of a parent. Later, after another loss—often one that seems much less significant (e.g., the death of the turtle at the group home)—the person will experience and express the grief that he did not with the first and more significant loss.

We often see people with DS show their grief in alternative ways (not that there are only certain ways that grief can be experienced). As noted with other issues above, they may express their grief through changes in behavior. They may also express grief through physical complaints. It is important to understand these possible ways of expressing grief when assessing a person with DS who has experienced a loss. This may be true even (or especially) several months after the loss has occurred.

DEVELOPMENTAL AGE VERSUS CHRONOLOGICAL AGE
◆ ◆ ◆ ◆ ◆ ◆ ◆ ◆ ◆ ◆ ◆ ◆ ◆ ◆ ◆ ◆ ◆ ◆ ◆ ◆

Due to the intellectual disability associated with DS, a teen or adult's developmental age generally is lower than his chronological age. However, for many of our patients, this difference is not the same for all aspects of their personality. In other words, there can be unevenness. For example, some adults with DS may have the typi-

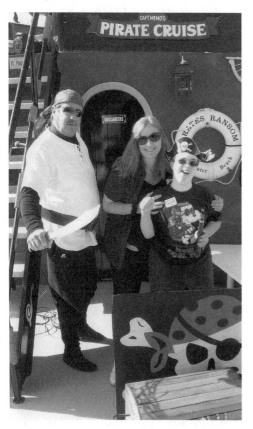

cal adult dreams and desires of getting married and getting an apartment but lack the skills to do this on their own. Others may want to work as cashiers in grocery stores, but be unable to handle money successfully because of difficulties understanding basic math concepts.

Sometimes this disparity between developmental and chronological age results in actions that affect an adult's health and well being—particularly if the person is allowed to make decisions and control aspects of his life when he doesn't have the skills or judgment to do so. Perhaps the best illustration of this problem we have seen involved four women with DS who were roommates in an apartment. Despite a high level of skill, three of the four were gaining significant amounts of weight. All were failing in their jobs (two of the four had excellent jobs in the community). All four were also showing signs of depression such as lethargy, listlessness, and fatigue.

These women were thought to be quite capable (and in most respects they were). They had been assigned intermittent supervision, and, as a result, had no supervision in their apartment after 11 p.m. The dramatic changes in their mood and behavior were a mystery until it was learned that all were staying up until very early in the morning. Apparently they were watching beloved horror movies and binging on favorite junk food. This, of course, did not allow the women to get adequate sleep, and they were paying a steep price for their emotional and vocational functioning and weight management. All four of these women had excellent skills, but they all had a need for help in one key area—decision-making about going to bed at an appropriate time. Once the right supervision was arranged, this problem was solved.

Another common issue involving developmental delays is that receptive language skills are often greater than expressive language skills. Because of this, many people with DS have a fairly good sense of what is going on around them, and an understanding of physical, emotional, or environmental problems they are experiencing. But their expressive language difficulties may limit their ability to communicate problems to others. This communication may be especially important to caregivers who may help them to solve whatever problem they are facing.

This unevenness of communication skills may affect people with DS in other ways. For example, we have found that people sometimes assume that adults with DS who have more intelligible speech have greater abilities than they actually do. Despite excellent verbal skills, they may not be able to conceptualize and communicate the presence of more complex issues and concerns. For example, at least two of the women in the above example had excellent verbal skills but still were unable or unwilling to communicate that their problems were related to nightly movie and eating binges. In short, when an adult with DS has good intelligibility, parents and other caregivers may assume that the person can communicate problems and issues, when in fact this may be beyond his capability.

On the other hand, we have seen the opposite assumption for people who are nonverbal or limited in their use of verbal speech. These individuals may be assumed to have less skill or understanding than they actually have. As a result, people may ignore or discount the individual's nonverbal communication even when it is quite creative and explicit in describing the presence of a problem. For example, we have had people brought to us with what caregivers and other mental health professionals described as severe behavioral problems and even the diagnosis of "psychosis" because of "self-injurious behavior." In fact, the behavior may have been severe and disturbing to others, but often it was also a very clear way to communicate the presence of a problem (if we were able to listen to this). For example, several people who were hitting their heads were found to have problems such as severe sinus infections and major dental problems. The individuals were clearly showing the locus of the problem, if others had been listening.

CONCLUSION

On one hand, it is important not to fall into the trap of labeling all symptoms of people with DS as "just the Down syndrome." On the other hand, it is also very important to understand that there are some common (albeit not universal) characteristics of people with DS. Understanding these characteristics will improve the ability to understand, diagnose, and treat health issues in people with DS.

Chapter 2

Promoting Health
at Home and
in the Community

Ruth, a 35-year-old woman with Down syndrome, visited the Adult Down Syndrome Center for her annual examination. She was 5 feet, 1 inch (155 cm) tall and weighed 193 pounds (89 kg). She did not exercise regularly. She was, however, looking forward to a trip to Europe with her mom in nine months to see her grandmother. She complained of aching in her knees when she walked even short distances. Other than her being significantly overweight, there were no abnormalities on the exam or the labs.

I discussed Ruth's weight with her and she was evaluated by our nutritionist. Like many people with Down syndrome (DS), she enjoyed following a routine and did well with a regular schedule that she wrote out for herself each week. She followed our guidelines and began to lose weight. However, her weight loss was slow and she wanted to lose much more weight before seeing her grandmother. Ruth started to go with her mother to Weight Watchers. She enjoyed the routine and could comprehend and follow the Weight Watchers' system of counting food "points." She also began to walk in the pool at the local park three days a week with a friend. Her knees did not bother her when she walked in the pool.

Ruth came into the office eight months later complaining of a cough. In the 35 weeks since we had seen her, she had lost 40 pounds (18 kg). Shortly afterwards, she went to Europe and was not bothered by pain in her knees when walking around sightseeing. Over the next year, she lost another 35 pounds (16 kg). She is still counting points, although she only goes to Weight Watchers once every few months. She continues to exercise regularly, her joints no longer hurt, and she is maintaining her weight.

The activities of anyone's daily life can promote either health or illness, depending on the person's lifestyle and habits. In addition, there are a number of aspects of care received in the medical office that can promote health (immunizations, health screening for early detection of disease, etc.). This chapter will focus on those lifestyle issues and habits that are part of life "outside the office." These include issues such as exercise, nutrition, cigarette smoking, drinking alcohol, and sleep. In addition, family and friends can play a significant role in the health of an adolescent or adult with Down syndrome.

ENCOURAGING SELF-PROMOTION OF HEALTH

The sibling of one of the authors called home from college years ago and proclaimed, "Jill and I exercised day after day and after two days we stopped." That was obviously not a very successful program.

For all of us, health promoting activities seem to work best if they become part of our life. Making the activity or the behavior part of our usual, customary day encourages us to "stick with it." For most healthy behaviors, we need to do them over and over to achieve success. Often it doesn't take great big changes, but rather, little changes done repeatedly.

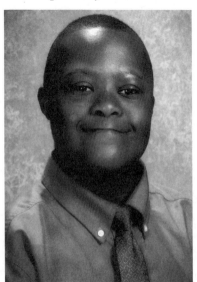

It is often no small challenge for us to make small, but consistent changes in our own routines. It can be an even bigger challenge to help someone else change her behavior. When the motivation comes from within, then the motivator is with us at all times. This is not the case when the motivator is outside us. Therefore, developing a program that helps the individual become self-motivated will often have better results.

How can you help an adolescent or adult with DS with self-promotion of health? This varies from person to person and depends on the individual's personality as well as her capabilities. We have, however, developed some guidelines that we have found helpful. These are explored below.

PROMOTING SELF-CARE SKILLS

We have found that many adults with DS are able to do self-care skills very well and consistently, once they have learned the task. This may be due, in part, to "the groove" and strong visual memories (discussed in Chapter 1), which are characteristic of many people with DS. Some need tasks broken into "doable" pieces and some need help organizing tasks. For many people with DS, being "organized" means developing a schedule or calendar. For example, the person may have six things she needs to do before going to bed. She uses the bathroom, brushes her teeth, changes her clothes, says her prayers, drops her clothes down the clothes shoot, and sets out her clothes for the next morning. For some, this series of tasks becomes routine, once learned. For others, making a schedule is helpful.

We have found that a schedule with pictures of the activities works best for most of our patients, even for those who read. For example, the schedule might have a picture of the toilet, a picture of the person brushing her teeth, a picture of her saying her prayers, etc. Generally, we find that a photo of the person herself doing the activity (when appropriate) works best (rather than a schematic picture or a photo that shows someone else). It also helps to have the person participate in developing the schedule.

Calendars for the week are also helpful. These help a person keep track of what she needs to get done, can remind her to initiate the activity (which often then allows the groove of doing the activity to "kick in"), and assists her in taking personal responsibility for the activities. Both weekly calendars and daily schedules promote repetition of the desired behavior.

HYGIENE

Hygiene is an important self-care skill that is essential to promoting health. Many adults with DS are very capable of taking care of their own hygiene. However, reminders are sometimes necessary. The following are a few pointers:

- Washing, rinsing, and drying are all important. Many adults with DS seem to have the "zip-zip" approach to drying and don't get in between toes, in folds, etc. Washing and rinsing are obviously important, but often completely ineffective if the drying is left out. Fungus and bacteria love to grow in warm, moist, dark places. It can be helpful for someone else to demonstrate good drying techniques. A videotape of the individual (when appropriate) drying herself (e.g. between her toes) that she can watch regularly can also trigger appropriate drying behavior. In addition, a timer can be used to help the person devote a reasonable amount of time to drying.

- Moisturizing cream is never effective if it stays in the bottle. Many people with DS don't like the sensation of moisturizing creams, so they have to be encouraged to use them. Putting cotton gloves or socks on for a few minutes after applying cream to hands and feet sometimes makes the sensation more tolerable.

◆ To ensure that the person spends enough time brushing her teeth, try using a timer. (This can capitalize on a person's tendency to follow grooves.) Some electric toothbrushes even come with built-in timing devices that directs the user to brush for a certain length of time (e.g., two minutes).

◆ To assist with taking medication, pill cases with compartments for the time of day and day of the week can be very beneficial. Many people with DS cannot tell time in the conventional sense (by looking at a clock and saying it is 3 o'clock). However, many seem to have an innate sense of time. They seem to know that it is 3:00 and time to take the medication. If not, timers (on watches or cell phones, for instance) can be used to prompt them to take medicine. It might also be appropriate for someone to learn to take medicine at breakfast, at supper, or at bedtime, if she has a regular schedule.

More specific tips on promoting self-care will be discussed in the chapters on different health problems.

EXERCISE AND RECREATION

Exercise and recreation are crucial to physical and mental health. In addition, they help make life enjoyable. While some of the benefits of exercise realized in other people may not be as apparent in people with DS, exercise is nevertheless still an essential part of a healthy lifestyle. Recreational activities often provide much of the benefit of exercise and can be most enjoyable.

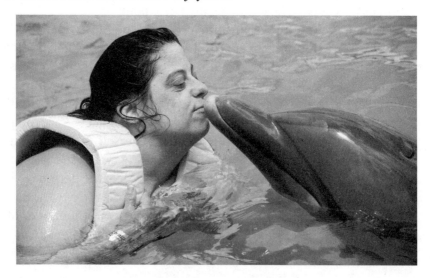

BENEFITS

For people without DS, exercise reduces the incidence of atherosclerotic heart disease (heart attacks and strokes), reduces blood pressure, helps in maintaining ideal body weight, increases bone density, reduces osteoporosis, helps prevent diabetes mellitus, may reduce the risk of some forms of cancer, and benefits mental health by decreasing stress.

For people with DS, atherosclerotic heart disease and hypertension (high blood pressure) are much less common. Therefore, the benefit of exercise in reducing these conditions is less clear than in people without DS. However, adolescents and adults with DS can, and should, definitely reap the many other benefits of exercise.

WEIGHT CONTROL

One of the most important benefits is that exercise can help people with DS control their weight. One study demonstrated that children with DS have a lower resting metabolic rate than children of similar size and age without DS (Luke et al., 1994). Over a 24-hour period, children with DS burn approximately 200 to 300 fewer calories during times when they are not doing any physical activity. Over the course of a year, this difference equals approximately 73,000 to 110,000 calories, or 20 to 30 pounds (9 to 14 kg). Small differences over a long period of time can add up to a very large change in weight. In addition, the study found that if the child with DS tried to avoid this weight gain purely by decreasing calories, then she was at greater risk for missing essential nutrients in the diet. At least some of the difference in the metabolic rate had to be compensated for by increasing the calories burned through exercise.

In 1998, we participated in a study that confirmed that weight problems continue into adulthood (Rubin, Rimmer, Chicoine, Braddock & McGuire, 1998). We looked at the weights of 283 adult and adolescent patients with DS for whom we had data at the time. We confirmed previous studies and the general sense that adults with DS are often overweight. We determined that 45 percent of our male patients and 56 percent of our female patients were overweight. These figures were higher than for the general population (33 percent of men and 36 percent of women). Although not statistically significant, we found a trend toward heavier weights for adults with DS who lived at home than for those who lived in residential facilities. We found that adults with DS were more likely to be closer to their ideal body weight if they had opportunities for recreational and social activities (not necessarily exercise).

Therefore, we recommend social activities such as shopping, visiting museums, dancing, etc. that involve walking or movement. We also encourage adults with DS to build a schedule that includes at least 20 to 30 minutes of exercise or activity 3 to 5 times per week. Working physical activity into daily life by parking a little farther away, taking the stairs, and doing chores in the house and yard is also helpful. Generally, turning off the television and being more active is beneficial. (The first author, a regular marathon runner, says that the hardest part of training for a marathon is pushing the red button on the remote to turn off the TV so he will get off the couch and go run.)

In our study, the people living in group homes may have had less of a tendency toward obesity because they had more opportunities for activity. Previous studies by other investigators have found that people with intellectual disabilities who live in group homes often have greater involvement in community skills training. Perhaps greater opportunity for social activities played a role in the trend we found in our study.

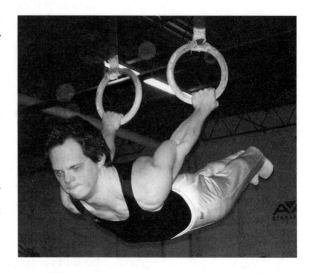

Determining Whether Someone Is Overweight or Obese

Body mass index (BMI) is a measurement that compares weight to height. For example, a person who is 5 feet 5 inches tall (165 cm) and weighs 150 pounds (68 kg) has a BMI of 25.

BMI is used to calculate the definitions of obesity and overweight:
- *Overweight* means a BMI greater than 25.
- *Obesity* means a BMI great than 30.
- *Severe obesity* means a BMI greater than 40.

Body mass index calculators can easily be found on the Internet by entering "body mass index calculator" into a search engine. Sex, height, and weight can then be entered and BMI will be calculated.

Another way to look at a person's weight is to compare his or her weight to Ideal Body Weight (IBW). IBW can be roughly calculated as follows:
- For women, start at 100 pounds (45 kg) for the first 5 feet of height (152 cm) and add 5 pounds (2.3 kg) for each additional inch (approximately 2.5 cm). A woman's IBW is within +/- 10% of that number.
- For men, start with 106 pounds (48 kg) for the first 5 feet (152 cm) and add 6 pounds (2.7 kg) for each additional inch (approx 2.5 cm). IBW is within +/-10% of that number.

In addition, there are weight tables for people with DS. However, these aren't very useful in determining whether a person with DS is overweight since the weight tables just reflect the actual weights of the individuals with DS in a research group, not the ideal weights.

SLOWING OR PREVENTING OSTEOPOROSIS

In addition to helping maintain ideal body weight, exercise has other benefits for people with DS. Osteoporosis (thinning of the bones) is more common in people with DS. This is associated with a greater incidence of fractures. Weight-bearing exercises such as walking, running, dancing, weight lifting, and sports that involve those activities strengthen bones and reduce the chance of developing osteoporosis. Osteoporosis is discussed further in Chapter 13.

PROMOTING MENTAL HEALTH

Exercise and recreational activities also play an important role in promoting mental health. In people who don't have DS, exercise has been shown to reduce stress, improve a person's sense of well-being, and even reduce depression. We have found these same benefits in adults with DS. We encourage exercise as part of general mental health maintenance. We also stress exercise and activity for our patients who are depressed to help reduce the depressive symptoms and improve mood.

Strategies for Encouraging Regular Exercise

Like many of us, adults with DS often resist doing repetitive exercises alone on an exercise machine such as a treadmill. Making the activity fun is an important part of an exercise program—otherwise the person is unlikely to sustain it over time. In addition, it is clear from our study that the activity does not need to be what has been traditionally considered exercise. Activity is the important piece.

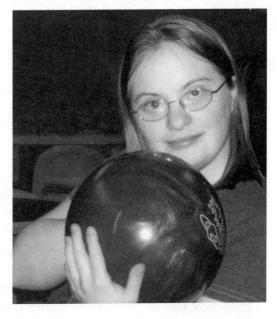

Social activities seem to be particularly successful at motivating adults with DS to exercise. Activities that involve walking, as noted above, are helpful. In addition, dancing, participating in drama groups, and other fun activities that involve movement can all be beneficial. We have found that many adults with DS particularly enjoy dancing. The second author often quips that "if there were a wedding reception every week with dancing we would never see an overweight person with DS."

Many of our patients enjoy watching TV and have been successful using exercise videos. The National Association for DS produced a wonderful exercise video several years ago that is a hit with many of our patients (see www.nads.org). Videos of Richard Simmons are huge favorites as well. We have recently begun to recommend playing games such as DDR (Dance, Dance Revolution) and Wii sports and fitness games. Although we have less experience in the use of these newer activities, they seem to be promising ways to promote exercise. Exercise videos and sports and fitness games may be particularly beneficial if the adult has difficulty getting transportation to a place to exercise or if the weather limits outdoor activities for parts of the year.

Variety as well as repetition can promote ongoing participation. For example, some of our patients tell us with pride, "On Monday night I bowl, Tuesday I exercise to my aerobics video tape, Wednesday I go to my drama group, Thursday is my relaxation night, Friday I go to activities like dances at the Special Recreation Program, Saturday we go shopping, and on Sunday we do a family activity like the museum." While the variety helps maintain interest and improves the fun, the repetition is reassuring, easier to follow, and helps the person with DS keep track of her activities on her own and remain self-motivated to participate.

Persistent life-long participation in exercise is important. Sometimes as parents naturally slow down with age or as the adult with DS ages out of the school system, fewer activities are available. These are particularly important times to seek other reliable people who can help the adult participate in recreational activities. We encourage participation in a mentor program or some similar program. Typically, a mentor program involves pairing an adult with DS with another adult to participate in activities together. Mentors might include volunteers from a local college, parents of younger children with DS, or other people.

Points to Remember about Exercise

- It doesn't have to look like "exercise" in the traditional sense. Physical activity is good in whatever form.
- Turn off the TV and get off the couch.
- Make if fun.
- Make it social.
- Small changes that are intended to be done over time are more beneficial and more sustainable than large (unrealistic) changes.
- Dancing is good exercise and is as close to being the universally loved activity for people with DS that we have found.
- Be realistic about exercise benefits. A two-mile walk (that burns 250 calories or so) to Dairy Queen will not lead to weight loss if 800 calories of ice cream are eaten at the destination.
- Make exercise and activity a part of life. Do more active family activities, park farther away in the parking lot, take the stairs, walk to the store, etc.

NUTRITION

Good nutrition is an important part of good health. Poor nutrition can lead to many diseases and/or can worsen their effects. Paying attention to nutrition can help prevent diseases as well as lessen their impact. It can also help people feel better and function better.

In the United States, the federal Department of Agriculture (USDA) provides recommended guidelines for good nutrition via the Food Pyramid (see below). The current Food Pyramid shows the relative amounts of different categories of foods (grains, vegetables, fruits, etc.) that should be eaten each day via bands of color of different widths. The pyramid does not, however, depict the number of servings of each food type that should be eaten each day, as the recommended quantity varies depending upon a person's age, gender, activity level, etc.

To help our patients select the appropriate number of servings, we recommend considering use of a board to check off servings as they consume them each day. Many people with DS are better able to comprehend the Food Pyramid concept with this visual aid. They can then make good choices for their diets, giving them a sense of personal ownership of good nutrition. This makes it more likely they will continue making good choices. The board we recommend at the ADSC is

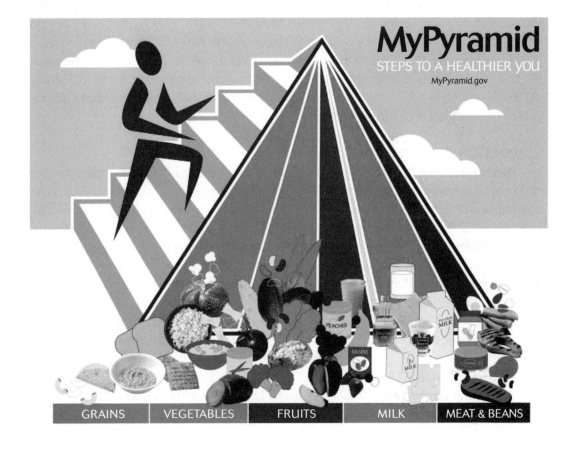

called the MyPyramid NutriScore Board and is available from Health Promotion Services (www.healthpromo.com).

Another possible alternative for keeping track of servings is to use some of the online tools provided by the USDA on its website: www.MyPyramid.gov. For Example, "My-Pyramid Plan" under Interactive Tools allows you to enter your current height, weight, and activity level in order to find out how many servings from each food group you need to eat to maintain your weight. The website also enables you to print out daily Meal Tracking worksheets to record how many servings from each food group you actually eat. In addition, for avid technology users, there are "apps" available for the iPhone that let you electronically check off the quantities of each food group you have eaten.

As discussed earlier, many people with DS have a preference for repetition or sameness (the Groove). Parents and other caregivers can take advantage of this tendency when helping a teen or adult learn to follow a consistent pattern of healthy eating. Teaching the teen or adult to check off foods as they are eaten (on a board or another visual aid) can capitalize on the person's fondness for routines.

MANAGING CALORIC INTAKE

Obesity is the most common nutrition-related disorder for people with DS. Many people with DS appear to have an impaired sense of satiation—that is, they have trouble determining when they feel "full." If food is available, these individuals will consume it. Others, as mentioned above, gain too much weight mainly because they do not get enough physical activity relative to the quantity of food they consume.

Unfortunately, there are no quick and easy fixes to calorie control for people with DS. The sections below briefly describe the cardinal principles. For more guidance, you may want to consult *The Down Syndrome Nutrition Handbook* by Joan Guthrie Medlen or consult a registered dietitian.

PORTION CONTROL

Portion control is an essential part of healthy eating for all of us. Helping teens and adults with DS internalize "correct" portion sizes and amounts of food groups is particularly important. Showing the person models of an appropriate portion can be helpful. For example, a deck of cards may be shown as the appropriate size for a piece of meat.

Also, determining the appropriate portion size and showing the person with DS what it looks like can help her choose appropriate portion sizes. For example, if one serving of a particular cereal is one cup, it is helpful to measure that amount out with the adult.

It can also be helpful to purchase smaller bowls that cannot hold much more than one serving. *The Down Syndrome Nutrition Handbook* has further information about helping people with DS select healthy choices and appropriate portions.

TAKING SMALL STEPS

Unfortunately, you are not likely to find a large, "quick fix" solution to helping an adult with DS reduce her caloric intake. You are much more likely to succeed in encour-

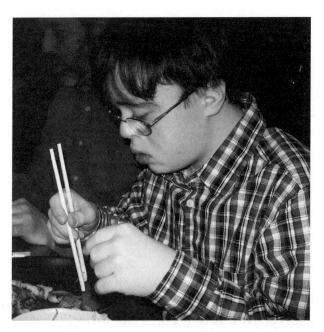

aging healthy eating through encouraging small changes consistently over time. These are lifelong issues.

Consistency and constancy are important aspects of the nutrition regimen. Drinking a can of soda (180 calories) or eating a candy bar (250 calories) every day can contribute greatly to weight gain over an extended period of time. Over a year's time, one can of soda per day adds up to 65,700 calories, and one candy bar a day equals 91,250 calories. These represent 18½ and 26 pounds (8.4 to 11.8 kg) respectively.

Conversely, small changes over time can result in significant weight loss. For example, eliminating a glass of apple juice every day (about 150 calories) and replacing it with a glass of water would result in eliminating calories equal to more than 15 pounds (6.8 kg).

Reducing calories is not enough by itself. The human body does a wonderful job of preventing starvation. As we decrease our caloric intake, the body conserves the calories that we do consume. Therefore, good nutrition must go hand-in-hand with regular exercise and activity as described above.

Dietary changes should be made both at home and as part of the person's social life. Better results can be obtained if the entire family agrees to try to eat healthy foods, limit problematic food choices in the home, and support each other. For example, if the adult with DS is being encouraged not to eat potato chips as a snack, then ideally, other family members should find an alternative healthy snack as well. Families should also seek out activities they can do together that aren't centered on food.

Some adults with DS enjoy and benefit from social activities that are proactively designed to teach and encourage healthy eating, cooking, shopping, etc. One example would be participation in Weight Watchers or similar programs. Like Ruth at the beginning of the chapter, some adults with DS can benefit from the structure and socialization of Weight Watchers.

WHAT ABOUT VITAMIN SUPPLEMENTS?

If people were able to follow the eating recommendations on the Food Pyramid to the letter, they would eat not only the appropriate amount of calories, but also the right nutrients. However, given the many choices of foods available and personal food

Insatiable Eating

As noted above, some people with DS don't seem to ever reach satiety. That is, they don't seem to have a shut-off switch when it comes to eating. For some, eating is truly like an addiction.

Unfortunately, there is limited information on how to "turn off appetite." Much research is being done on this topic in people who don't have DS, as well as in those who do. A variety of issues are being studied that will, hopefully, one day lead to better treatments to limit overeating and obesity. Although at present it is certainly enticing to consider using medications to suppress appetite, the available medications do have significant side effects and, therefore, we have had limited experience in using them.

Until better treatments are developed, the most successful approach for those individuals with compulsive-like, addiction-like eating is limiting access to food. This can include putting locks on cabinets, the refrigerator, and the pantry, and providing very close supervision. While taking these steps can be challenging and frustrating for family members and other caregivers, sometimes it is the only way to limit the person's intake and prevent uncontrolled obesity.

---

preferences, most people—with and without DS—are unable to eat everything on the Food Pyramid each day. Consequently, we recommend considering a daily multiple vitamin—generally without added iron—for teenagers and adults with DS. A calcium supplement might also be needed, depending on the person's needs and dietary intake. (See Chapter 13.)

There has been a great deal of interest in determining whether large doses of vitamins are of benefit to people with DS. Several different regimens have been recommended at different times over the years. These regimens have often been touted as improving cognitive and other developmental skills in people with DS. To date, no studies have demonstrated clear benefit of these treatments beyond those associated with vitamin C and zinc supplementation discussed below. Further information is being gathered regarding some regimens that some practitioners are currently recommending. Presently, there are no data that support us recommending these high-dose multivitamin regimens for our patients. There are, however, studies that support the use of some aspects of vitamin therapy, as discussed below.

The question of whether it is possible to reduce infections with supplements is often asked. There are some data that suggest that it might be so. A study in children with DS found that many had ascorbic acid (vitamin C) deficiency. The deficiency was associated with an increase in a variety of infections. The authors of this article suggested considering vitamin C supplementation for people with DS (Colombo et al., 1989).

Another study looked at the effects of oral zinc supplementation on infections in children with DS. These researchers saw an improvement in some laboratory parameters of immune function, as well as a reduction in the number of infections in the children who were given zinc supplementation (Franceschi et al., 1988).

Although the data from these two studies are not overwhelming, the studies certainly suggest that we consider supplementation with vitamin C and zinc. This would be particularly true if recurrent infections are a problem for someone with DS. We recommend evaluating the person's personal health history before considering supplementation. For our patients who have problems with recurrent infections, we generally recommend 1000 mg daily of vitamin C and 100 mg daily of zinc gluconate (about 14 mg of elemental zinc). This is in addition to a good multiple vitamin.

DRINKING ENOUGH FLUIDS

Another component of healthy nutrition is appropriate water consumption. While there is some debate about the right amount of water to drink, we recommend 6 to 8

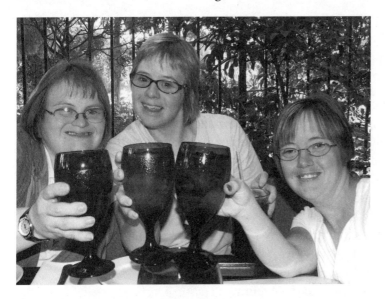

glasses (48 to 64 ounces) of water per day. Not only is drinking water a healthy habit, but drinking plenty of water can help reduce caloric intake.

We have noticed that many people with DS seem to have an impaired thirst mechanism. That is, unless encouraged to drink, they will not drink enough because they don't seem to feel thirsty. At the Adult Down Syndrome Center we have seen about 4500 patients. As part of the evaluation, we ask about the person's medical history, do a physical exam, and review lab studies. We have come to the conclusion that many people with DS go through their day at least mildly dehydrated. They are not drinking enough fluids.

Our bodies don't work as well when we don't drink enough fluids. We are more susceptible to getting dizzy, lightheaded, and passing out. We have less energy and tend to become constipated.

Addendum 1 has recommendations to help people with DS drink adequate fluids. These are recommendations for a typical day. If the person is exercising, it is important to drink even more. Using the nutrition score board (see above regarding the Food Pyramid) to encourage improved water consumption can also be helpful.

Healthy Eating and Exercise at Work

At the Adult Down Syndrome Center, we frequently encounter adolescent and adult patients who have serious challenges with weight control.

One of the problems we face with our patients is the availability of high-fat, high-caloric, and low-nutritional foods in vending machines, particularly in work settings. We encourage employers to help people with DS make good food choices. We also encourage the employers to review the contents of their vending machines. It's difficult to make good food choices if there are no good choices available. We suggest that employers consider including some higher-nutritional, lower-calorie, and lower-fat types of food and drinks in their vending machines.

In addition, where possible, we encourage employers to think of ways to increase their employees' activity. For example, during "down time," workers can be encouraged to participate in activities such as walking, dancing, or exercising to aerobics videos.

SLEEP

Sleep is another crucial aspect of health. Generally, adults with and without DS require 7 to 8 hours per night of sleep. Adolescents need 8 to 10 hours.

Poor sleep, which includes both inadequate sleep and poor quality sleep, can lead to difficulties with both physical and mental health. Good sleep hygiene can help people optimize their sleep. The elements of good sleep hygiene include:

- a nightly bedtime routine,
- regular sleeping hours,
- sleeping quarters that are free of bothersome noise or light,
- regular exercise and activities,
- avoidance of caffeine in the evening, and
- avoidance of exercise into the evening.

SLEEP HYGIENE

Sleep problems are more common in people with DS. The sleep centers (that guide our sleep) are in the brain. Since there are abnormalities in the brains of people with DS, it is probably not a surprise that sleep is commonly affected. In addition, sleep apnea is more common in people with DS. Sleep apnea is characterized by intermittent, temporary pauses in breathing while sleeping. (Sleep apnea is discussed in greater detail in Chapter 18.)

It is certainly important to be aware of these potential underlying causes of sleep problems. However, something that is often overlooked—by people with and with-

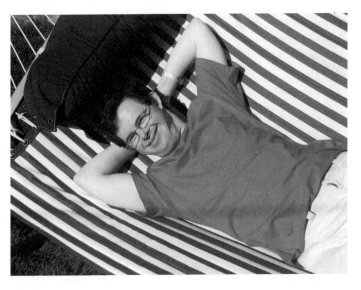

out DS—is the day-to-day sleeping habits known as "sleep hygiene." Just as good dental hygiene involves a set of planned activities such as brushing and flossing your teeth, the choices and plans you make during the day can affect the soundness of your sleep at night.

One night without good sleep does not have much effect on our performance the following day. Add together a string of bad nights, however, and you start seeing effects. It can become difficult, if not impossible, to stay awake during the day (especially for "boring/repetitive" tasks), tempers are shorter, creativity suffers, and you can start feeling "run down" all the time.

Here are some suggestions for improving the quality of normal sleep—to have good sleep hygiene:

1. Set a daily bedtime and a wake-up time. Stick to this schedule, even on weekends.
2. Exercise daily, but not within an hour of bedtime, if possible. Late afternoon may be the best time for exercising.
3. No caffeine after lunchtime. It would be best to avoid it altogether (it stays in the body 12 to 15 hours), but this habit is hard to break. Caffeine is found in coffee, black tea, chocolate, and many varieties of soda pop (but not usually fruit flavors). Herbal tea is okay.
4. Minimize sleep interruptions. Keep noise/light levels at an absolute minimum (snoring roommates can be a problem); make sure the room is not too hot or cold; don't drink a lot of water before bedtime; make sure the bed is comfortable.
5. No big meals within 1 to 2 hours of bedtime. A light snack is okay.
6. No smoking—ever.
7. Wind down toward the end of the day. No challenging or upsetting activities (if possible) in the evening. This can mean setting aside time earlier in the day for thinking through difficult issues or problems or for watching scary movies (although several of our patients don't sleep well if they watch scary movies at any time of the day).
8. Avoid taking naps during the day, especially in the evening. If you do nap, don't sleep more than 20 to 30 minutes.

9. Use your bed only for sleeping. No TV, reading, homework, or eating in bed. People will often stay awake longer doing these activities in bed and get inadequate sleep.

10. Try taking a warm shower or bath before bedtime.

We have found that it helps many of our patients with DS to follow a picture schedule for the sleep routine. Photographs taken of the person doing the activity herself, when appropriate, often work best. For example, the person may select six tasks that she needs to do before going to bed:

◆ Change into pajamas.
◆ Use the toilet.
◆ Brush her teeth.
◆ Set out clothes for the next morning.
◆ Put dirty clothes in the hamper.
◆ Say her prayers.

Next, take photographs of the person doing the activity or take a picture of the setting where the activity takes place (e.g., a picture of the bathroom). Put the photos in a small photo album or arrange them sequentially on a piece of paper (either left to right or top to bottom) to remind the person of the routine. A schedule can

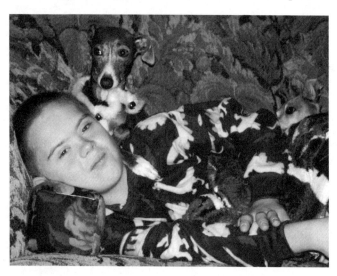

also help the person initiate the activities and can often eliminate the need for reminders from others.

As with all people, there will be differences among individuals on the amount of sleep needed (6 to 9 hours per night seems to be the average), the activities that help or hinder sleep, and just how much chocolate actually counts as a caffeine risk. It is also normal for anyone to have sleeping problems when going through difficult or stressful times in life. If the person with DS has a sleep disturbance that continues for weeks, however, it is time to get help.

The direct impact of DS on sleep is not fully known. There are some tendencies and environmental issues, however, which keep many people with DS from sleeping as well as they could:

◆ A group home environment or having roommates may lead to more disruptions of sleep.

- It may take adults with DS more time and effort to sort through complex problems or emotional, stressful issues. This can lead to increased time lying awake "just thinking."
- Some adults with DS do not get regular exercise and so may not be physically tired at bedtime.

Finally, as every human ages, there are expected changes in sleep habits. Staying asleep is more difficult; older adults wake up more frequently during the night and early morning. The amount of deep sleep is less than in young adults. With these changes comes an increase in daytime sleepiness and napping. Other medical problems can begin to interrupt sleep and the natural body sleep cycles become irregular. Since early aging occurs in people with DS, we suspect that these changes may occur earlier in people with DS.

If you suspect that a teen or adult with DS needs help with her sleep hygiene, start keeping track of bedtimes, wake-up times, and environmental issues that could be contributing to sleep difficulties. Try to make some of the suggested sleep hygiene modifications to fit the individual's particular needs. If difficulties persist, have the person see her primary care provider. Additional referral may be needed to a sleep specialist, a mental health provider, or others, depending on the cause. Sleep issues are further addressed in Chapter 18.

How Social Health Affects Physical Health

The important role of friends and family in helping a person achieve and maintain health is often overlooked. And yet, a sense of well-being generally requires a sense of connection to others. As discussed in the definition of health in the Introduction, health is based on physical, mental, and spiritual well-being. We believe these three are linked. A positive connection to others can therefore positively affect health.

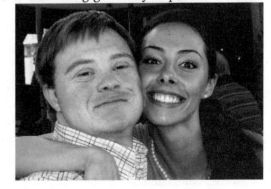

A study that assessed the impact on people with intellectual disabilities who moved from a state facility that was closing found that those who moved to the new facility with a fellow resident had better health than those who did not move with a fellow resident. Those who moved with a fellow resident even had a lower chance of dying. This was true even for the people with limited verbal and interacting skills who had not seemed to have significant interactions with the other residents in the state facility. Clearly, even for those individuals, social contact played an important role in their survival (Heller, 1982).

For all of us, having friends and family who love, support, encourage, and advocate for us, no matter what our age, stage, or situation, is critical to our health and well-being. Family support and advocacy may be especially important to people with DS because of limitations that may make it difficult to advocate for themselves. Peer friends are equally important but for different reasons than family members. Peers share common interests. They struggle with similar developmental tasks and issues. They also serve an important mirroring role in identity formation.

It is particularly important to ensure that adults with DS continue to have meaningful, consistent relationships in the face of changes that occur as they age. Relationships with parents and staff at a group facility are not enough, since staff often leave to take new jobs and parents grow older and die. It is crucial to ensure the support of additional people who have a committed, ongoing relationship. These relationships can broaden the adult's sense of connection with others as well as soften the impact of future losses.

For more on family support and peer friendships, especially on how to make and maintain friendships, please refer to *Mental Wellness in Adults with Down Syndrome* (Woodbine House, 2006).

OPPORTUNITIES FOR ACCOMPLISHMENT AND SENSE OF WORTH

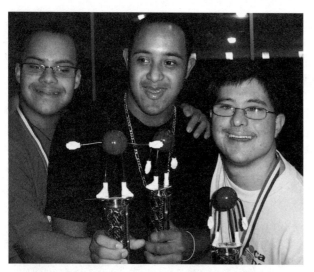

Adults with DS have the same need as others to feel a sense of accomplishment and self-worth. For some, that may mean getting and keeping a repetitive job that fulfills a need for order and regimen. For others, that may mean feeling needed as the result of doing things for others. For still others, it may mean working or volunteering in a field that they are passionate about. We recommend that people with DS be assessed to determine what they need to get from a job, as well as what their skills are to do the job. This can help ensure that the person feels a sense of accomplishment and worth, which, in turn, plays a role in improved health.

SELF-ESTEEM

Self-esteem is one's overall sense of value and self-worth (Rosenberg, 1965). There are many dimensions to self-esteem, but perhaps the two most important include social

The Dennis Principle

In business, the Peter Principle describes the phenomenon in which an employee is recurrently promoted until she reaches a position for which she is not qualified. We have seen a similar phenomenon for a number of our patients. We have named it the Dennis Principle (not because Dr. Dennis McGuire has reached a position for which he is not qualified, but rather because he was the first to describe it).

A number of our patients with DS have been recurrently "promoted" to less restrictive residential or work environments until they have reached a level that they cannot manage. Often we find that they can manage the actual tasks. For example, they can cook for themselves at home or can do the actual job at work. However, they may not be able to develop a plan to use these skills without assistance or direction. In addition, when they reach the level they cannot manage, the emotional challenge can overwhelm their coping skills.

At times, it is an issue of lacking the self-initiation skills to use the appropriate behavior. It can also involve difficulties in handling roommate issues or interpersonal problems. Often the issue is that the person does not know how to use "downtime" or relaxation time. The individual may not be able to decide on and initiate a recreational activity when there isn't a structured event. This can lead to isolation, frustration, or unhappiness when the person spends time without anything to do. She may not have the skills to use her time in a fashion that allows for healthy relaxation.

If these issues are not addressed, it can become a progressively stressful situation. We have seen patients who are struggling with these issues become depressed. Some have become overwhelmed and have lost skills in several areas, even to the point of not being able to do the tasks they could previously do.

In these situations, we have found that the people usually have the necessary skills. For example, they can cook, clean, plan nutritious meals, participate in a regular exercise program, etc. However, the abstract piece of their cognitive skills "to put it all together" is not adequate. They need assistance in making their schedules and figuring out how to constructively use "downtime," as well as some guidance and direction. While some of our patients do live quite independently, many require this little piece of organizational assistance. With this relatively small amount of help, they are able to live far more independently than they are able without it. The tips on helping a person self-promote health (discussed earlier in this chapter) can help avoid the pitfalls of the Dennis Principle.

*(Reprinted from McGuire, D. & Chicoine, B. **Mental Wellness in Adults with Down Syndrome: A Guide to Emotional and Behavioral Strengths and Challenges.** Bethesda, MD: Woodbine House, 2006.)*

health—described previously as support and connectedness to family, friends, and important others—and competence. Competence is a person's ability to do for herself in order to have some sense of control or mastery of the world (Bandura, 1977).

How do social health and competence relate to physical health? In general, people who are valued by significant others, and who value themselves, will ussually take the initiative to care for their own physical health, such as through good nutrition, exercise, and seeking medical care when necessary. This is as true for people with DS as for people in the general population.

However, one problem that people with DS may have in maintaining good health is that they may have trouble understanding and verbalizing to others that a health problem exists. This limitation may be minimized if the person with DS can use a variety of communication methods (verbal and nonverbal) and if parents or other caregivers are open to this type of communication. For example, many parents become astute observers and interpreters of a person's subtle changes in behavior. They often understand that a specific behavior is a clue to pain or discomfort associated with some health condition. In these cases, the person with DS will have some confidence, based on previous experience, that her parents are receiving her message, even if delivered in behavioral form. The major drawback with this form of communication is that it is not as specific as verbal communication. Still, caregivers may act on the person's nonverbal message by taking her to a doctor.

For the person with DS, communicating that a problem exists, and then getting the help she needs, is not only a boast to her self-confidence but an essential means to stay healthy. For more on these issues, please see the chapter on self-esteem in the Mental Wellness book.

CONCLUSION

Health promotion starts outside the medical office. It has many aspects, including healthy diet, regular exercise or activity, appropriate sleep, social connection to others, and activities that promote self-esteem. Individuals with DS need different types and levels of assistance to successfully carry out these health-promoting behaviors, depending on their level of skill and experience. However, we encourage parents and other caregivers to help the person with DS learn how to be as independent as possible in pursuing healthy behaviors.

Chapter 3

Promoting Health

· · · · · · · · · · · · · · · · · ·

in the

· · · · · · · · · · · · ·

Medical Office*

· · · · · · · · · · · · · · · · · ·

Jane, 23 years old, was brought to the Adult Down Syndrome Center by her mother. Jane had been receiving excellent health care, including annual evaluations with blood tests for thyroid screening, from her internist at home, 75 miles from the Center. At the Center, Jane had a history and physical by a medical practitioner, update of immunizations, discussion of health screening testing, and a consultation with the psychosocial practitioner. Jane's mother reported that Jane had talked to herself for years and did not think it was anything to be concerned about. Still, she was reassured to learn that it was common behavior for people with Down syndrome.

After discussion with Jane and her mother, a pelvic exam and PAP smear were performed, the first time Jane had had this exam. Jane also had blood testing for celiac disease. The need for a lateral neck x-ray was discussed. Since Jane was going to be starting a karate class in the near future, she had a lateral neck x-ray done. Finally, because she was considering a move into a group residential facility in the next year, hepatitis B vaccination was discussed and her first shot was given.

---

* This chapter is based partly on work we have done as part of the Down Syndrome Medical Interest Group Adult Health Working Group (for Health Care Guidelines).

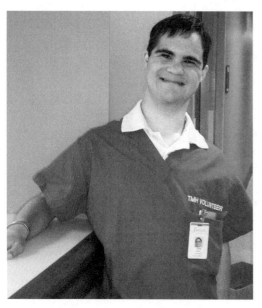

There are several important pieces of health promotion that can and should take place in the medical office. First, the medical office can be a resource for health education for the adult with Down syndrome (DS) and his family. Second, health screening and health assessment can detect issues before they become problems, and health problems can be detected early before they cause significant impairment. Third, preventive measures such as immunizations can help prevent illness before they occur. All of these aspects of a medical visit can help people with DS learn about their health needs and encourage healthy behaviors.

Still, it is worth remembering that patients spend a comparatively short period of time in the medical office. What is done in the medical office cannot replace attention to a person's health outside the office.

EDUCATION

Education is a primary tool in health promotion. For example, just learning that many other people with DS talk to themselves and that we generally consider it a healthy, normal behavior was very important for Jane and her mother. This knowledge helped eliminate her mother's anxiety. Hopefully it will also prevent Jane's family and others who interact with her from trying to change the behavior—which could potentially cause problems.

The office visit provides an opportunity to discuss issues of healthy (or unhealthy) behaviors done outside the office. Many people find it helpful to prepare a list of questions to discuss in advance of their visit. The health care provider may answer your questions directly, offer you written material, or direct you to other sources such as books, the Internet, or support groups for a particular issue. Both the person with DS and his family or caregiver may ask questions. It may be helpful for the family or caregiver to review concerns with the person with DS in preparation for the visit.

If your physician does not have answers to your questions, one solution is to seek out information in books, the Internet, and at conferences. You can then review this information with your practitioner. Our webpage for the Adult Down Syndrome Center (www.advocatehealth.com/adultdown) has information as well as links to additional sources. Additional helpful resources are listed at the end of this book.

HEALTH ASSESSMENT AND HEALTH SCREENING

The purpose of health *screening* is to find conditions before the person develops symptoms. The goal is to treat the condition while the outcome can still be improved. Improved outcome can include reducing pain and suffering, secondary complications, possibilities of transmitting the condition to someone else, the need for treatment, and even the chances of death from the condition. The goals of health *assessment* are similar, but involve assessing symptoms (complaints a patient expresses) to diagnose a condition as early as possible and then improve outcome. Health screening and health assessment are done through:

1. the history,
2. physical exam, and
3. lab tests, x-rays, and additional tests, as needed.

The following sections describe these three general parts of the evaluation for health screening and health assessment. As you proceed further through the book, more specifics about disorders (including how often they occur in people with DS) will be discussed. Hopefully, this additional information will help clarify why we recommend certain evaluations and don't recommend others.

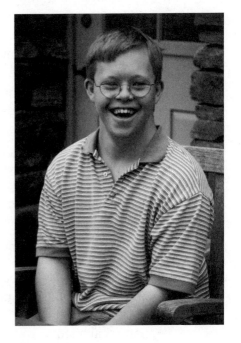

The screenings and assessments may be done by a physician, nurse practitioner, or other practitioner who is familiar with adults with DS. If a practitioner familiar with adults with DS is not available locally, you might want to consider a visit to the nearest DS clinic. A list of clinics is available at www.ds-health.com or www.ndss.org. Alternatively, if the adult has a practitioner who is willing to care for adults with DS but has limited knowledge, a copy of the Down Syndrome Medical Interest Group Health Care Guidelines can be provided for the physician. These are available at the above websites.

HISTORY

The importance of a good health history cannot be overstated. Some people with DS are able to provide important personal health information. Others, however, are not able to provide much, if any, health information. To the extent possible, we encourage practitioners to obtain the history from the patient himself. This helps the patient learn to advocate and speak for himself, empowers him, and gives the practitioner an opportunity to assess interpersonal skills.

Preparing the person with DS in advance for his appointment may improve his ability to provide his own medical history. You may want to suggest that he write down his concerns and questions prior to the appointment. Or, if he communicates better with pictures, you could develop a set of pictures he can use to communicate his health concerns.

Depending on the adult's communication abilities, parents or other care providers may need to confirm the person's medical history or give more details. Family and caregiver observations of the individual with DS are obviously essential when the person with DS is not able to provide his own history.

Some important issues to cover in the person's history include:

- healthy (and unhealthy) behaviors including exercise, cigarette smoking, alcohol consumption, etc.;
- support system (family, care providers, etc.);
- residence;
- occupation;
- opportunities for volunteer work and other activities that promote self-esteem and/or give the person an opportunity to help others;
- participation in recreational activities;
- change in skills (cognitive, activities of daily living, etc.);
- loss of or gains in independence;
- memory impairment;
- swallowing difficulties, choking;
- change in gait (walking), unsteadiness;
- hearing or vision concerns;
- dental health and concerns;
- arthritic discomfort, neck discomfort;
- changes in motor (muscle) function or new neurological impairments such as numbness or headaches;
- incontinence of urine and/or stool;
- other changes in stool/bowel movements or urination;
- menstrual history;
- testicular masses, undescended testicle;
- change in appetite;
- change in weight;
- sleep and sleep apnea;
- fatigue;
- behavioral issues;
- psychological concerns such as
    - mood changes,
    - less interest in life, or
    - mental confusion or reduced sense of reality.

Physical Exam

The physical exam is an important means of gathering health information about the person, discovering concerns the person did not mention in the history or the family was not aware of, and developing rapport and trust between the patient and practitioner.

The first time an adolescent or adult with DS sees a health care provider, it can be very helpful for the family or caregiver to provide information about examination techniques that have worked in the past. If needed, family may also need to help hold the person briefly (or give approval for others to hold him) to allow part of the exam to be performed. For example, it may be helpful for a family member to hold the person's head while his ears are being examined.

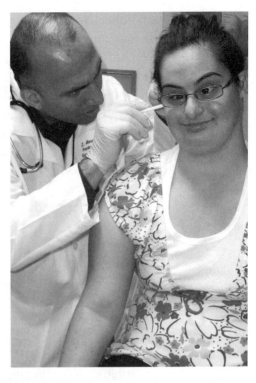

Here are some important parts of the physical exam and findings/problems that the practitioner should cover in a thorough exam. You should expect all these areas to be covered at least annually:

- ◆ General physical exam: Does the person look well or in distress? Assess weight and height; check vital signs.
- ◆ Assess the person's verbal skills, ability to participate in the interview, and behavioral issues (both in general and related to the exam).
- ◆ HEENT (head, eyes, ears, nose, throat)—check for the presence of:
  - ➤ cerumen impaction (ear wax),
  - ➤ hearing impairment,
  - ➤ chronic sinusitis and/or allergies,
  - ➤ evidence of GERD (gastroesophageal reflux),
  - ➤ cataracts, keratoconus, vision impairment, and
  - ➤ small airway ("crowded oropharynx").
- ◆ Neck—check for:
  - ➤ thyromegaly (enlarged thyroid),
  - ➤ thyroid nodules, and
  - ➤ the position in which the person holds his neck/head.
- ◆ Lungs—check for:
  - ➤ abnormal lung sounds (that might indicate pneumonia or other lung problems) and
  - ➤ abnormalities in breathing effort.

- ◆ Heart—check for:
  - ➤ murmur,
  - ➤ cardiomegaly (enlarged heart),
  - ➤ cyanosis (blue discoloration) of skin and lips,
  - ➤ unrecognized congenital heart disease,
  - ➤ acquired heart disease, including:
    - • mitral valve prolapse or
    - • aortic regurgitation.
- ◆ Abdomen—check for:
  - ➤ tenderness,
  - ➤ findings suggesting liver problems (such as hepatitis B or C), or
  - ➤ hernias.
- ◆ Genitourinary—
  - ➤ Male—check for:
    - • testicular masses (possible cancer),
    - • absence of testicle
  - ➤ Female (see health screening, below).
- ◆ Extremities—check for:
  - ➤ arthritic changes,
  - ➤ subluxation (slippage in joints),
  - ➤ hallux valgus (bunion), and
  - ➤ pes planus (flat feet).
- ◆ Neurological exam—check:
  - ➤ reflexes and
  - ➤ muscle strength.
- ◆ Skin—check for:
  - ➤ texture (dry skin),
  - ➤ boils,
  - ➤ seborrheic dermatitis, and
  - ➤ fungal infections of the skin and nails.

ADDITIONAL TESTING

At the conclusion of the physical exam, the doctor will typically recommend screening tests based on the patient's age, gender, family history, and risk factors. For adults with DS, many of these screening tests are the same ones recommended for any adult at their annual physical. But there are also some additional tests that should routinely be ordered for people with DS because they are at a higher risk of developing certain disorders.

Here are some screening tests that may be considered:

- ◆ *Thyroid*—We recommend annual blood testing of TSH, with additional testing if indicated. (See Chapter 15 for information on thyroid disorders.)

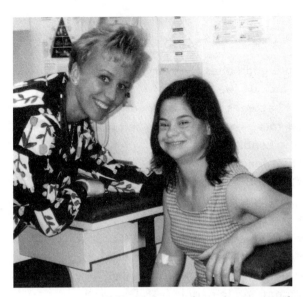

◆ *Celiac disease*—We recommend blood testing based on symptoms suggestive of celiac disease (anti-tissue-transglutaminase antibody; total IgA). Even if a previous test has been negative for CD, the test should be repeated if symptoms occur. (See Chapter 11 for information on celiac disease.)

◆ *Neck x-ray* to screen for atlanto-axial instability and other cervical subluxation (slippage of the vertebrae in the neck). There have not been studies to indicate how often the x-rays should be done. We recommend that they be done at least once in a lifetime and believe it may be reasonable to consider repeating them every ten years. However, if the person has symptoms or if signs of subluxation are noted on the exam, additional neck x-rays should be done even if previous x-rays were normal. Some organizations require that participants have the x-rays more frequently. For example, an organization providing horseback riding might require annual x-rays for participants with DS. (Further information on the cervical spine can be found in Chapter 13.)

◆ *Pap smear*—We recommend this test to check for cervical cancer every three years (after two normal annual tests) for women who are not sexually active and asymptomatic. If the woman is sexually active, the recommendation is every one to three years.

◆ *Mammogram*—See the section below.

◆ *Testicular exam*—We recommend an annual exam to screen for cancer of the testicle and that male patients be taught to do a self-exam (if possible). See Chapter 12 for information about testicular cancer.

◆ *Prostate screening*—See the section below.

◆ *Vision test*—We recommend an exam with an optometrist or ophthalmologist every one to two years.

◆ *Hearing test*—We recommend that an audiologist test the person's hearing every one to two years.

◆ *Bone density testing*—We recommend testing for women every other year at the onset of menopause. Consider testing for men and earlier for women if they are on medications that put them at higher risk for osteoporosis (thinning of the bones).

Elements of a Good Screening Test

Not all screening tests available are good ones for every given patient. Elements of a good screening test include the following:

- ◆ It detects a condition before it becomes a disease or early in the course of the disease before there are symptoms (before the person is aware that he has the condition).
- ◆ The test screens for a condition for which intervention is available that can alter (improve) the outcome. (A test that finds a disease for which there is no treatment that will improve the outcome is not a good screening test.)
- ◆ The costs are acceptable when compared to the benefits. Cost refers both to the financial cost as well as the potential for complications from the test or possible follow-up testing. For example, disease X is very uncommon in people with DS. In the general population, there is a recommendation to do a test every five years to screen for disease X. However, this test is very challenging for many people with DS, and often requires that the person undergo general anesthesia to have the test done. Consequently, the cost of this test is relatively high (a greater potential for complications because of the need for general anesthesia) and the benefit is relatively low (a lower likelihood of the condition being found because the disease is rare in people with DS). Therefore, we would generally not recommend this particular test for people with DS. (Specific examples will be discussed in later chapters.)

A test or exam done to assess symptoms (even early symptoms) is not a screening test by definition. We refer to those tests or exams as health assessments and they are discussed in subsequent chapters describing health problems.

MAMMOGRAMS

Discussion and study of the recommended frequency of mammograms continues for all women. Breast cancer appears to be less common in women with DS. Therefore, we recommend discussing the frequency of mammograms with the health care provider. Currently, we recommend a mammogram annually for our patients after age 40. If a woman cannot cooperate for a traditional mammogram, we consider ultrasound screening for breast cancer. Bear in mind, however, that published studies of ultrasound screenings have been based on using ultrasound as an adjunct to mammography rather than as a substitute for mammography. Ultrasound alone is limited by its dependence on the experience and skill of the technologist/radiologist and by its failure to visualize calcifications, which are often the only manifestation of early breast cancer.

The official position of the American College of Radiology and the Breast Imaging Society is that mammography is the only modality proven by large-scale, long-term studies to reduce mortality from breast cancer. The decision as to whether to screen a patient via ultrasound instead needs to be made on an individual basis after considering factors such as the patient's other conditions, life expectancy, and ability to undergo breast biopsy and breast cancer treatment should a lesion or malignancy be discovered. If the patient is otherwise healthy and screening is deemed appropriate, a screening ultrasound can be considered with the understanding that it yields an incomplete evaluation that nonetheless may represent the best imaging alternative under the circumstances.

PROSTATE SCREENING

In men and boys, the prostate is a gland that sits below the bladder. The prostate contributes fluid that mixes with the sperm from the testicles to form semen (the substance released when a man ejaculates). While prostate cancer is the most common cancer in men without DS, it is uncommon in men with DS. Therefore, the benefit of screening for cancer of the prostate is less clear in men with DS. Screening for prostate cancer includes both:

- ◆ An exam of the prostate, which a physician performs by inserting his finger into the patient's rectum: Abnormalities may include an asymmetry of the prostate, a nodule (mass), or a change in texture (increased firmness or hardness).
- ◆ A blood test for prostate specific antigen (PSA): An elevated PSA level is abnormal.

Currently, the benefits of PSA testing in men without DS are being further investigated, as there is debate as to whether PSA and/or digital exam testing improves survival. Some organizations recommend PSA testing if:

- ◆ The man is age 50 or over (age 40 for men with a family history of prostate cancer), and
- ◆ The man has a life expectancy of at least 20 more years. (Prostate cancer is often a slow-growing tumor. Treating a man for prostate cancer if he has a life expectancy of less than 20 years is often not recommended because of the likelihood that he will die sooner from health issues other than prostate cancer.)

If an abnormal PSA is found, the next step is usually a referral to a urologist and a consideration of an ultrasound and a biopsy. The ultrasound is done by passing the ultrasound device into the rectum. The biopsy is also performed through the rectum (transrectally). These tests are usually done in the urologist's office without anesthesia and produce some discomfort. If a man with DS is referred for these procedures, the ultrasound and the biopsy often must be done under anesthesia because the person usually has difficulty tolerating or cooperating with the procedures. Anesthesia increases the risk of the procedure.

At the Adult Down Syndrome Center, our approach to screening prostate cancer is generally less aggressive in men with DS for the following reasons:

- ◆ Prostate cancer is less common in men with DS.
- ◆ The life expectancy of an adult male with DS at age 50 is less than 20 years.
- ◆ If an abnormality is found, the follow-up testing has the potential for more complications due to the need for anesthesia often required for men with DS.

For these reasons, we generally don't recommend prostate cancer screening.

If prostate cancer is found, the treatment is surgical removal of the prostate. Additional or alternative treatment may be needed if the cancer has spread beyond the prostate. Little information is available as to the survival rate of prostate cancer in men with DS.

SEDATION AND/OR ANESTHESIA FOR TESTING AND PROCEDURES

Some people with DS cannot cooperate with certain tests. As noted above in the section on mammograms, sometimes it becomes necessary to use a different test to optimize health screening. As is the case with using ultrasound instead of mammography, the replacement test may not be as good as the one that is ordinarily used.

Sometimes testing is more successful if the person is sedated. While we have not found sedation to be of benefit for mammography (because it limits the person's ability to cooperate as needed to do the test), we have found it to be of benefit for some other tests. Sometimes, however, adding sedation or anesthesia may significantly increase the risk of the test (by adding the risk of anesthesia/sedation) and raise the risk: benefit ratio so the test is no longer advisable (see above).

The risk of sedation or anesthesia must be minimized. At times we use small amounts of a benzodiazepine such as diazepam (Valium) or lorazepam (Ativan) to reduce anxiety and help the individual with DS successfully participate in the testing. These medications are prescribed to be taken a few hours before the exam.

If greater sedation is needed, we prefer to have the test done in a monitored setting, often with an anesthesiologist present. One reason is that the risk of aspiration (of saliva, stomach contents, or food) into the lungs while sedated appears to be greater for people with DS. Another reason is that the person with DS may be injured if he fears the procedure and fights back or uses some other unexpected behavior in response to his fear. Finally, sleep apnea (both recognized and undiagnosed) is more common in people with DS and can lead to cessation of breathing while sedated. For all these reasons and others, we don't use sedation without an anesthesiologist present (other than the small doses noted above to reduce anxiety). In a monitored and controlled setting, the proper amount of sedation can be given safely and allow testing to be effectively completed.

Normal vs. Abnormal Lab Results

Lisa, age 27, is a generally healthy young woman with DS who developed a fever and was evaluated in the emergency room. As part of her evaluation, she had some blood tests done, including a CBC (complete blood count). Lisa and her family were told there were no concerning abnormalities on her lab tests. She was discharged and subsequently completely recovered.

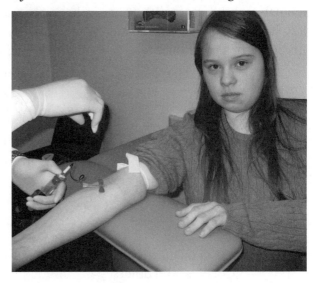

Lisa's mother obtained a copy of the lab results and at her next visit to the Adult Down Syndrome Center asked about a value that had been reported as abnormal on the CBC. The MCV (mean corpuscular volume—size of the red blood cells) was elevated. We discussed the meaning of an abnormal MCV in a person with DS (see below). Lisa and her family were reassured and no further testing was performed.

Lab tests can be very beneficial in diagnosing health problems and assessing effectiveness or complications of treatment. Sometimes lab tests in people with DS may have values that are different from the normal values. Some of those values truly are abnormal and need further assessment and/or treatment. Some differences, however, are common findings in people with DS and may not indicate any health issues of concern. Two tests where abnormalities are often not a reason for concern are described below. Other lab tests that are helpful in diagnosing, treating, and monitoring medical conditions in people with DS are discussed in later chapters.

MCV

One lab test in which results are commonly elevated in people with DS is the MCV. MCV (mean corpuscular volume) is a measure of the size of red blood cells. A change in the size of red blood cells can be indicative of a number of health problems. However, in people with DS, it may be more a variant than a true abnormality.

Red blood cells are made in the bone marrow. As red blood cells mature in the bone marrow, they become smaller. If red blood cells are released from the bone marrow before they mature, the cells will be larger and the MCV will be elevated.

It is thought that red blood cells are often released early from the bone marrow of people with DS. One theory is that red blood cells die more quickly in people with DS, so less mature cells are released in order to replace them. Another theory is that there is an abnormality in folic acid metabolism in people with DS that may lead to larger red blood cells.

An elevated MCV is generally not considered an abnormality that requires additional assessment in a person with DS, so long as he has a normal blood count (hemoglobin and hematocrit). (That is, he is not anemic.) However, if the person has a low hemoglobin and/or hematocrit (anemia), or if there are additional concerns or findings, then additional assessment is recommended.

ESR

The erythrocyte sedimentation rate (ESR) may also be elevated in people with DS. The ESR is determined by how quickly red blood cells settle in a column of blood and is a nonspecific indicator of inflammation. (That means it indicates that there is inflammation somewhere in the body, but not the source of the inflammation.) An elevated ESR can be an indication of:

- infections,
- autoimmune diseases,
- malignancy,
- use of medications such as some anti-seizure medications, birth control pills, and others,
- anemia.

Fairly often, the ESR is elevated in people with DS without a clear cause. Whether additional testing is done depends on findings in the history, physical exam, or other tests, and on whether the health care provider suspects an underlying problem. If there are other findings to suggest one of the above conditions, additional testing may be done. In some people, no additional testing may be required at that time, but regular follow-up may be in order. Again, an elevated sedimentation rate in someone with DS often turns out not to be an indication of any kind of disease.

IMMUNIZATIONS

◆ ◆ ◆ ◆ ◆ ◆ ◆ ◆ ◆ ◆ ◆ ◆ ◆ ◆ ◆ ◆

Immunizations are an important piece of health promotion and disease prevention. Our recommendations for adolescents and adults with DS assume all childhood immunizations were given appropriately. If so, we recommend the following schedule of immunizations:

- *Tetanus-diphtheria (Td)*—A tetanus-diphtheria shot is recommended every ten years. However, the TdaP (tetanus-diphteria-acellular pertussis) is recommended one time to replace the next Td for those

18 to 64 who have not previously had the TdaP during that age range. In 2005, The Advisory Committee on Immunization Practices recommended that the next time an individual was due for the Td, he receive TdaP. In addition to being given every 10 years, a Td should also be given whenever someone suffers a "dirty wound" (e.g., steps on a rusty nail). If the person is due for the TdaP, that can be given at that time instead of the Td.

◆ *Influenza*—We recommend that our patients consider getting a flu shot each fall, especially if they spend time around many people. It is recommended annually for people with certain other health problems such as diabetes, heart disease, lung disease, etc. It is recommended for all people over age 50. The recommendation changes from year to year, so we recommend consulting the web page of the Center for Disease Control (www.cdc.gov).

◆ *Pneumonia*—We recommend considering the pneumonia vaccine at age 50 for adults with DS. It is also recommended at a younger age for adults with certain other health problems (see influenza) and then should be repeated in 5 years or at age 50 if it has been less than 5 years since the first pneumonia vaccine. (Our recommendations are similar to our recommendations for influenza. For people without DS, the recommendation is to begin receiving the vaccine annually at age 65, but we recommend that adults with DS begin receiving it at age 50 due to early aging.)

◆ *Varicella (chickenpox)*—We recommend testing adults with DS for immunity via blood tests if there is no history of having had chickenpox or they were not vaccinated previously. We recommend the two-shot series if the person is not immune.

◆ *Hepatitis B*—We recommend that this three-shot series immunization be given one time for people living in residential facilities. We also recommend it for adults who work in a group setting (e.g., workshop) and recommend considering it for all others. We usually do a blood test before administering the vaccine to an adult with DS to see if he has immunity (and thus does not need the vaccine). In addition, we recommend drawing a blood test (hepatitis B surface antibody) to document attaining immune status four to six weeks after the third shot.

◆ *Hepatitis A*—We have not been recommending hepatitis A vaccine for all our patients, but we do recommend it for patients with liver disease (including hepatitis B) and for other high risk individuals as indicated for those without DS. We also recommend it for individuals who live or work in a place where hepatitis A has been a problem.

◆ *Human papillomavirus (HPV)*—This is given to women (preferably before they become sexually active) to prevent HPV infection (the virus linked to cervical cancer). Recommendations are to give it to young women before age 26. Currently, there are not data to help in making recommendations for women with DS who are older than 26 and have never been sexually active but might become sexually active.

◆ *Measles-mumps-rubella*—We recommend giving one dose of this vaccine if the person's immunization history is unreliable. A second dose may also be recommended for others based on their immunization history. (The usual recommended schedule is one dose at age one year and the second between 4 and 6 years of age.)

◆ *Meningococcal (meningitis)*—This immunization is usually recommended for children aged 11 to 12 or for students before entering high school. It is also recommended for those entering college who have not had it previously. At this time, there are no recommendations for meningitis vaccine for individuals moving to residential facilities.

CONCLUSION

◆ ◆ ◆ ◆ ◆ ◆ ◆ ◆ ◆ ◆ ◆ ◆ ◆ ◆ ◆ ◆ ◆ ◆ ◆ ◆

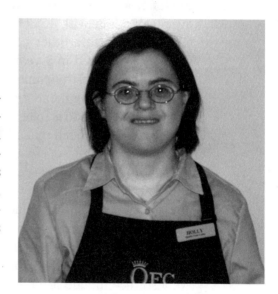

Health promotion in the office includes a variety of activities, including patient education, taking a good history, and doing a physical exam, lab tests, and immunizations. Much of this information is summarized in table form in Addendum 2, at the back of the book. Further information is provided in the following chapters that address specific health issues.

Chapter 4

Health Concerns:
• • • • • • • • • • • • • • • • • • • •
Introduction
• • • • • • • • • • • •

Thomas, age 45, had been experiencing chest pain intermittently for one month. The pain was in the center of his chest and often woke him at night. He couldn't give a good description of the pain, but he was clearly worried about it. He likes to watch the medical television show, ER, and he indicated a concern regarding characters in the show who had chest pain and then needed CPR.

Thomas had recently started working in the evening and was eating after work just before bed. He had also been drinking more cola because it was available at work. He had gained five pounds in the last month because of the cola and because he could no longer attend his evening exercise classes.

After examining Thomas, I discussed the low incidence of coronary artery disease in people with Down syndrome with Thomas and his father, which reassured them. I diagnosed gastroesophageal reflux disease (which is more common in people with Down syndrome) and recommended weight loss, not eating just before bed, reducing caffeinated cola beverages, and a six-week course of ranitidine (Zantac). Thomas's symptoms completely resolved and he is once again much more comfortable watching ER.

When we started the Adult Down Syndrome Center, one of the questions we were frequently asked was, "Why do you need a clinic for adults with Down syndrome? I didn't know there *were* any adults with Down syndrome." While

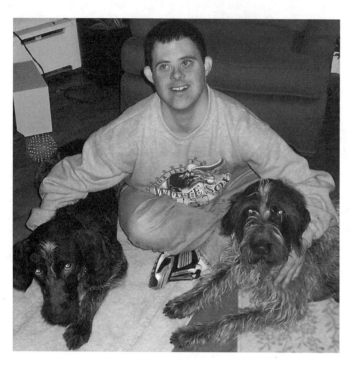

this may have been true in the past, the situation has changed dramatically in the last century, even the last 30 years. The life expectancy of people with Down syndrome (DS) in the United States is now up to 56 years. In 1900, the life expectancy was about 9 years.

To put this in perspective: The life expectancy of people in the U.S. in the general population was in the mid-50s in 1900. If the life expectancy of people without DS had increased by the same percentage as for people with DS since 1900, the average life expectancy would now be about 300 years for people without DS. Even as recently as 30 years ago, the life expectancy for people with DS was only in the 20s to 30s. As people with the condition are living longer, the need to address health issues of adulthood has become more important.

HEALTH PROBLEMS THAT OCCUR MORE OR LESS FREQUENTLY

There are problems that are more common in people with DS than in other people, and there are problems that are less common. There are also problems whose incidence does not seem to be affected by having DS.

Among the health issues that are thought to be *more common:*

- ◆ infections (including skin infections),
- ◆ cataracts,
- ◆ keratoconus (abnormal curvature of the lens of the eye),
- ◆ cerumen impaction (wax blocking the ear canal),
- ◆ diabetes mellitus (types 1 and 2),
- ◆ hypothyroidism (underactive thyroid),
- ◆ hyperthyroidism (overactive thyroid),
- ◆ mitral valve prolapse,
- ◆ sleep apnea,
- ◆ gastroesophageal reflux disease (GERD),

- celiac disease (sensitivity to gluten),
- constipation,
- urinary retention,
- osteoarthritis,
- osteoporosis,
- cervical subluxation (slipping of the vertebrae in the neck)—particularly but not limited to atlantoaxial instability (slippage of the first cervical vertebrae on the second),
- cancer of the testicle,
- cancer of the ovary,
- leukemia (the higher incidence seems to last only until the end of the teen years, however),
- dysphagia (swallowing dysfunction),
- some psychiatric disorders,
- obesity
- seizures,
- gum disease,
- autism.

There are also some problems that are more common at a younger age (or occur at a younger age) in adults with DS, such as dementia (including Alzheimer disease) and high frequency hearing loss.

In addition, some health problems are *less common:*

- Atherosclerotic heart disease (narrowing of the arteries)—the primary cause of myocardial infarctions (heart attacks), strokes, and peripheral vascular disease—occurs less frequently.
- Hypertension (high blood pressure) is uncommon.
- Asthma, which is increasing in the rest of the population, appears to be less common in adults with DS.
- Most types of cancer (other than those listed above) are less common.
- Dental cavities seem to occur less often. This was especially true when people with DS often lived in institutions and had less access to sugary food, but still seems to be true today.
- Suicide attempts are less common.
- Substance abuse problems, including drug and alcohol abuse, are less common.

THE PRESENTATION OF MEDICAL PROBLEMS

◆ ◆ ◆ ◆ ◆ ◆ ◆ ◆ ◆ ◆ ◆ ◆ ◆ ◆ ◆ ◆ ◆ ◆ ◆

There are not just differences in the incidence of specific health problems among adults with DS. There are also sometimes differences in the way these medical problems "present." That is, the complaint a person describes or the changes someone else observes may be different than for someone without DS. Often times, the difference is that the person is not able to say, for example, "I have this pain." Rather, it may be noted as a change in mood, behavior, or function.

To better promote health in people with DS and to diagnose and treat medical problems, it is imperative to understand that medical problems may present differently in people with DS. To the best of my knowledge, there are no disease states that are completely unique to people with DS. However, there is clearly a difference in incidence, as outlined above. There are also differences in combinations of health issues and in the way that they present.

Due to differences in frequency of health issues, a person with DS may have a combination of autism, diabetes, and celiac disease. The diagnosis of diabetes and celiac disease and the dietary restrictions required to treat them may be particularly challenging for this person who also has autism, a limited ability to change, and a strong reliance on continuing patterns of behavior (and sometimes dietary preferences).

It can also be very challenging to diagnose a physical health issue when the presentation is atypical, behavioral, or completely unique. For example, William, a 32-year-old man with limited verbal skills, presented with aggressive behavior. He was diagnosed with significant allergies that were making him feel poorly. We investigated the social settings where he was having the most problems and found that he was having difficulties tolerating the most stressful situations. However, his behavior in these settings improved dramatically with the treatment of his allergies.

As in William's case, differences in presentation are often related to difficulties communicating the symptoms. When someone feels poorly but is not able to communicate her concerns, she is more likely to communicate through behavior changes. Likewise, if an illness or disorder is affecting a person's ability to function, but she is unaware that something is wrong or she doesn't realize she should seek medical attention, others may not notice the problem until it affects her behavior. The next chapter will discuss the interaction between mental and physical health in more detail.

AGING AND EARLY AGING

Aging is not synonymous with health problems. There are, however, some physical changes that are commonly a part of aging. There are also some health problems that occur more often with aging but are not directly a part of aging. Some of the changes that occur with aging in people with DS are the same as in people with DS; others occur more often or at an earlier age.

Glucose intolerance, reduced muscle mass, increased body fat percentage, a general physical slowing down, and difficulties with near vision are all examples of changes seen as people *without* DS age. These changes—which are considered a normal part of aging—are also commonly seen in people with DS. Likewise, cataracts, diabetes mellitus, osteoarthritis, dementia, gum disease, and high frequency hearing loss are health problems that occur more often with aging in people both with and without DS. However, these problems are not a part of normal aging.

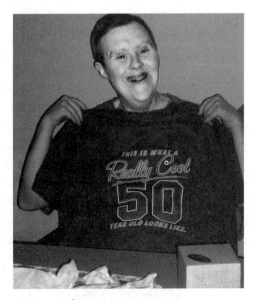

Some reduction in cognitive (thinking) abilities is a part of normal aging in people without DS. Similarly, in one study published in 1996, researchers showed a small decline in function with age in adults with DS (Devenny et al., 1996). This decline was comparable to that seen in healthy adults who do not have an intellectual disability.

How Is the Aging Process Different in Adults with Down Syndrome?

People with DS appear to age earlier than other adults. In our experience, many people with DS appear younger than their chronological age until about their mid-30s, but then appear to age more rapidly. This premature aging pattern appears to affect both their physical appearance and the onset of health issues that occur more frequently as people age.

As adults with DS enter their mid- to late thirties, we find it is helpful to think of them as 5, 10, 15, even 20 years older than their chronological age. For example, we would think of a 70-year-old person with DS as being comparable to a 90-year-old person without DS.

Certainly there is variability in all people, with or without DS. For example, some people without DS in their 80s need to use a walker or a cane due to arthritis. Others are still running the marathon (two men in their 80s completed the Chicago Marathon in 2006). We have certainly seen a wide range of aging patterns in people with DS as well.

Diseases that tend to occur at higher frequency with age occur at a younger age in people with DS. For example, cataracts, osteoarthritis, osteoporosis, and gum disease all occur more frequently in people with DS and occur more frequently at a younger age.

Dementia is a condition that may not occur more frequently overall in adults with DS, but it clearly occurs at a younger age. Further study is being done to determine the overall incidence of dementia in people with DS. Our data suggest a similar incidence of dementia for people with DS when compared to people without DS. However, when it does occur, it occurs, on average, 20 years earlier (which is similar to the extent of early aging described earlier). In the general population, dementia occurs in approximately 10 percent of adults in their 60s, 20 percent in their 70s, and 40 percent in their 80s. The data for our patients with DS show a similar increase of dementia with increasing age, but the starting point is earlier in life. Thus, approximately 10

Do Adults with Mosaicism or Translocation Age Differently?

The oldest person in our practice—who had not developed any signs of Alzheimer disease when she died at age 83—had mosaic DS. While her long life suggests that there may be a reduction of certain health issues associated with aging or even an overall slowing of the aging process in adults who have mosaic DS, there are limited data to make a more generalized statement.

In our practice, we do not have chromosome studies for most of our older patients, and, therefore, are not aware whether they have trisomy 21, mosaic DS, or DS due to translocation. Nor has there been any research into differences in aging in people with mosaic or translocation DS compared to those with trisomy 21. For now, our best recommendation is to ensure that adults with these types of DS have the same preventive care and health screenings as other adults with DS.

percent of adults with DS develop dementia in their 40s, 20 percent in their 50s, and 40 percent in their 60s.

Although there has been a great deal of focus on dementia (particularly Alzheimer disease) as part of aging in people with DS, it is also important to consider other issues that can cause an adult to lose cognitive skills. Often these issues are not considered for people with DS when there is a change in abilities or behavior.

For example, for a number of reasons, the need for an adult with DS to retire is often overlooked. For some adults with DS, this is a funding issue. They may live in a supported residential facility where there is no staff available during the day, so the residents are required to work or to go to a day program. While some agencies have developed senior programs or retirement programs, many have not. Therefore, as people slow down with age and want to do something different than the work they have been doing (a normal social development with age), there is no opportunity for them to retire. For other older adults, it is not an issue of funding. Rather, those who are supporting the person with DS don't appreciate that people with DS go through the typical life cycle at a faster rate and may be ready to retire in their 40s.

Other problems may occur if health issues impede the person's ability to work or slow her down significantly, leading to conflicts. For example, if an adult begins producing less at work, it may be misinterpreted as a behavioral issue, "noncompliance," or depression, when in fact the person is slowing down physically with age and no longer able to work as quickly as she did in the past.

It is very important to understand and appreciate the differences in normal aging in people with DS. Understanding these differences will increase your effectiveness in assisting and guiding adults with DS, as well as in interpreting changes in health or behavior.

The next chapter will discuss the interaction between physical health issues and mental health issues. The rest of the book will then highlight specific physical health issues that are more common or problematic in adults with DS.

Chapter 5

The Interaction between Physical and Mental Health

Jason, age 23, had been a model employee at the grocery store. He did an excellent job bagging groceries and gathering shopping carts, and had great rapport with the customers and his coworkers. Recently, however, he had begun to have difficulty staying on task and would move away from his aisle before he finished packing the groceries. He had also become anxious and irritable with customers. Jason's parents were concerned that he would lose his job and brought him to the Adult Down Syndrome Center for evaluation. The history and physical exam revealed no clues to the cause of the changes. However, thyroid blood tests demonstrated that Jason had hyperthyroidism (overactive thyroid). Anxiety is a known symptom of hyperthyroidism. With treatment for hyperthyroidism, Jason's mood and behavior once again returned to normal.

At the Adult Down Syndrome Center, we take a multidisciplinary approach to evaluating and treating our patients' health problems. That is, professionals with expertise in a variety of different fields often work together to try to figure out the causes for a problem and to devise the best way of treating it.

The reason we use this approach is that a complex interplay of biological, social, and psychological factors can be involved in causing or maintaining a problem. Teasing out all the factors at play is vital to effective treatment.

For example, Jason, above, initially appeared to have a change to his mental health (mood change) that was affecting his social functioning (his ability to perform his job). However, a blood test revealed that a physical problem—a thyroid disorder—was the root cause of his mental health difficulties.

That is not to say that all physical problems in adolescents and adults with Down syndrome (DS) have an effect on the person's mental health and vice versa. But it happens often enough that we have found it is essential to always consider the possibility that a problem may be more complex than it at first appears.

THE BIO-PSYCHO-SOCIAL APPROACH

Technically, the approach we use at the Adult Down Syndrome Center to diagnose and treat physical health, mental health, or behavioral problems is known as the bio-psycho-social approach. What this simply means is that we consider all the biological, psychological, and social factors that may be contributing to an individual's problem.

- ◆ *Biological problems* are physical problems that are affecting the person's body and may include pain or discomfort, a sensory difficulty (such as trouble seeing or hearing), broken limbs, or a problem with any organ or part of the body.
- ◆ *Social or environmental problems* are changes in the person's interactions or the settings where she lives, works, or pursues leisure activi-

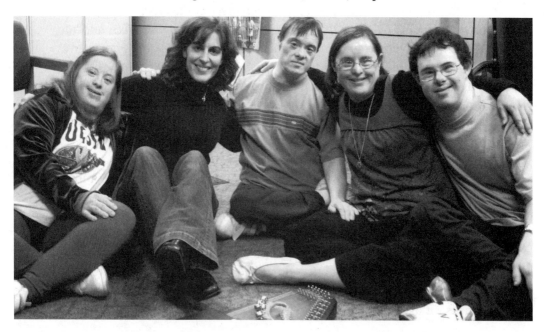

ties. This may include the loss of a family member or caregiver, conflicts with others, or changes in routine that are experienced as stressful.

◆ **Psychological or mental problems** involve difficulties with thoughts and emotions and may include depression, obsessions and compulsions, anxiety, behavior issues, and more serious disorders such as psychosis.

The bio-psycho-social issues that are present or active in any human situation may have a compounding effect on each other. To look at just one of many possible scenarios, let's imagine that a hypothyroid medical condition has triggered symptoms of depression in an adult with DS. If this person has a tendency for negative thoughts, he may overreact to the hypothyroidism, which may intensify the symptoms of depression. Once the symptoms begin, the person may also become, in effect, "depressed about being depressed." That is, he becomes embarrassed or stigmatized by his depressive symptoms. This may further intensify his negative thoughts, which then worsens his symptoms and reduces his chances of recovering from the problem.

THE MULTIDISCIPLINARY APPROACH

At the Adult Down Syndrome Center, a variety of professionals are available to assist in diagnosing and treating our patients' health problems. These professionals include:

◆ medical doctors,
◆ certified nurse practitioner,
◆ doctor of social work,
◆ nurses or certified medical assistants,
◆ advocate (who provides educational information and assists with connections to other sources of services),
◆ nutritionist,
◆ audiologist, and
◆ other medical specialists as needed.

All patients attending the Center see the medical doctor or the certified nurse practitioner, the social worker, advocate, and the nurse or medical assistant, and many see the nutritionist, and/or audiologist. Other specialists, such as an ear, nose, and throat specialist, are enlisted to share their expertise as needed.

Having professionals available from so many disciplines makes it more likely that we will uncover all the biological, social, and psychological factors that are contributing to an individual's problems. We have found that if we ignore any of the key bio-psycho-social influences on a behavior, then the problem may continue. We have to be careful, though, because we all have biases that may tend to point us to certain causes while we ignore others. What we get wrong, if we are not careful, is that we assume we know the sole cause and explanation of a problem. We have learned

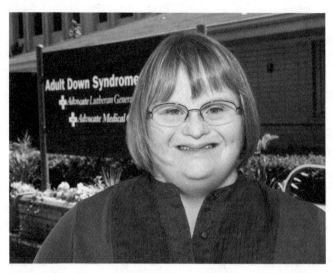

the hard way to keep looking for issues and concerns even when we have identified some possible precipitants.

This is why a multidisciplinary team is so important. A multidisciplinary team views each person from many different perspectives—examining health, nutritional, social, and vocational issues, and even looking at the person's thought processes, if possible. Each practitioner on the team is like a detective scrupulously searching for causes related to his or her areas of specialty, be that health, mental health, nutrition, a lack of programs and services, negative thoughts, or environmental stressors.

If you live in a community where there is not a multidisciplinary team, you should consider working with a trusted professional (such as a family doctor, internist, or nurse practitioner) who will help to coordinate the care of the person with DS. When a problem occurs, you could ask him or her for a referral to other medical specialists or to behavioral or mental health practitioners (social workers, psychologist, or counselors) as needed. Your primary doctor could then receive and interpret reports from these specialists or practitioners.

THE MULTIDISCIPLINARY APPROACH IN ACTION: CASE STUDIES

In this section we will describe three individuals with DS who were all diagnosed with depression and obsessions or compulsive behaviors at the Adult Down Syndrome Center. Although they all shared the diagnosis of depression with obsessions/compulsions, they each had different biological and social problems intertwined with their mental health issues. As a consequence, they had previously received less than optimal treatment because these issues had not been identified and treated. These practical examples should illustrate the value of using the multidisciplinary approach to evaluating and treating health issues in people with DS.

GEORGE

The first patient, George, was a 29-year-old man with DS who lived with his parents in a mid-sized town in Illinois. His parents brought him to a psychiatrist in his town because they were concerned about a change in his mood and behavior. He had become uncharacteristically dragging and lethargic at his job, and had barely enough energy or motivation to socialize with others. Although George was previously known for being friendly and outgoing, he was avoiding family and friends and had little to say when he encountered them.

At home, George's parents noted that he had little interest in beloved free-time activities, such as listening to music, playing video games, or watching favorite movies. His parents stated that he had always talked to himself in the privacy of his room, but now his self-talk seemed to occupy more and more of his free time and the tone was uncharacteristically angry and self-deprecating. He had also lost interest in his favorite foods and he seemed to be restless at night. In addition, he was no longer meticulous about his appearance, or about keeping his room neat or orderly. His parents noted too that he had become obsessed with certain concerns that had not bothered him before such as whether there would be rain or thunderstorms.

The local psychiatrist diagnosed George with major depression with obsessive compulsive features and started him on an antidepressant medication, escitalopram (Lexapro). George's mood and behavior improved for about six weeks, but then his symptoms returned and even seemed to worsen. Neither an increase in his medication nor a trial of a second antidepressant medication helped. While George was trying the second antidepressant medication, his parents arranged a consultation at the Adult Down Syndrome Center.

ANITA

Coincidentally, at about the same time that George's parents first brought him to the Center, the parents of a 32-year-old woman named Anita also sought out the Center for an appointment. Anita's problems had begun six months before George's, but ran a similar course.

Anita had been successful in an assembly job and had been active in social, recreational, and church activities prior to the start of her symptoms. Like George, she had begun to withdraw from family and friends and had little energy or motivation for things she had enjoyed. Also like George, she had begun talking to herself more, and her self-talk included more angry and self-critical comments. She also had begun to talk to herself in public, especially when not engaged in some type of activity. She was becoming increasingly obsessed about placing certain objects in her house "just so." Although she had always been particular about her bedroom, she was now extending this behavior to the family room and she was very rigid about where certain items could go. Additionally, Anita had become less flexible with changes or disruptions in her routine and she tended to repeat certain questions over and over. Although she had had these types of behaviors before, they became more intense and more problematic for her family and others in her life.

Like George's parents, Anita's parents sought the assistance of a psychiatrist in the community and Anita was also diagnosed with depression and compulsive behaviors. Unlike George's psychiatrist, however, Anita's psychiatrist viewed self-talk as a form of psychotic behavior. As a result, Anitia was treated with an antipsychotic medication, olanzapine (Zyprexa), as well as an antidepressant medication, sertraline (Zoloft) for her depressive and compulsive symptoms.

Like George, Anita showed an initial improvement in her mood and behavior, but her improvement did not last, despite a trial of a number of different antidepressant and antipsychotic medications. To complicate matters, her parents observed two new problems. First, Anita seemed to be "driven and obsessed with food." She quickly gained a significant amount of weight, which seemed to aggravate her depressive symptoms. The heavier she got, the less energy or motivation she had to do activities. Second, Anita developed a problem with sleep involving loud snoring and gasping for breath, whereupon she would wake up. Anita's parents watched with growing concern as her depression seemed to worsen and she developed major new problems with sleep and weight. Out of desperation, they scheduled an appointment at the Adult Down Syndrome Center.

COLLEEN

At about the same time that George and Anita were being treated for depression and compulsive behaviors, Colleen, age 32, was having similar symptoms. Like George and Anita, she was lethargic at home and work, despite previously enjoying her free time and job activities. She began to refuse to participate in social or recreational activities and Special Olympics, although she had previously enjoyed these activities immensely. Like the others, she was tired and had little energy or enthusiasm for much of anything. She was also talking to herself more, and doing it in public settings, which she had not previously done. In addition, her compulsive behaviors had increased. She was a little less flexible with changes in her schedule and routine and was more anxious about changes in weather, especially when thunderstorms were a possibility.

Increasingly concerned about the changes in Colleen's mood and behavior, her parents took her to a psychiatrist in a nearby city. She was treated with an antidepressant medication, sertraline (Zoloft). At the psychiatrist's suggestion, she also began weekly sessions with a clinical social worker who had some experience working with people with DS and other disabilities.

Colleen's social worker and psychiatrist had also suggested a thorough physical exam, which was conducted by her regular physician (a family practitioner who had experience working with people with intellectual disabilities). This exam showed that she had hypothyroidism (underactive thyroid), for which she was treated. (See Chapter 15.)

The evaluation also showed that Colleen had celiac disease, which meant that she could not process gluten, a protein that is in wheat and many processed foods. (See Chapter 11 for more on this.) The treatment for this condition involves eliminating all gluten from the diet. Although the dietary restrictions are hard for most people, whether or not they have DS, Colleen's parents had already developed a gluten-free diet for her father, who also had celiac disorder. Thus, they did not find it hard to adapt to Colleen's dietary needs. They had already found some local stores that sold gluten-free food and had found tasty substitutions for many wheat products. This made it that much easier for Colleen to adapt to her new diet.

Over the course of several months of treatment by her psychiatrist, social worker, and family doctor, Colleen began to perk up. Within six months, her mood and behavior had improved considerably. Although she was not 100 percent back to her old self, her parents were very pleased with the improvements that she had made. Still, her family doctor, psychiatrist, and social worker encouraged them to follow through with the appointment they had scheduled for Colleen at the Adult DS Center.

MULTIDISCIPLINARY ASSESSMENT AND DIAGNOSIS FOR GEORGE, ANITA, AND COLLEEN

At the Center, George, Anita, and Colleen were scheduled for multidisciplinary assessments, which included a complete physical exam with extensive lab work, x-rays and other testing, and referrals to specialists as needed. All were also seen by the second author for a psychosocial evaluation, and a nutritional evaluation by the clinic's licensed nutritionist. Additionally, they all met with the Center's resource specialists to discuss possible programs and services in the community that could be of use.

The multidisciplinary team at the Center diagnosed all three patients with major depression. The diagnosis was based on DSM IV-R criteria for major depression which had been adapted to meet the needs of people with intellectual disabilities. (See our previous book, *Mental Wellness in Adults with Down Syndrome,* for more on this.) Although the primary diagnosis for each of them was depression, clinic staff also noted the presence of obsessive compulsive behaviors that were significant enough to interfere with normal functioning. In short, the clinic supported the diagnoses of depression with obsessions and compulsive behaviors made by the three patients' psychiatrists.

Additionally, each psychiatrist had noted certain life events that they believed may have aggravated or precipitated the onset of symptoms. The ADSC staff also believed that these events may have played a role in triggering symptoms, although from our perspective, life events represent only one type of influence on a behavior. Still, they represent an important type of stress and should therefore be considered as part of the total picture or approach.

All three individuals had experienced some type of loss prior to the onset of symptoms. For example, one of George's best friends had moved out of state with his family. According to George's parents, he had taken this loss rather hard. George also had a coworker who had been teasing him, and this, too, was stressful for him. For her part, Anita lost two very close and positive relationships in the year preceding her diagnosis with depression. Both her job supervisor and her coach at Special Olympics had moved on to different pursuits. For Colleen, there had been a recent significant loss and one that may have been overlooked. Recently, she had lost her dog, who had been a close companion for over fifteen years. This loss seemed to remind her of another loss that had been difficult for her as well—her grandfather's death. Even though he had died over five years ago, her dog's death seemed to bring back this loss very intensely. (This is not uncommon for people with DS; see the discussion in *Mental Wellness in Adults with Down Syndrome*.)

To summarize, when we did our evaluations at the ADSC, the case for depression with obsessions and compulsive behaviors appeared to be clear and well documented by family observers and by the three adults' respective psychiatrists. We also believed that stressful life events were possible precipitants to the depression and obsessive compulsive symptoms.

There was one diagnosis we disagreed with, and that was the diagnosis of a psychosis given by Anita's psychiatrist. A psychosis is a serious mental health disorder evidenced by delusions, hallucinations, disorganized speech, or grossly disorganized or catatonic behavior (American Psychiatric Association). We understood how this diagnosis was reached, however. We find that many mental health practitioners view self-talk as evidence of a psychosis. But self-talk is quite common in adults with DS and should not be automatically considered a symptom of psychosis, even when the person is expressing anger or self-critical comments through his self-talk. Anita did not seem to have been delusional, hallucinating, or out of touch with reality, which would be the more accurate gauge of a psychosis.

Because of the psychiatrist's diagnosis, Anita had been prescribed an atypical antipsychotic medication, olanzapine (Zyprexa). This class of antipsychotic medication may be used for more extreme forms of agitation or for obsessive compulsive symptoms that do not respond to treatment from other classes of medications (such as antidepressants). While Anita was anxious, her anxiety was not extreme, and she did not have a more extreme form of obsessive compulsive behavior, so we did not find that her symptoms justified the use of an antipsychotic medication.

These types of antipsychotic medications may be "wonder drugs" for people who need them, but they also have some negative side effects. For example, olanzapine (Zyprexa) can affect some people's metabolism adversely and it also makes many people obsessed and driven for food. When this occurs, as it seemed to for Anita, the individual will often gain a significant amount of weight in a very short time. The only way to counteract this problem is for the person to remain very active with sports and recreation activities. Unfortunately, this is not easy for people who are already depressed and who tend to resist these types of activities. They often have much less interest or energy in doing essential or beneficial social, recreational, and vocational activities.

Following from this, the main goal of any treatment of depression is to get the person moving again (or "un-depressed") by doing essential or normal life activities. Doing activities may then serve as a natural antidepressant. The more the person moves, the better he feels, and the better he feels, the more he moves—until he gets back to a more normal "un-depressed" state.

Antidepressant medications such as the sertraline (Zoloft) Anita was prescribed can reduce lethargy and increase energy and motivation, but this may be counteracted by other influences, such as weight gain that may result from taking an anti-psychotic medication. This seemed to be the case for Anita. As she gained more weight, she became more sedentary and less active, thus making it more difficult for her to become less depressed.

THE ROLE OF HEALTH ISSUES IN THE DEPRESSION OF GEORGE, ANITA, AND COLLEEN

Of the three adults who came to the Center with diagnoses of depression, only Colleen had had a physical exam to look for other health issues. This section describes the medical issues that were eventually uncovered, how they contributed to each person's emotional issues, and how treatment resolved the medical and emotional problems.

COLLEEN'S MEDICAL AND EMOTIONAL HEALTH

The medical issues identified by Colleen's family physician were quite important. They included hypothyroidism and celiac disease, both of which may contribute to the development, continuation, or severity of depression. At the Center, several additional issues were pinpointed. We may have identified these issues simply because of our many years of experience with adults who have DS. For example, we found that Colleen had several painful boils in sensitive areas. While this may seem like a relatively small concern, it may have created a great deal of discomfort for her, especially when added to the other issues that were bothering her. We also discovered that Colleen had some hearing loss, which may have led to frustration or miscommunication for her in various situations.

Our treatment recommendations for Colleen:

A) We recommended that the antidepressant medication, sertraline (Zoloft), be continued. It seemed to be very successful in reducing symptoms and Colleen tolerated it well. We suggested that if she continued for at least one year without symptoms her medication could be reduced and possibly discontinued, if symptoms did not reemerge. If, however, her symptoms returned, she could easily go back on the medication. In fact, when she was weaned off the medication after one year, her symptoms did return and thus she was restarted on the medication. However, one year later (two years from the start of treatment), we again tried to discontinue the medication, and this time the symptoms did not return.

B) We suggested that Colleen continue seeing her social work counselor since the counseling seemed to help her develop a more positive attitude about herself and her competence in dealing with the world. This is especially important when someone is depressed, because negative thoughts and beliefs about oneself, the world, and one's ability to affect the world are often at the heart of a depression (Scott, 1996; Beck and Rush, 1995).

C) Our only suggestion to her social work counselor was to consider using Colleen's propensity for self-talk to help her develop positive thoughts and phrases she could use throughout the day. For example, she could praise herself or tell herself that she did something well at work or during daily living tasks. She could use previously rehearsed positive phrases and pronounce them out loud in private or very quietly in public settings. This would serve as a substitute for the negative or critical thoughts she had been communicating to herself. This treatment strategy is a modification of the model called cognitive behavioral therapy (CBT), which is a very successful treatment approach for depression.

D) Our medical team suggested her treatment for celiac disease and her hypothyroidism not be changed because of the success of the treatment.

E) Regarding her boils, we gave Colleen's family very detailed instructions about cleaning procedures, creams, medications, and other steps to try to control the outbreaks (see Chapter 6).

F) Her hearing was evaluated by the audiologist. Her problem did not require hearing aids, but strategies were discussed to improve her hearing (see Chapter 7).

G) Finally, we recommended that Colleen and her family return in approximately three months so we could check her progress and to call if there was any change in the mean time.

Summary and Update: Three years after the start of her depressive symptoms, Colleen had no new bouts of depression. She had had several bouts of sadness, however, when others in her life experienced losses. These losses reminded her of her grief over the deaths of her grandfather and her dog. She also had a crisis after a boyfriend dropped her. Still, she weathered these life stresses without developing full-blown depression.

GEORGE'S MEDICAL AND EMOTIONAL HEALTH

During his physical exam at the Center, George was found to have at least one major health issue that could have easily aggravated or led to his depressive symptoms. This health issue was discovered when his mother reported that he seemed to have "restless sleep." His parents were actually not sure how long this restless sleep had been going on, but had first observed it when they started paying closer attention to him as a result of his depression. Upon further questioning, George's family reported that when he did sleep, he snored loudly and sometimes appeared to stop breathing.

The Center's medical staff referred George to have a sleep study done by a neurologist who was also a sleep specialist. This study showed that George had significant sleep apnea (see Chapter 18). The sleep deprivation that results from sleep apnea can have an enormous impact on physical and mental functioning and is strongly associated with depression. After his diagnosis, George was treated for sleep apnea with a CPAP machine. Fortunately, he was able to tolerate the CPAP mask after some adjustments, and, after several months of treatments, he was definitely showing more energy and life.

Like Colleen, George also had various skin problems. He had boils under his arms and in his groin, as well as cracked lips, and a problem with acne rosacea on his face. (For more on all these conditions see Chapter 6.) These skin conditions can be very uncomfortable and sometimes embarrassing. The rosacea may be especially difficult to deal with since it can cause large, unsightly blotches on the person's face.

Our treatment recommendations and strategy for George:

A) George had one major health issue—sleep apnea—which was not diagnosed or treated prior to coming to the Center. Fortunately he was able to tolerate the CPAP mask prescribed for him after diagnosis, and his sleep improved significantly. After three or four months, his level of daytime alertness and energy had markedly improved. He also rarely complained of fatigue or problems sleeping and no longer needed naps during the day.

B) As with Colleen, we recommended that George receive treatments to clear up or better manage his skin problems, as described in Chapter 6.

C) We initially recommended that George stay on the antidepressant his psychiatrist had prescribed, escitalopram (Lexapro), until it was clear how treating his apnea and skin conditions would affect his mood. George's symptoms of depression showed significant improvement once his sleep improved. His family reported, however, that he still continued to move somewhat slowly at his grocery job, compared to his previous performance. He also still sometimes resisted going to social or recreation activities and was quite often standoffish when he did go. In addition, he continued to have some angry self-talk, although the frequency and intensity of his self-talk had greatly decreased.

We discussed with George's family that depressive symptoms often continue even after treating some of the possible precipitants. Also, as explained below, we believe there is often more than one cause of a mental health condition. For example, George had skin problems that may have been an irritant to him, and he had experienced several losses that may have had a profound effect on him. There may also have been other stresses that we did not know about. This is often an issue for people with DS whose expressive and articulation limitations prevent them from communicating problems to others. We also could not rule out the cumulative effect on George of all of his possible health or environmental stresses. Furthermore, people with DS may be less able to comprehend why or how their depression happened, which may frighten or even traumatize them. This, too, may lengthen or intensify the symptoms.

D) Having discussed why George's depression may have continued, we agreed to try a different antidepressant medication, at the family's request. We began a trial of venlafaxine (Effexor). Over time, George's depression gradually improved. It was not clear that this medication was more effective than the other, but at the very least, the family felt that we had listened to them and that they were able to do what they could to help George improve.

E) George did not have a counselor, but his family helped him replace negative thoughts about himself and his ability to affect the world whenever they observed self-criticism or negative thinking. As with Colleen, his self-talk became a simple and easy means for helping him to make positive comments to himself.

Summary and Update: Over the course of several years, George continued to improve. After two years, his family said he was almost back to the way he had been before the onset of his depression. There were, however, several periods when his family noted that his symptoms were returning. The first time this occurred, his CPAP machine was not working correctly, but this was not discovered for at least three weeks. By the end of the second week, George was becoming moody and was resisting going to social activities, as in the past. Once the CPAP problem was fixed, he began to improve and within several months was back to what his family described as his "good-natured self."

A second bout of depression occurred when a bully began teasing him at many of his social and recreation programs. George was unable to articulate the problem and he began to show more and more of the symptoms that had previously concerned his family. Fortunately, a staff person saw the bully targeting George and informed his family. A meeting with staff and the families of both men was arranged to discuss solutions. Once the bullying stopped, it took George some time to get back on track, but he did bounce back fairly quickly once the problem was solved.

ANITA'S MEDICAL AND EMOTIONAL HEALTH

At the Center, Anita was found to have a vitamin B12 vitamin deficiency, which occurs more frequently in people with DS. This deficiency is treated either with B12 injections or, sometimes, B12 tablets. If undiagnosed and untreated, the vitamin deficiency can result in physical symptoms as well as mental health symptoms such as depression.

Anita also had some significant premenstrual discomfort, for at least one week out of the month, which could also have made her depression appear more severe during that time of the month. We also found that she had gained a considerable amount of weight. We suspected that this was due to the use of the antipsychotic medication olanzapine (Zyprexa). As discussed previously, her weight gain aggravated her symptoms of depression.

As with George, we suspected that Anita had sleep apnea, based on symptoms reported by her parents, including snoring, restless sleep, and apparent pauses in her breathing while asleep. We referred her for a sleep study, which revealed that she had obstructive sleep apnea. This condition had likely developed or worsened due to her obesity.

Our treatment recommendations and strategy for Anita:
A) At the Center, we treated Anita for her vitamin B12 deficiency with monthly injections of B12.
B) As mentioned previously, we agreed with her psychiatrist's diagnosis of depression. We recommended that Anita continue on the antidepressant medication sertraline (Zoloft) as prescribed by this psychiatrist. Later, we increased the dosage of this medication, but not in the first months of treatment. We believe that, as much as possible, it is better to make only one medication change at a time; otherwise it is impossible to tell which medication caused which results. In Anita's case, we were

more concerned about the effects of the antipsychotic medication, so we began by tapering it off. As mentioned previously, we believed that this medication was not appropriate given her symptoms, and, more importantly, that it may have caused her dramatic weight gain, thereby aggravating her depression.

C) We strongly supported treatment of Anita's sleep apnea, since this may have a major negative effect on both mental health and health. It can also be much more difficult to treat depression if the person is fatigued and lethargic as a result of sleep deprivation.

Unlike George, Anita was not comfortable with a CPAP device, but she did eventually tolerate apnea treatment with adjustments and a shift from CPAP to BiPAP (one pressure for inhalation and one for exhalation). What helped with her acceptance of the BiPAP was strong encouragement from her family and clinic staff and a behavior plan that allowed her to earn rewards for wearing the mask. The behavior plan capitalized on her regular use of calendars, her family support, and her love of music. Each morning she had successfully worn the mask, she was given a star on a large calendar in the family kitchen. She also received copious praise from any family members present, as well as fifty cents toward the purchase of music CDs. (Her family put the money in a large glass jug that was just out of reach, so that she would not use this money to buy unhealthy snacks at her job.) After several months of wearing the mask, Anita's level of energy was back to a more normal state and she was not showing any fatigue in the course of her day.

D) Anita's sleep and her general health were also at risk from the weight gain, so ADSC Staff helped her to develop a plan to reduce her weight. Once she was weaned off the antipsychotic medication, she did not seem to lose weight but she also did not gain any additional weight. On the plus side, her family noted that discontinuing the medication greatly reduced her obsession and driven behavior around food. We explained to Anita's family that it is very difficult to lose weight once it is put on. We explained our long-term strategy for weight management (see Chapter 2). Her family listened carefully and then worked very hard and patiently over the next several years to solve this problem. They worked with our nutritionist to make sure Anita's diet was healthy. Equally important, they developed a regular exercise plan for her. As Anita's depression began to slowly lift and she began to lose weight and sleep more normally, she had more energy for sports and recreational activities. With much effort, she gradually lost most of the weight she had gained.

Summary and Update: After her health and mental health problems were identified and treated, Anita gradually regained her sense of health and well-being. Two and a half years after the onset of symptoms, she had lost the excess weight and staved off any new bouts of depression or problematic obsessions or compulsions. She was working productively at her job, she was active in social and recreational activities, and she had regained her sense of pride and self-esteem. One thing that helped her in regaining and maintaining her health and well-being was a newfound interest in a unique past time—belly dancing. This was offered as a class by the park district and taught by a very good and encouraging instructor. Not only did belly dancing provide Anita with a fun way to exercise, but it introduced her to many interesting people and boosted her confidence and passion for life—all of which helped reduce her risk of depression.

SUMMARY

This chapter presents a rationale for, and case examples of, the Adult Down Syndrome Center's multidisciplinary approach. We believe this approach is the most effective means of dealing with the complex biological, psychological, and social influences on people with DS, just as it is for all others. We believe that approaches that only target one influence or cause of behavior are less effective than a more holistic approach that looks at multiple influences. For example, treatment for mental health problems may only target the person's behavior through behavior modification approaches. Others may only target biochemical differences in the brain through the use of psychotropic medications such as antidepressants.

In our experience, a host of influences, such as health, environmental, and personal thought processes, are usually involved. We have found that the influences on people with DS are actually quite complex. There are many reasons for this. First, people with DS often have fewer adaptive skills with which to manage or solve problems they encounter in their lives. Second, they may have trouble conceptualizing and communicating the source of a problem. This may lead to a delay in the identification and treatment of problems. Third, problems that fester untreated may affect other areas, leading to negative thoughts or further stress. Finally, as discussed at length in this book, people with DS are more susceptible to many physical and sensory problems. Given the complexity of the lives of people with DS, we have found that a multidisciplinary approach is the most likely to identify and resolve problems when they arise.

Chapter 6

Skin and Nail

. . . .

Problems

. . . .

When I was looking at his feet during the physical exam, James, age 25, suddenly asked me what time it was. I told him it was 11:35. He said, "Pronounce them." He was referring to his toenails, which were yellow, thickened, and ridged. I discussed with him that they were not dead, just infected with a fungus and the infection was called onychomycoses. We discussed treatment options and James opted to try Vicks VapoRub applied to his toenails nightly. Several months later, James reported he was glad we didn't "pronounce them" at the previous appointment.

S kin problems are common in people with Down syndrome (DS). These problems include fungal infections of the nails and skin such as onycho-mycoses and tinea pedis (athlete's feet), conditions that cause dry or flaky skin, and acne, boils, and other inflammations of the skin.

There appear to be several reasons for the prevalence of skin problems among people with DS. First, dry skin is common in people with DS, and that seems to be a starting place for a number of skin infections. Dry skin that tends to crack allows bacteria and fungus to get through the natural skin barrier. In addition, the immune system of people with DS is often impaired. This limits the person's ability to resist infection. Furthermore, adolescents and adults with DS don't always have the self-care skills

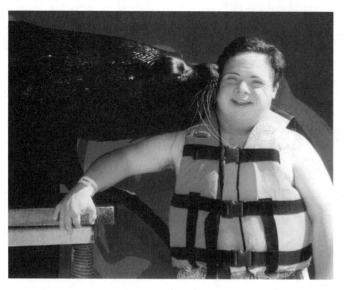

needed to take care of their own hygiene adequately. We tell our patients that they may not "get away with the average hygiene" and may need to spend extra time and effort in keeping their skin clean and healthy.

In general, most of the skin conditions common in DS can be diagnosed and treated by a primary health provider. Consider a consultation with a dermatologist if treatment is not helping or if the person has persistent physical discomfort or emotional distress because the condition is unsightly.

ESSENTIAL ELEMENTS OF SKIN CARE

Excellent hygiene certainly starts with good washing. We recommend washing daily with antibacterial soap, although there is some debate as to the effectiveness of this soap. We find that an antibacterial soap that has a moisturizer (e.g., Lever 2000 or

Itchy Skin

Dry skin is a common cause of itching. Many other skin problems can also itch. Unfortunately, scratching often makes the situation worse and can lead to secondary bacterial infections. Being vigilant with treatment of dry skin or other causes of itching is the first step. Additional steps may include:
- ◆ covering the area
- ◆ keeping fingernails cut short
- ◆ having the person wear cotton gloves
- ◆ redirecting the person (we often recommend having a subtle "secret signal" that others can use to remind the person not to scratch. This helps avoid the embarrassment of audibly reminding the person.)
- ◆ trying oral antihistamines; e.g., chlorphenamine (Benadryl) or loratadine (Claritin)

Dial with moisturizer) provides the antibacterial benefit but doesn't dry the skin like most soap does. Our other recommendations for skin care include:

- Use a soft brush on a handle or a loofah to help the person reach areas and "buff off" some of the dry skin.
- Rinse thoroughly. Some people with DS don't give rinsing the attention it needs, and leaving soap on the skin causes the skin to become drier.
- Dry thoroughly. Many of our patients have the "zip-zip" approach to drying. Their skin remains wet after they do cursory drying. Folds, crevices, and other places where skin touches skin are particularly problematic. Fungus and bacteria like to live in warm, moist, dark places, and areas that have not been dried are perfect sites for the development of infections.
- Apply powder, such as unscented baby powder, to help keep moist areas dry, especially in warm weather.

CONDITIONS THAT CAUSE DRY OR FLAKY SKIN

DRY SKIN

Dry skin is extremely common in people with DS. Although it is generally not a serious condition, it can be quite bothersome. Many people tend to be more affected in the winter when the air is dry and the cold winds can increase the dryness of the skin. To treat and reduce dry skin, try these strategies:

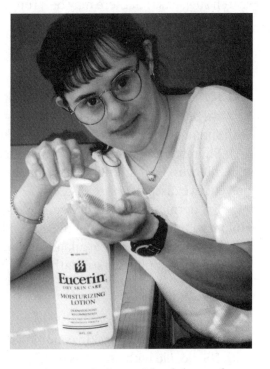

- Liberally apply moisturizing cream or lotion. Creams tend to be better. Using the cream after a shower or bath when the skin is still moist can optimize the skin's moisture.
- If the skin is particularly dry and thickened, use a moisturizing cream that loosens the dry skin; e.g., Eucerin Plus cream or Jergens lotion with alpha and beta hydroxy acids
- Use a mild soap such as Lever 2000, Dove, or Dial with moisturizers.
- Decrease the frequency, length, and temperature of showers, especially in the winter (use lukewarm water instead of hot).

◆ In the winter, avoid exposure of the skin to the cold, dry, winter air by covering as much of the skin as possible when outdoors.
◆ Humidify the air in the house in the winter.
◆ Use sunscreens (30 SPF or higher) and light, protective clothing to protect the skin from the burning and drying effects of the sun.

SEBORRHEIC DERMATITIS

Seborrheic dermatitis is a skin condition characterized by flaking, redness, scaling, and greasy skin that can include patches and thick plaques of skin and oil. It can occur at any age, and is more common in males than females. In infants, it is known as cradle cap. It can also occur on the face, eyebrows, chest, and back (hairy regions of the body) and can be a source of dandruff on the scalp.

Seborrheic dermatitis is not curable but is generally manageable. Exposure to sunlight may help reduce the condition. Anti-dandruff shampoos such as Head & Shoulders, Selsun Blue, or Denorex are beneficial. If the problem persists, consider the use of ketoconazole (Nizoral) shampoo, which is an antifungal shampoo. (Some research suggests that there may be a fungal component to some seborrheic dermatitis.) We usually recommend using an anti-dandruff shampoo five days a week and Nizoral shampoo twice a week.

It is important to gently but firmly rub the scalp while shampooing and to rinse well. Cutting the hair shorter may make cleaning easier.

If the scales or plaques on the scalp are thick or resistant to shampoo, placing baby oil on the scalp and gently combing the scalp can help loosen the scales. Follow with shampooing to remove the oil and further treat the condition.

Shampoo can also be used for seborrhea on the eyebrows, taking care not to get it in the eyes. Half-strength baby shampoo can be used around the eyes if needed to prevent eye discomfort.

For dermatitis on the back and chest, try one of the anti-dandruff shampoos. Selenium sulfide, the ingredient in Selsun Blue, also comes in a lotion that can be applied to areas of the body. It is available without a prescription in lower strengths and with a prescription for higher strengths.

PSORIASIS

Psoriasis is another skin condition that appears to be relatively common in people with DS. People with psoriasis develop dry, scaling patches with well-defined papules and plaques. The knees and elbows are common locations for the patches, but they can also be scattered across other parts of the body.

Psoriasis is more common in adults but can also occur in younger people. It is a condition related to immune system dysfunction and people who have it will often have flare-ups followed by periods of remission.

Treatment consists of applying:

- emollients—thick, moisturizing creams such as Vaseline (the petroleum jelly is thicker and more effective for most people with psoriasis, but it is often messier and may be less acceptable to the individual than some lotions)
- topical steroids—prescription or nonprescription creams that contain hydrocortisone or stronger steroids
- retinoids—such as tazarotene (Tazorac), a prescription cream
- calcipotriene (Dovonex, a vitamin D derivative), a prescription lotion, cream, or ointment that is applied to the skin

Exposure to sunlight may sometimes help reduce psoriasis, but for more severe cases, light therapy in a medical office may be necessary. Different types of ultraviolet radiation are used based on the recommendation of the dermatologist. Home light therapy may also be an option. Light treatment can have serious side effects, however, and is therefore usually reserved for more serious, resistant cases. Oral medications that suppress the immune system (such as methotrexate) can also be used for more difficult-to-treat cases of psoriasis.

FUNGAL INFECTIONS

ATHLETE'S FOOT, JOCK ITCH, AND RELATED INFECTIONS

Fungal skin infections occur when a fungus, a microscopic organism, invades the skin. Fungus thrives in warm, moist, dark places. Sometimes people get fungal infections from being in a warm, moist place, such as a communal shower. More commonly, they develop fungal infections from paying inadequate attention to warm, moist, dark places on the body.

Athlete's foot (tinea pedis) is a common fungal infection of the feet that can develop if a person does not dry well between her toes. Symptoms include peeling, itching, and redness of the skin. The skin between the toes is particularly susceptible. Treatment involves cleaning the area with soap and water and drying it well two to three times a day and then applying an antifungal agent, such as Lotrimin Cream, Desenex, or Tinactin, until the infection has cleared up. The spray powders of these products are particularly convenient. Keeping the feet as dry as possible is also recommended; so sometimes it is necessary to change the socks in midday to keep the feet dry.

Fungal infections are also common in other areas of the body, particularly in folds or where skin surfaces oppose each other. If the infection appears in the groin, it is called tinea cruris ("jock itch"). Patches on other areas of the body are called tinea corporis. Fungal infections are also often seen along the belt line, under breasts, and in the axilla (armpits). In the folds, when the skin stays moist, the skin may macerate (develop cracks or open sores), which makes it a prime target for invasion of fungus (and bacteria). These are often referred to as intertrigo infections. Treatment is the same as for tinea pedis—including cleaning, rinsing, drying, and using an antifungal cream or powder. Keeping the area dry, with powder, if necessary, can help prevent the infections. If a rash in these areas does not improve with good hygiene and antifungal treatment creams or powders, an evaluation by a medical practitioner is recommended.

TOENAIL INFECTIONS

As mentioned above, onychomycosis—a fungal infection of the toenails (and less often, the fingernails)—is common among adults with DS. The toenails tend to be thick, yellowed, and dystrophic (abnormal appearing).

Since this condition generally does not cause any bothersome symptoms, consider treating it conservatively. That is, if the person with DS is not bothered by the condition, it may not need treatment other than regular hygiene. Cutting the nails may be the most difficult aspect of care. Cutting the toenails after bathing or showering, when they are a little softer, makes trimming a little easier. Sometimes, however, it may become necessary to seek care from a podiatrist—a medical professional specializing in diagnosing disorders of the feet and ankles for toenail-cutting maintenance. A manicurist may also be helpful with toenail-cutting maintenance.

The treatments available for onychomycosis take months to resolve the problem because they kill the fungus at the nail bed and then the toenail must grow out (and toenails tend to grow slowly).

Oral medications such as terbinafine (Lamisil) or itraconazole (Sporanox) are effective. They have to be taken for three to four months, however, and can affect the liver. It is, therefore, important to consider monitoring liver function through blood tests if one of these medications is prescribed.

Topical products (e.g., lotions or ointments used externally) are another option. These are generally less effective than oral medications. Clotrimazole (Lotrimin), econazole (Spectazole), ketoconazole (Nizoral), and others can be placed on the toenails under an occlusive dressing (such as gauze). We have not found these to be particularly successful. Another preparation is ciclopirox (Penlac) lacquer, which is painted on the toenails daily and wiped off with alcohol once a week. While most adults with DS tolerate this well, we have not found ciclopirox to be successful very often either.

Interestingly, one topical preparation that we have had some success with is Vicks VapoRub. The ointment is thicker and probably more effective, but the cream may be better tolerated. We recommend applying it to the toenails nightly before bed. While the mechanism of action is not understood, if the person can continue to use the VapoRub nightly, we have had a number of people with DS successfully treat their onychomycoses this way. It has minimal side effects and most adults with DS can tolerate it. As with other treatments, it does take months to successfully eliminate the abnormal toenails.

A more immediate treatment is surgical removal of the toenails. Ordinarily the toenails will grow back slowly over several months. Then there is a possibility that the infection may recur. To prevent recurrence of the infection, the doctor may sometimes use a surgical procedure that prevents the toenails from growing back.

Because the discomfort and side effects of some of these treatments would seem to outweigh any benefits to be gained from treating this asymptomatic condition, observing (not treating) the infection is an option. Of course, the toenails should still be regularly trimmed if the persons opts not to pursue treatment.

ACNE, BOILS, AND OTHER INFLAMMATIONS OF THE SKIN

Adults with DS are prone to developing red or inflamed pimple-like bumps on the skin. Some of these bumps actually *are* pimples, but some are other types of inflammations. It's important to have the skin condition properly diagnosed because the treatments are not all the same.

The primary care practitioner is usually a good person to assess the condition to start. Under some circumstances, a dermatologist—a medical doctor who specializes skin care—can help with diagnosis and treatment recommendations. If the condition is not responding to the treatment prescribed by the primary care doctor, consider requesting a dermatology consultation.

FOLLICULITIS

Folliculitis is an infection or inflammation of the hair follicles caused by bacteria or sometimes fungus. It results in small red lesions in the hair follicles, especially on the back and chest, but can occur wherever there is hair. The inflammation is sometimes itchy, less commonly uncomfortable, and often without symptoms.

Folliculitis is a fairly common problem in adults with DS and very difficult to eliminate. We recommend treating it with antibacterial soaps, such as Lever 2000 or Dial Soap with Moisturizer. In addition, since folliculitis is often in harder-to-reach places such as the back, consider purchasing a soft brush on a long handle and teaching the adult to use it to help reach these areas. Sometimes oral antibiotics or oral antifungal medications can eliminate folliculitis, at least temporarily. However, these medications aren't always successful, and when they are discontinued, the infection tends to recur. Folliculitis can lead to recurrent boils (see below).

Shaving sometimes seems to aggravate the condition. It may make shaving uncomfortable. Shaving may need to be temporarily discontinued until the condition improves.

BOILS

Boils are painful skin infections that occur when bacteria or other organisms get beneath the skin, leading to the formation of pus. When the pus collects under the skin, red tender bumps form, anywhere from the size of a pinhead to several inches or more across. Boils may appear singly or in clusters.

Recurrent boils are common in adolescents and adults with DS (and may sometimes appear at a younger age). The armpits, groin area, the buttocks, along the waistband or bra line, and the thighs are common sites where this problem occurs.

As mentioned above, boils may result from folliculitis, but can occur wherever bacteria are able to invade beneath the skin. In people with DS, dry, cracking skin often offers bacteria a place to invade. Hormonal changes also contribute to boils. This can become a bigger problem at adolescence. In girls and women, boils often increase just before or during menstruation. Extra attention to hygiene at this time may help.

We recommend the following steps to prevent and treat boils:

1. Gently but thoroughly wash the area of concern daily with an antibacterial or soap. A loofah sponge is often helpful.
2. Thoroughly rinse the area.
3. Gently but thoroughly dry the area.
4. Consider applying baby powder to help keep the area dry, particularly in hotter, humid weather.
5. When a small boil occurs, apply a triple antibiotic cream such as Neosporin. Prescription-strength acne medication is also sometimes helpful (e.g., Clindamycin lotion).
6. A few studies have suggested that zinc and vitamin C supplements may improve the immune function of some adults with DS and help prevent infections. We recommend Vitamin C 1000 mg daily and Zinc gluconate 100 mg daily. This is in addition to a good one-a-day vitamin.
7. Using the prescription soap Hibiclens on the problem areas (from a few days a week to daily) may be helpful.
8. If the boils continue to be a problem, some of our patients have benefited from using a daily antibiotic such as amoxicillin or tetracycline, similar to the way persistent acne is treated.
9. Some women benefit from taking oral contraceptives (birth control pills). Some birth control pills have an FDA-approved indication for treating acne and may help reduce boils. These include Trinessa and Orthotricyclen.
10. Warm compresses can help the boils drain. Squeezing and sticking unsterile needles, etc. into the boil can worsen the infection.
11. When a boil occurs, sometimes they require oral antibiotics and sometimes incision and drainage of the pus in the doctor's office.
12. When the boils burst on their own, which they often do, washing the area with antibacterial soap to prevent spread is important. Covering the draining wound also helps.
13. Topical anesthetic (pain relief) ointments that contain lidocaine can reduce discomfort.

Picking or Scratching Boils and Pimples

When boils occur, it is very important for the person to limit touching or scratching the area. Touching the affected area can spread the infection to other parts of the body or to other people. If the boil or pimple is draining, it should be covered to help prevent it from spreading. The area should also be covered if the person cannot stop touching it. To prevent scratching, consider the ideas discussed on page 66 for itchy skin.

If the boils become larger, are surrounded by redness, are persistent, or are associated with fever, it is important to see a doctor. He or she can make sure there is not a more serious infection going on, and can prescribe antibiotics and/or drain the pus. One of the more serious concerns is when boils are due to infection with MRSA (methicillin resistant staph aureus). Treatment requires specific antibiotics—often oral antibiotics—but sometimes requires intravenous antibiotics and surgical drainage.

ACNE VULGARIS

Acne vulgaris is the name for the acne typically associated with adolescence. It is an inflammatory disorder of the sebaceous (oil) glands. Typical skin symptoms include comedones (whiteheads and blackheads), papules (raised red bumps), pustules (raised bumps with pus inside), and, sometimes, scarring.

Acne seems to be about as common in teens and adults with DS as in other people. Treatment is the same as recommended for those without DS. Cleansing with a mild soap will control oily skin. Lotions and ointments that may help include those that reduce the bacteria that causes acne (including peroxide, clindamycin, erythromycin, and others), as well as tretinoin and adapalene. Oral antibiotics can also be beneficial, but are not usually used unless the lotions and ointments are not enough. Some oral contraceptives can also help treat acne in women and girls, as discussed under "Boils."

Despite popular belief that foods such as chocolate or French fries cause pimples, diet does not play a role in acne. The known factors that do contribute to acne include:
  ◆ family genetics (it runs in families),
  ◆ hormonal issue (acne can increase during puberty, at different times of the menstrual cycle, and with use of some birth control pills),
  ◆ some medications (e.g., steroids, phenytoin/Dilantin, phenobarbital)
  ◆ oily cosmetics and rubbing or covering the skin surface (such as with sports equipment).

Most cases of acne are relatively mild and pimples disappear on their own without damaging the skin. Occasionally, however, people with DS develop cystic acne (inflamed cysts or pustules). For severe cystic acne with scarring that has been resistant to other treatments, isotretinoin (Accutane) may be prescribed. Only physicians who participate in the manufacturer's training program can prescribe this medication. This precaution is taken because of the concern that Accutane may cause birth defects in babies born to a woman who becomes pregnant while taking it. In addition, there are a number of other possible side effects that require careful monitoring.

ACNE ROSACEA (OR ROSACEA)

Acne rosacea is a separate condition from acne vulgaris. It is a chronic skin eruption with flushing and dilatation of small blood vessels in the face, especially in the nose and cheeks. It may also cause pimples. The condition is generally not uncomfortable but can lead to self-consciousness or embarrassment. The condition is common in women who don't have DS and may be even more common in women who have DS. Acne rosacea can be complicated by rhinophyma—dilated (enlarged) follicles ("pores") and thickened skin of the nose and inflammation of the eyes and surrounding structures.

Factors that may increase symptoms include:
- alcohol, coffee, tea, spiced food,
- exposure to cold or hot temperatures,
- emotional stress, and
- exposure to sun and wind

Treatment includes:
- avoiding the triggers listed above,
- taking oral antibiotics (tetracycline, doxycycline, minocycline),
- using sulfur-containing lotions such as sulfacetamide-sulfur (e.g., Sulfacet-R) or urea-sulfacetamide (e.g., Rosula),
- using prescription lotions (metronidazole, erythromycin, clindamycin), and,
- for severe cases, the prescription of isotretinoin (Accutane).

HIDRADENITIS SUPPURATIVA

Hidradenitis suppurativa is a painful condition that occurs in areas of the body that contain certain types of sweat glands (apocrine glands). These sweat glands are in the armpit and groin areas. For unknown reasons, the hair follicles in these areas become blocked and cyst-like abscesses form. This may cause scarring, nodules (firm, thickened areas of tissue under the skin), and sinus tracts (small channels from the skin surface that go into the tissue under the skin and often drain liquid or pustular material).

Hidradenitis suppurative is relatively rare but may be more common in adults with DS than in other people. It can be misdiagnosed as recurrent boils. In contrast to boils, however, there are more and larger swellings and the infections are a secondary problem. Hidradenitis suppurativa tends to cause persistent changes, and more scarring than boils. Anyone with repeated large boil-like swellings in these areas of the body should consult a medical practitioner to get the proper diagnosis and treatment. Consultation with a dermatologist (and possibly a surgeon) may be necessary.

Common treatments include:

- keeping the areas clean as described above, under the section on "Boils,"
- taking antibiotics for acute infections,
- applying topical clindamycin to the affected areas,
- surgical removal of the obstructed hair follicles,
- prescription of low-progesterone oral contraceptives (for women) or isotretinoin (Accutane), or
- injection of steroids.

ALOPECIA AREATA

Alopecia areata is a condition in which hair is lost rapidly in round or oval patches. Usually this hair loss occurs on the scalp, the beard area, eyebrows, or eyelashes. The patches are usually from 1 to 5 centimeters in diameter and have short broken hairs at the periphery. The condition is more common in people with DS. It may begin in childhood but sometimes does not appear until adulthood.

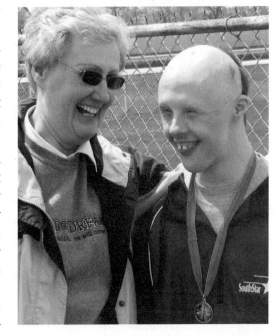

The cause of alopecia is not known but it is believed to be an autoimmune disorder. "Autoimmune" refers to the body attacking itself, and in this case it is probably the body's own antibodies attacking the hair follicles.

How the condition affects any given person can vary quite a bit. The hair that has been lost may spontaneously grow back in a few months, more patches may occur, or when hair grows back in one patch, hair loss may occur in another area. Even if hair grows back after one episode, the condition frequently recurs.

Sometimes the hair loss progresses to total loss of hair on the scalp or even all over the body. When all hair is lost, the condition is called *alopecia totalis* or *alopecia universalis.* However, most people with alopecia—especially those with minor cases and those who develop the condition after puberty—spontaneously recover.

Effective treatments are still being investigated. Topical steroid creams, steroid injections into the hair loss area, and oral steroids have all been used with mixed results. Some have proposed using minoxidil (Rogaine), the same preparation that is used for male pattern baldness. Bear in mind, though, that there is a good chance that the hair will spontaneously grow back if alopecia first occurs after puberty and if there are only one or a few patches. Consider consulting with a dermatologist to discuss treatment options.

CONCLUSION

Good skin care is extremely important for teens and adults with DS. Skin problems can cause physical discomfort and also affect the person's self-esteem. Many skin problems are more common in people with DS, and adults and teens who have these problems need guidance or assistance to optimize care and to develop good hygiene and skin care routines.

Chapter 7

Ear, Nose,

& Throat and Dental

Concerns

Ray, 42, was seen at the Adult Down Syndrome Center because the support staff from his apartment thought he might be developing Alzheimer disease. The staff reported that when they asked Ray to do something, he often did not do as they had asked. They were concerned that he was not processing what was being said or was forgetting what he was asked to do in the middle of the task. This was a much more significant problem at work than in his home. His place of employment tended to have a high noise level. During the interview, it was apparent that Ray understood what was being said much better if the words were spoken loudly and slowly in a room with little other noise.

During the exam, a large amount of cerumen (ear wax) was found in Ray's ears and was successfully removed. His hearing test, however, showed that he still had a high frequency hearing loss in both ears. Ray was prescribed and received hearing aids. His ability to follow instructions improved dramatically, although he still had difficulty hearing when he was in noisy places.

DIFFICULTIES WITH THE EARS AND HEARING

Hearing loss is more common in people with Down syndrome (DS) of all ages. Sometimes it results from reversible causes such as cerumen (ear wax) or serous otitis (fluid behind the eardrum). It can also be due to permanent causes such as inner ear problems or damage. Other problems are not necessarily permanent but can be more challenging to treat. These include perforation in the tympanic membrane (eardrum) or damage to the small bones in the middle ear.

As was the case with Ray, above, hearing problems may be difficult to detect in adults with DS. If the person does not or cannot complain of discomfort in his ears or of his difficulties hearing, behavior changes related to hearing loss may be attributed to psychological and other causes. Because of the high prevalence of hearing problems in people with DS, we recommend that adults with Down syndrome have their hearing checked every one to two years.

EXCESSIVE EARWAX

People with DS tend to have more problems with wax build-up in their ears. Smaller ear canals, tortuous canals, and dry skin all contribute to an increase of earwax (cerumen) or difficulties with the natural clearing of wax. These difficulties can lead to cerumen impaction (hard plugs of wax that stop up the ear canal). This can be a cause of hearing loss, discomfort in the ear, and tinnitus (ringing in the ear), and can contribute to poor balance or worsen hearing loss from other causes.

Wax softening drops can be used to help remove the wax. Debrox or other similar over-the-counter products can be dropped into the ear to soften and loosen wax. We find that these drops tend to dry out the skin, however, and persistent use is often not beneficial. Baby oil or mineral oil can also be used to soften earwax. We often recommend placing 3 to 4 drops in each ear twice a week to keep the wax soft and help the body's natural processes. To keep the drops in the ear, the person should lie on his side or tilt his head for several minutes while the drops are working.

Warning: Do not use earwax softening drops or baby and mineral oils if the person has a perforation or an ear tube in the eardrum. Never use a cotton-tipped swab (Q-tip) to try to remove impacted wax because it tends to push wax in further and it could damage the eardrum.

Despite the above measures, some people still build up too much wax. These people may need to see a doctor to have the wax suctioned out or irrigated with a mixture of warm water and hydrogen peroxide. Again, irrigation should not be done for someone who has a perforation or a tube in his eardrum. A health practitioner, usually an ENT (ear, nose, and throat physician), can suction the wax.

Some people with DS find it very difficult to cooperate with removal of ear wax. If the wax is causing significant hearing loss and discomfort, it may be worth removing it under anesthesia in the operating room. These individuals often find other testing or treatment challenging as well. Therefore, while the person is under anesthesia, it may be a good opportunity to do other invasive medical procedures that are needed, such as drawing blood, giving immunizations, performing a gynecological exam including PAP smear, or removing a skin lesion.

OTITIS EXTERNA

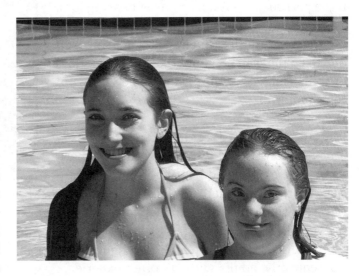

Otitis externa is an infection of the ear canal. Water that gets in the canal during swimming, showering, or through other means can lead to an outer ear infection. The condition is painful, so ear pain warrants an investigation for otitis externa. Sometimes redness in the canal or drainage from the canal can be seen without the use of an otoscope. Otitis externa seems to be more common in teens and adults with DS because of their small ear canals and wax build-up—both of which may trap water.

Prevention and treatment include:

- ◆ Avoid putting objects (such as Q-tips) into the ear canal. Trauma to the canal can lead to infections.
- ◆ If the person with DS has recurrent infections, consider using ear plugs during swimming and showering.
- ◆ Another way to prevent recurrences of otitis externa is to use products to dry the ear canal after swimming (or even showering, for some individuals). Commercially available products such as Swimmer's Ear can help. Or try a mixture of equal parts of rubbing alcohol and white vinegar, dropped in the ear with a dropper. Three or four drops after swimming helps return the correct acid status of the ear canal and dry the moisture, both of which help prevent infections.
- ◆ Topical antibiotic or combination drops may be helpful. Antibiotic drops such as ofloxacin Otic (Floxin Otic) or combinations such as hydrocortisone/polymycin/neomycin Otic (Corticosporin Otic) or ciprofloxacin/hydrocortisone Otic (Cipro Otic) can treat the infection.

HEARING LOSS

Hearing loss is more common in people with DS of all ages. Hearing loss that develops in adulthood may be temporary and due to treatable medical conditions such as fluid behind the eardrum. Or hearing loss may be permanent, due to the normal aging process.

Since hearing loss is so common in adults with DS, it is important to schedule a hearing test at least once every two years; more often, if the person has possible signs of hearing loss. The individual may complain of hearing loss or others may notice that he is not hearing well due to changes in behavior or an apparent loss of skills (such as with Ray at the beginning of the chapter).

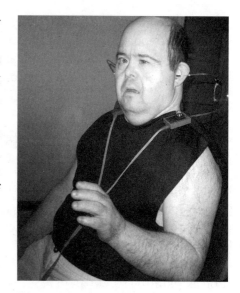

AGE-RELATED HEARING LOSS

As we age, all of us will eventually experience some age-related hearing loss (presbycusis). As we grow older, we lose our ability to hear higher-pitched sounds because these hearing cells are damaged more by the loud sounds that everyone is exposed to over a lifetime.

As discussed in Chapter 4, early aging is common in people with Down syndrome. Consequently, adults with DS often experience age-related high frequency hearing loss at younger ages. Sometimes this occurs as early as the 20s. High frequency hearing loss often impairs a person's ability to discriminate sounds. Distinguishing consonant sounds can be a particular problem, since sounds such as "s" are higher pitched than vowel sounds. Although the person may still be able to hear the sounds, he may not be able to discriminate what is being said.

Many people with hearing loss get tired of asking others to repeat what they have said. In addition, like Ray at the beginning of the chapter, many people with Down syndrome are "people pleasers." They don't like to disappoint or bother others. In Ray's situation, he was hearing the sounds, but was unable to discriminate the exact words and didn't want to annoy the other person by asking her to repeat her requests. So he would take his best guess and do what he thought was being asked. Unfortunately, he was often not correct and others jumped to the conclusion that he was unable to follow directions.

High frequency hearing impairment is usually worse in noisy environments. In addition, since female voices are often higher pitched, it may be more difficult to discriminate what women are saying.

If an adult with DS has trouble hearing high frequencies:
- ◆ Speak to him in a quieter environment, when possible.
- ◆ Speak slowly and loudly, but not too loudly.
- ◆ Make sure he can see your face when you talk to him.
- ◆ Use clear gestures that support your verbal communication.

Hearing aids can help when the hearing loss is significant enough to cause problems in daily life and the other measures are inadequate (see box on page 82).

EAR INFECTIONS AND FLUID

Hearing loss due to fluid behind the eardrum (serous otitis) is very common in children with Down syndrome. Often, as children with Down syndrome become adults, they become less prone to middle ear fluid. This is because as a person's skull grows,

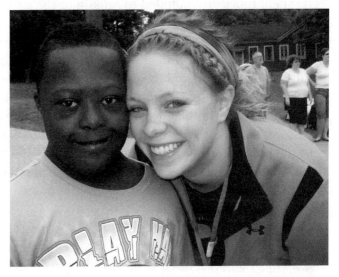

the anatomy of the middle ear and the Eustachian tube (the tube between the middle ear and the pharynx) changes, allowing the middle ear to drain better. However, some adults with Down syndrome continue to have problems with middle ear fluid. This is often because they have Eustachian tube dysfunction and/or other anatomical differences.

One of the most common causes of middle ear fluid is a middle ear infection (otitis media). This can be caused by an infection (viral or bacterial). Often the infection gets better on its own without treatment, but sometimes antibiotics are required. After the acute infection is over, residual fluid may be trapped behind the eardrum for weeks to months. (Even if there has not been an infection, fluid may also accumulate if the Eustachian tube becomes blocked due to allergies or other causes of Eustachian tube dysfunction.)

Middle ear fluid can muffle and distort the sounds that an individual hears, resulting in what is known as a *conductive hearing loss*—so called because the sound cannot be *conducted* normally from the outer ear, through the middle ear, and to the part of the brain that interprets sounds. Antibiotics, decongestants, antihistamines, and other medications have not been found to successfully remove the fluid. Generally, the fluid clears on its own.

Signs that someone might have middle ear fluid, with or without an infection, include:
- ◆ holding or rubbing the ear,
- ◆ banging the head against furniture or a wall,
- ◆ balance problems,
- ◆ general irritability,
- ◆ impaired hearing.

If there is an ear infection, an exam by a physician or other medical practitioner can determine whether it would be better to treat with antibiotics or simply observe the infection.

If middle ear fluid remains for several months or more and is contributing to hearing loss, a ventilation tube (ear tube) might be inserted to drain the fluid. Ear tubes are surgically implanted in the eardrum while the person is under light anesthetic. Tubes are available in two general varieties—temporary and permanent. The temporary tubes are designed to work their way out of the eardrum over the course of months or a year, after which the hole that the tube has left in the eardrum closes up on its own. Permanent tubes are intended to remain in the eardrum for a longer period of time. They often have to be removed by the physician. For adults with persistent middle ear fluid, a hearing test and a consult with an ENT can help determine the best course.

Sometimes an ear infection can lead to a perforation (hole) in the eardrum if the fluid builds up behind the eardrum, putting excess pressure on it. This can cause significant hearing loss. Perforations will often heal on their own, but sometimes will not. To find out whether the perforation should be surgically repaired, the person may need to consult an ENT and get a hearing test. If at all possible, it is best to prevent the eardrum from becoming perforated in the first place. That means ensuring that the adult with DS has a way to communicate that there is something wrong with his ear, or making sure adults in the environment are alert to possible signs of an ear infection (see list above).

Whether it be due to a perforation or an ear tube, an ear that has an opening on the tympanic membrane (eardrum) should not get water or other fluids into it (unless it is medication prescribed by a medical practitioner). Getting water in an ear that has a hole in the eardrum can lead to middle ear infections. Ideally, earplugs should be used while the person is showering and swimming to keep water out of the middle

Hearing Aids

Hearing aids can be very beneficial for an adult with Down syndrome who has a hearing loss. Otherwise, impaired hearing can significantly reduce the person's ability to function in daily life. People with Down syndrome who have hearing losses generally have less cognitive ability to compensate for the loss. That is, they may be less likely to deduce what was really said if they cannot clearly distinguish others' spoken words.

Not all people with Down syndrome can use hearing aids. Some find the presence of the aid in the ear unmanageable or bothersome. Others have become used to the quiet and find the "noise" bothersome. This may be especially true in noisy environments.

Often it is best to gradually introduce the person to a hearing aid. Just inserting the aid without turning it on may help the individual adjust to its presence before having to adjust to the sound. Gradually turning up the aid over several days to weeks may also help him accept the device. It may also help to make sure that the person is hearing something rewarding to him, such as a DVD he likes, when he first tries out the hearing aids. "Bone conduction" aids, which rest entirely behind the ear, may be an acceptable alternative for someone who cannot stand the feel of an aid inside his ear.

ear. However, some people with DS cannot tolerate the feel of earplugs in their ears. They might, however, agree to wear a rubber headband over their ears to keep water out. It might also be helpful for them to avoiding swimming until the hole heals and to have someone wash their hair for them over a sink, ensuring that water does not get into the ears.

RECRUITMENT

Sometimes adolescents and adults with DS respond very negatively to louder noises. It is often assumed that they have overly sensitive hearing. Often, however, the problem is really that the individual has impaired hearing and is experiencing the phenomena of "recruitment."

In this situation, the person is not able to hear softer sounds. As the sounds get louder, more and more of the hearing cells in his ear are gradually "recruited" until suddenly the person will hear the sound. This sound can be startling because the person has been hearing very little and suddenly hears a loud noise. Although it may seem counterintuitive, these individuals may benefit from hearing augmentation (hearing aids).

NOSE, SINUS, AND THROAT PROBLEMS

◆ ◆ ◆ ◆ ◆ ◆ ◆ ◆ ◆ ◆ ◆ ◆ ◆ ◆ ◆ ◆ ◆

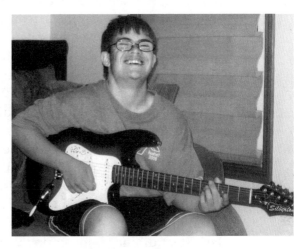

People with DS often have small or absent sinuses—the cavities or open spaces in the skull near the nose. They may be missing some or all of the eight sinuses.

Because of these anatomical differences as well as immune system problems that can persist into adulthood, *sinus and nasal congestion* and rhinorrhea (runny nose) frequently occur. These can result from infections (bacterial, viral, or less commonly fungal), allergies, irritants, or unknown causes. In addition, smaller openings to the sinuses may lead to the opening becoming plugged and the sinuses congested.

Preventative steps and treatment depend on the cause, but include:
- ◆ Advise the adult with DS not to smoke and to avoid exposure to cigarette smoke.
- ◆ Limit outdoor activity on days of high pollution or ozone alerts.
- ◆ Take steps to reduce mold in the person's home.
- ◆ Keep carpets cleaned and vacuumed.

- Avoid allergens (substances that trigger allergies).
- Change the furnace filter regularly and keep air ducts clean.
- Use nasal saline drops or saline inhalation to help flush out mucous and allergens or irritants.
- Irrigate the nasal cavity and sinuses with warm water or salt water with a Neti pot or sinus rinse kit
- Consider using a humidifier in the winter (or any season that is dry) but be sure to keep the humidifier clean so it doesn't spray irritants, bacteria, or viruses into the air.
- Try antihistamine medications such as loratadine (Claritin), diphenhydramine (Benadryl), and others to reduce allergy symptoms.
- Use decongestants to help reduce congestion and runny nose. Pseudoephedrine (Sudafed) is one example. There are also topical decongestants such as oxymetazoline (Afrin nasal spray). We generally don't recommend the sprays because use for more than a few days can cause rebound congestion and runny nose. That is, when the product is stopped, the blood vessels dilate beyond normal, causing a feeling of stuffiness and runny nose as a rebound effect of coming off the medication. This can lead to a chronic "need" for the medication to prevent the rebound.
- Instead of decongestant sprays, try topical nasal steroid sprays or inhalers, as they can be very effective. Fluticasone (Flonase), mometasone (Nasonex), and others reduce congestion and inflammation. These are generally well tolerated, but some people with Down syndrome resist having them squirted in their nose. They may also have difficulty sniffing upward at the right time or with sufficient force when the spray is administered. In this case, it might work to have the person lie down and squirt the medication into the nose so it trickles down into the right place.
- Use oral antibiotics only when the cause of the sinus problem is a bacterial infection. (Antibiotics are not helpful and can cause the emergence of more antibiotic-resistant bacteria if over-used). Note that the type of nasal drainage (cloudy, etc.) does *not* indicate a bacterial infection, as viral infections and allergies can also be cloudy. Persistent drainage, increasing discomfort, lack of response to the above treatments, and persistent fever can all be indicative of bacterial infections.

For persistent sinus symptoms that don't respond to the above measures, it is a good idea to look for underlying causes for the problem. For example, a screening CT of the sinuses may reveal that the cause of persistent sinus infections is enlarged adenoids, polyps, small sinuses, or other problems. An Ear, Nose & Throat physician can use an endoscope to examine the upper nasal passages, sinuses, and adenoids, and other areas that are not visible on a physical exam. Using an endoscope to look into the nose and sinuses is an invasive procedure. To help the person tolerate the procedure, see the suggestions at the end of this chapter under "Dental Care for Those Who Find It Challenging," pages 91-92.

Often the same problems that lead to sinus problems can also lead to a ***persistent cough.*** Common causes include: congestion and postnasal drip (drainage of mucus down the back of the throat). Less commonly, a persistent cough can be due to bronchospasm (asthma).

Another cause for persistent cough is ***gastroesophageal reflux (GERD),*** in which acid or other stomach contents come out of the stomach into the esophagus—the tube between the mouth and the stomach. The refluxed material can be irritating to the back of the throat and can also be aspirated into (breathed into) the lungs. Either of these can cause a cough. Treatment of GERD is discussed in Chapter 11.

LIP AND MOUTH PROBLEMS

Many adolescents and adults with DS develop ***chelitis***—an infection or inflammation at the corner of the mouth. This condition can result when saliva collects at the corner of the mouth, causing irritation. The accumulation of saliva can also lead to fungal skin infections, or, less often, bacterial infections. A barrier cream or ointment such as Vaseline petroleum jelly can reduce irritation from the saliva. Sometimes an antifungal agent such as clotrimazole (Lotrimin) cream is helpful. Since these lotions are recommended for use outside the mouth, they should only be used if the individual can refrain from licking them.

Cracked lips can occur for similar reasons. Some people with DS may habitually protrude their tongue, exposing the lips to persistent saliva that can dry out the lips. Others may lick their lips when they feel dry, such as during the winter. Encouraging and instructing the person with DS to work on keeping his tongue in his mouth may help. Frequent use of lip balms, especially thicker ones like Vaseline petroleum jelly, may help. Some people have used lip balms with candula oil with success. Antifungal agents also are beneficial for some individuals.

When the crack is deep and won't heal, we suggest applying antifungal cream three times a day. In between the application of the antifungal creams, regular use of moisturizing ointment or oils is helpful. Since inadequate fluid consumption probably contributes to this problem for many people with DS, we recommend increasing fluid intake, especially water, to help improve the hydration of the lips. Adding moisture to the air with a humidifier should also help.

DENTAL CONCERNS

. . . .

Stephanie, age 46, had become more irritable and moody and seemed to be losing her appetite. Even though a physician had prescribed an antidepressant for assumed depression, her symptoms persisted. An appointment was made at the Adult Down Syndrome Center, where she

was found to have a few very loose teeth that were causing her discomfort. Once Stephanie visited her dentist and got appropriate treatment, her pain went away, and her mood and eating improved.

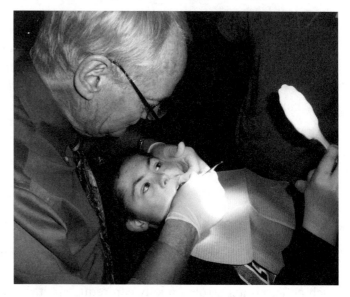

People with DS have some developmental differences in the face and mouth compared to those without DS. These include:

- ◆ The palate, or upper part of the mouth, is usually narrow and high or V-shaped.
- ◆ The nose, midfacial bones, and maxilla (jaw) tend to be smaller.
- ◆ The nasal passages are smaller, which can lead to mouth breathing. So, too, can enlarged adenoids and tonsils.
- ◆ Teeth are often smaller, unusually shaped, or missing, and often do not align properly.

All of the above problems can lead to difficulties with dental care. These problems are compounded if the person with Down syndrome has fine motor or cognitive problems that make it harder for him to care for his own teeth, or if he resists letting other people help him with dental care.

MOUTH BREATHING

Over time, mouth breathing can cause cracks and fissures of the tongue that can contribute to halitosis, or bad breath. For this reason, teens and adults with DS should be instructed to brush their tongue when they brush their teeth. Generally, the patients we see at the Adult Down Syndrome Clinic don't complain of discomfort when brushing their tongues, but the sensation can take some getting used to.

Chronic mouth breathing also decreases the amount of saliva in the mouth and increases dryness of the lips and skin surrounding the mouth. Saliva is a natural cleanser of the mouth; with less saliva, patients can develop caries (cavities). In addition, people who mouth breathe are more likely to get periodontal (gum) disease, and at an earlier age than usual. For these reasons, adults with Down syndrome who breathe through their mouths should be taught to be even more vigilant about brushing their gums well, and to use dental floss. More frequent visits to the dentist for professional cleaning may also help.

MISALIGNMENT OF TEETH

Due to the palate shape and relatively small mouth, tongue protrusion is relatively common among adolescents and adults with DS. Some people may habitually keep their tongue out of their mouth, resting it between the top and bottom incisors. Some individuals only poke out their tongue briefly when chewing or swallowing.

The tongue pressing against the teeth can help to create malocclusion and misalignment of the teeth. This, in turn, can sometimes lead to an "open bite," in which the top teeth extend abnormally beyond the bottom teeth.

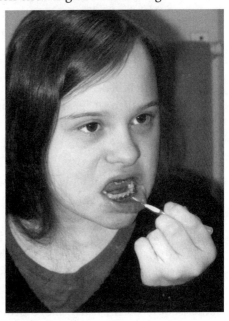

Tongue protrusion is not the only cause of misaligned teeth. Teeth may also be misaligned because they erupt in unusual positions in the mouth, or because some or all of the teeth are too small or missing. In addition, the jaws may be too small or misaligned. Some people with DS have an "underbite" in which the lower teeth protrude beyond the upper teeth.

Malocclusion, or misalignment of the teeth, may make it harder to chew food thoroughly. It may also cause plaque buildup, since it is more difficult to clean the misaligned tooth surfaces completely.

Like other people with malocclusions, adolescents and adults with DS may benefit from orthodontic care. Types of dental appliances that may be recommended include:

- ◆ palate expanders to make the palate larger (generally not used in adults when the palate has stopped growing),
- ◆ braces to align teeth,
- ◆ retainers to help maintain alignment,
- ◆ surgical interventions to move teeth that are significantly out of place.

However, before embarking on expensive orthodontic treatments, it is important for families to assess how well their child will be able to tolerate the frequent visits to the orthodontist, having molds of the teeth and x-rays taken, and the feel of the braces, retainer, or other mouth appliance. It is also important to assess how well the person with DS will be able to clean his own teeth and gums, since braces complicate tooth brushing and flossing. There are also physical considerations, such as whether the roots of the teeth are long enough to support braces. All of these concerns should be discussed thoroughly with the orthodontist to determine whether treatment will do more good than harm.

CAVITIES

People with Down syndrome generally have fewer cavities (dental caries) than usual. There are many theories for this reduced rate, including:

- delayed tooth eruption (so the teeth have less time to be exposed to mouth bacteria);
- congenitally missing teeth;
- higher salivary pH (their saliva is more basic—less acidic) and bicarbonate levels (which provides better buffering), which helps prevent acids from eroding the teeth;
- smaller teeth;
- increased space between teeth; and
- shallower fissures on tooth surfaces.

Still, people with DS can and do get cavities—especially if they do not use good dental hygiene. Like everyone else, they need to learn the proper procedures for cleaning their teeth with fluoride toothpaste and a toothbrush. They also need to understand the importance of eating foods with less sugar content. At home, they may try using over-the-counter or prescription fluoride mouthwashes to reduce cavities. In addition, teens and adults with DS should visit the dentist every six months. It may be helpful for the dentist to apply a sealant to the chewing surfaces of the back teeth—which are harder to reach with brushing—to decrease cavities.

Due to misalignment of teeth, mouth breathing, or difficulties with oral hygiene, some people with DS are more prone to cavities. For these patients, oral antimicrobial rinses with 0.12 percent chlorhexidine are effective in controlling oral bacteria. Chlorhexidine is retained on the tooth surfaces for prolonged periods to prevent plaque buildup. However, chlorhexidine has a bitter taste, stains the tooth enamel and the tongue, and can encourage resistant bacteria strains.

GUM DISEASE

A much greater concern for people with DS than cavities is periodontal (gum) disease. This is the leading cause of tooth loss in adults with DS. One reason for this increased rate of periodontal disease is that people with Down syndrome often have impaired immune systems. Second, as previously noted, mouth breathing causes decreased saliva, which allows more bacteria to grow. Interestingly, dental cavities are much less likely to lead to tooth loss than is gum disease.

There are two forms of periodontal disease: gingivitis and periodontitis.

Gingivitis is a very common problem in children as well as adults. Its primary symptom is inflammation—swelling and redness—of the gingival or gums. The gums may bleed spontaneously and the person may have bad breath. This is a reversible condition and does not cause any damage to the underlying bone.

Periodontitis is a chronic inflammation and infection of the gums, tooth ligaments, and underlying bone. This can cause loss of bone, and teeth may fall out as a result. Other consequences of periodontitis can include:

- The infection can spread to adjacent structures, such as to bone and surrounding soft tissues in the mouth and face.
- The infection can spread through the blood to the heart. This can be of particular concern for those with a history of congenital heart disease or other structural abnormalities of the heart. It can lead to heart dysfunction and even death (see Chapter 9).
- The infection can spread to bones or joints anywhere in the body—especially to those that have been operated on and have hardware (artificial joints, rods, pins, etc.).
- The person may lose teeth. While loss of teeth is clearly a cosmetic issue, the complications can be much more problematic. Most importantly, loss of teeth limits chewing abilities. Although some people with DS successfully use dentures, others don't tolerate them, and some people

What Happens When Teeth Are Lost?

Clearly, the goal is to prevent gum disease and the loss of teeth to begin with. Once gum disease has caused either spontaneous loss of teeth or the need to pull teeth, treatment is more challenging.

As mentioned above, some people with Down syndrome cannot tolerate the sensation of dentures. Others have too much bone loss to be able to use dentures. If only some of the teeth are lost, a partial denture may be attached to adjoining teeth—but only if these teeth are not loose or significantly decayed.

If dentures are not possible, dental implants may be an option. In this procedure, metal posts are surgically implanted into the bone of the mouth and dentures are attached. Unfortunately, when the bone loss is too great, even this treatment is not successful because there is not enough bone to anchor the posts.

If an individual has no teeth, or very few teeth, it may limit his diet. It may be helpful for the person to visit a dietitian to make sure he is still getting enough fiber and nutrients from softer foods.

have had too much bone loss to be able to use dentures. Some people with DS are able to chew remarkably well without teeth. However, for most, loss of teeth can significantly impair chewing, swallowing, and digesting of food. Swallowing is further discussed in Chapter 11.

Treatment and prevention for both types of gum disease include:
- regular brushing and flossing of teeth (see below);
- limiting high sugar foods (especially processed foods like candy and cookies);
- regular dental visits—generally every six months, but some people benefit from visits every three months. Sometime alternating visits with a dentist and a periodontist—a specialist in the prevention and treatment of periodontal (gum) disease—every three months is recommended.

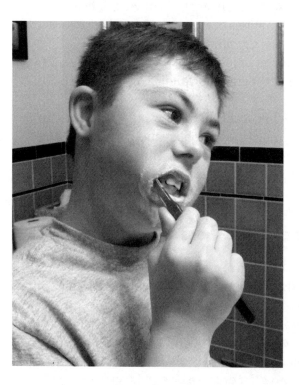

TEETH BRUSHING AND FLOSSING

Some people with Down syndrome resist brushing their teeth or flossing. Others actually cause gum damage by brushing too hard, too diligently, or too compulsively. Both situations are obviously not ideal for optimal dental hygiene.

As discussed in Chapter 1, many people with Down syndrome have a tendency to get in "The Groove." Order and repetition are part of their routine. If at all possible, figure out some way to help your adult child or client with DS use his grooves in fostering a good dental care routine.

For example, if the person uses a written or picture schedule to remind him of his bedtime schedule, add in a step or two that will lead to better hygiene. For example, add a photo of flossing to his schedule. It may help to encourage the person to develop a groove in which he immediately goes to the bathroom to brush after a meal or uses a checklist to record each brushing.

Be aware that even as adults, some people with Down syndrome may not have the fine motor skills to use a manual toothbrush effectively. Children can usually brush their teeth well enough by themselves when they are able to tie their own shoes, which is something some people with DS never do master.

We often recommend that our patients use an electric toothbrush and a timer (the timer may be built into the toothbrush or separate). Provided the teen or adult is taught to use the appropriate technique and pressure, the electric toothbrush will get the teeth cleaner than a manual toothbrush. The timer (set for 2 to 3 minutes) will ensure that the person brushes long enough. A song that lasts 2 to 3 minutes could also be used as a timer. Be sure the individual uses a toothbrush with soft bristles, especially if he has a tendency to brush too hard or too often.

For some people, picture or written cues may still be necessary to ensure that all surfaces of all teeth are brushed. Another technique is to use a rinse or pill that colors the teeth in places where there is plaque that needs to be brushed or flossed away.

Even though teens and adults with DS may have extra space between their teeth, it is still important for them to floss. Again, fine motor skills may be limited, impairing the ability to use dental floss. Sometimes it is easier for people with DS to use floss on a disposable plastic holder. Oral irrigators such as Water Piks may also be helpful.

Dental Care for Those Who Find It Challenging

Some people with Down syndrome find dental care quite challenging. They may fear dental care based on past experiences, dislike the feel of anyone touching them in or around the mouth, or have a painful condition that is aggravated by touch.

Some suggestions to help a teen or adult with Down syndrome with these problems get good dental hygiene:

- ◆ If mouth defensiveness (dislike of being touched) is a general problem, consider working with a speech therapist to desensitize the person.
- ◆ Optimize prevention and treat problems early to limit pain and fear of future dental exams.
- ◆ Start fresh with a new, gentler dentist who understands the need for the person to get accustomed to the office and dental chair before being asked to undergo any frightening procedures.
- ◆ Try using a Social Story to acquaint the person in advance with what he can expect in the dental office. Pictures are usually particularly beneficial. With the dentist's permission, you might take pictures of the waiting room, examination room, dental chair, hygienist, and dentist. Then write a simple story to go with the pictures, explaining step by step what will happen in the dental office.
- ◆ Look for a dentist who will use a light sedation, if necessary. For example, a dose of lorazepam (Ativan) a few hours before the appointment can reduce anxiety.
- ◆ If necessary, find a dentist who can use sedation in the dental office. Some dentists use midazalom (Versed) orally, intravenously, or by intramuscular injection. These may help the person relax, and, with heavier doses, significantly sedate him. It is important to do this in a safe, monitored setting to make sure the person is tolerating sedation.
- ◆ As a last resort, consider having dental care performed under general anesthesia (usually in a hospital). Some teens and adults with DS

can only tolerate dental care under anesthesia. While the person is under anesthesia, it is a good idea to do preventative as well as restorative work (and extractions, if necessary) during the same procedure to limit the number of times he needs anesthesia. Often the person who requires anesthesia for dental care also finds other medical procedures challenging. Therefore, to optimize use of the period under anesthesia, other procedures such as blood drawing, immunization, etc. may be done. Insurance may not cover anesthesia for dental care. In some instances, adding the dental care to a needed medical procedure under anesthesia may reduce the cost.

Chapter **8**

Eye and Vision

· · · · · · · · · · · · · ·

Concerns

· · · · · · · ·

Antonio's first appointment at the Adult Down Syndrome Center was made because he had fallen several times over the last year. His most recent fall had resulted in a fractured arm. Antonio, age 33, was also occasionally having urinary incontinence. He always seemed to be headed toward the bathroom when he had these "accidents." Upon further questioning, his parents noted that he was walking more slowly and cautiously. He would often walk close enough to the wall that he could touch it. Antonio's memory appeared to be fine, and no seizure activity had been observed.

During Antonio's physical exam, it was noted that the cornea of his eye appeared to have an increased curvature. Although Antonio was not able to complete a formal visual acuity test, his vision did appear to be impaired. Antonio was referred to an ophthalmologist, who confirmed our suspicion of keratoconus, a bowing or abnormal curvature of the cornea. After an unsuccessful trial with hard contact lenses, Antonio underwent a corneal transplant that dramatically improved his vision. He regained his former walking skills and he is no longer falling.

Good vision is extremely important to all of us in our daily lives. Without good vision, it is very difficult to take care of our own needs, get around in our homes and communities, work, and participate in leisure activities.

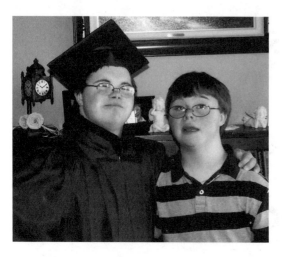

That said, it is surprising to note that not everyone appreciates exactly how important good vision is to people with Down syndrome (DS). This became apparent to me one day when an ophthalmologist called me about an adult with DS whom we had referred to his office. (This was the last patient we referred to him.) This doctor was recommending against removing the patient's cataracts, because, as he put it, "What does he do that good vision is that important for anyway?"

Although it was clear that we would not change this ophthalmologist's bias by giving him a detailed explanation of the beauty of Antonio's life, the question did cause us to think through our answer. While there was no need to sell *us* on the value of our patient's life, we took the time to think about the importance of vision for this man with DS. We concluded that, in some ways, good vision for adults with DS may be even more important because their intellectual disability limits their ability to compensate for a decline in vision. Therefore, paying close attention to maintaining good eye health is very important, as will be discussed in this chapter.

There are a variety of vision problems that become more common as all of us age. Adults with DS are just as likely, if not more so, to acquire these problems as anyone else. In addition, as with many other medical problems, adults with DS may develop these problems at an earlier age than usual, possibly due to the tendency to premature aging.

As Antonio's example, above, illustrates, many people with DS are not able to report that they are having difficulties with their vision. They may not notice the change, understand that what they are experiencing is a visual problem, or be able to express their concerns. That makes it especially crucial for teens and adults with DS to have regular eye exams to help detect vision change.

Eye Exams

◆ ◆ ◆ ◆ ◆ ◆ ◆ ◆ ◆ ◆ ◆ ◆ ◆ ◆ ◆ ◆ ◆ ◆ ◆

We recommend an eye exam by an ophthalmologist or optometrist at least every two years throughout adolescence and adulthood. For people who wear glasses or have some other known vision problem, more frequent exams may be warranted.

A complete eye exam consists of several components, including:

- ◆ testing of visual acuity (the ability to see clearly at near and distant range);
- ◆ testing for glaucoma (pressure inside the eyeball);

◆ an examination of the retina (back of the eye where the light is focused and where signals are sent to the brain);
◆ an examination of the tissue around the eyes.

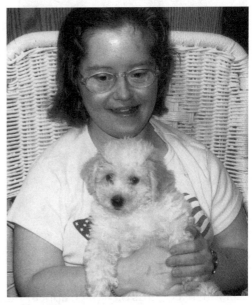

These exams may be completed either by an ophthalmologist—a medical doctor who specializes in diagnosing and treating problems with the eyes or vision—or an optometrist—a specialist who usually has a four-year degree but is not a medical doctor.

Families often express concern that the person with DS will not be able to cooperate with the eye exam. Only a small percentage of our patients are unable to comply at all with the exam. These individuals require anesthesia for an exam. More often, people with DS are willing to cooperate, but do not have the skills to participate in all portions of the exam. For example, in testing visual acuity, a patient is generally required to look at different pictures or letters and inform the examiner which is more clear. Many people with DS find this challenging. However, a patient examiner can often get the job done well. Fortunately, there are now instruments available that allow the examiner to get a pretty accurate prescription for corrective lenses even without the patient being able to identify letters or objects, or to report the clarity of objects or letters. This device can also be used when a person is under anesthesia.

CONDITIONS THAT AFFECT VISUAL ACUITY

In general, vision problems are more common in people with Down syndrome. Conditions that affect visual acuity (the clarity of vision) are especially common. These include:
◆ nearsightedness,
◆ farsightedness,
◆ astigmatism, and
◆ presbyopia.

NEARSIGHTEDNESS

People who have nearsightedness (myopia) are able to see objects that are close to them clearly, but objects that are far away appear blurry. This is a common condi-

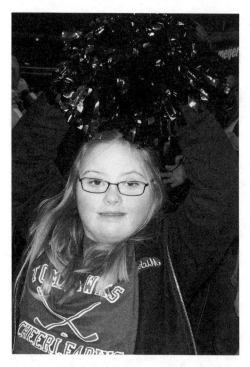

tion in both people with and without Down syndrome. Depending on the severity of the condition, the person may be able to see objects clearly at several yards away to only a few inches away. Myopia tends to run in families. It can develop gradually or quickly and often becomes worse in childhood or adolescence. It can be corrected with glasses, contacts, or surgery (e.g., Lasik (laser in-situ keratomileusis), PRK (photorefractive keratectomy), LASEK (laser in-situ keratomileusis, and others).

Farsightedness

People who have farsightedness (hyperopia) have the opposite problem to those with nearsightedness. They are able to see objects that are further away clearly, but closer objects such as words on a page appear blurry. The worse the farsightedness, the further an object has to be away from the person before it is clear. Farsightedness also tends to run in families, but is usually present at birth. Treatments include wearing glasses or contact lenses or surgery to correct the farsightedness.

Astigmatism

Astigmatism occurs when there is an imperfection in the curvature of the eye. There is a slightly different curvature in one direction from the other, which results in blurry vision at all distances. The curvature can affect the cornea (the front surface of the eye) or the lens. Astigmatism can accompany nearsightedness or farsightedness and is often present at birth. The treatment options are the same as for nearsightedness and farsightedness: glasses, contacts, or surgery.

Presbyopia

"Presby" means old and "opia" means eye, so presbyopia translates as old eye. As people age, whether or not they have previously had other problems with visual acuity, the lens of the eye loses its flexibility, so focusing on near tasks becomes more difficult. In people without Down syndrome, the need to correct this problem (with "reading" glasses) often becomes apparent around age 45. This may occur at a younger age in people with Down syndrome, so be alert to signs that the person is no longer seeing clearly up close.

GLASSES AND CONTACT LENSES

Wearing eyeglasses is diffi-cult for some people with DS. Some reasons for this include:

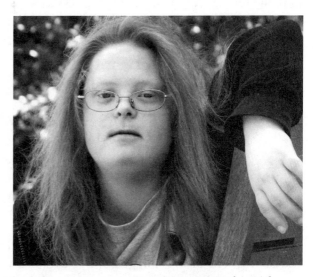

- ◆ The person may not want to wear the glass-es or may be tactilely defensive about wear-ing anything on her face or head.
- ◆ The person may have trouble accepting the change in vision that comes with new glass-es, even though she can clearly see better with the new prescription (Some people with DS seem to become comfortable with, or used to, abnormal vision. The correction is a change and, therefore, not tolerable.)
- ◆ In some cases, having a smaller, flatter nose, or differently placed ears makes it harder to keep the glasses on the face, or the glasses just don't fit comfortably because of the different dimensions of the person's face.

There are other options besides glasses for vision correction, including contact lenses and corrective eye surgery (see above). A few of our patients do successfully use contact lenses. These individuals have both good fine motor skills and are highly self-motivated to wear contacts. We are not aware of any of our patients who have had corrective eye surgery.

HELP IN ADAPTING TO A NEW PRESCRIPTION OR A FIRST PAIR OF GLASSES

If a teen or adult with DS has trouble tolerating a first pair of glasses or a new prescription, she may need a period of gradual adjustment to the new glasses. This can be achieved by:

- ◆ wearing the glasses for short periods of time initially and gradually increasing the time;
- ◆ initially only wearing the glasses at home and gradually increasing the range of places where they are worn;
- ◆ initially wearing glasses that don't fully correct the impaired vision; then, over time, increasing the prescription to provide more correction.

Adapting to bifocals, trifocals, and "progressives" can be particularly challenging. Some people may need to use two different pairs of glasses—one for close vision and one for far. Very few adults with DS drive, so there rarely is a need for bifocals or progressives to be able to see the road as well as the instruments on the dashboard. For most adults, in many situations, using two separate pairs of glasses for near and far vision may work.

Medical Problems That May Affect the Eyes

Keratoconus

As described in the case example at the beginning of this chapter, keratoconus is more common in people with Down syndrome. Keratoconus is a thinning of the cornea (the clear, curved part at the front of the eye) that results in irregular protrusion of the cornea. The protrusion gets worse over time and causes impaired vision.

Particularly in the early stages, the changes to the eye may not be noticeable to someone else (except an eye doctor). In the later stages, the cornea may get cloudy or the protrusion might be visible (especially if you look at the person from the side). The cause of keratoconus is not clear, but chronic rubbing of the eyes has been implicated as one possible cause.

Treatments include:

- eyeglasses to improve vision early in the course of the disease;
- hard contact lenses to reduce the abnormal curvature;
- identifying any medical problems that might lead the person to rub her eyes, such as allergies, dry eyes, or cataracts, and then treating the underlying problem;
- if no medical reason is found for the eye rubbing, figuring out why the person rubs her eyes (e.g., boredom or self-stimulation) and then finding a substitute behavior for her to do instead;
- teaching the individual to avoid rubbing her eyes;
- corneal transplantation for advanced cases.

Cataracts

A cataract is a clouding of the lens of the eye. It can affect one or both eyes. In the early stages, a cataract often doesn't affect vision, but as it grows larger and/or denser, it blocks more and more vision.

Cataracts are more common in people with DS. Some are born with cataracts (congenital cataracts), and others develop them later in life. When a congenital cataract is obstructing vision, it should be removed early in life. Otherwise, the vision centers of the brain won't develop appropriately, since there is only a window of time during the first several months of life that they develop. Cataracts that develop later in life can also obstruct vision. These cataracts tend to occur at a younger age in people with DS than in other people. We have seen cataracts develop in individuals with DS as early as their 20s.

Signs that an adult with DS is developing cataracts can include:

- a visible change (cloudiness) of the person's eye that others can see;
- turning the head to look at things out of the sides of the eye (if the cataract is central);
- rubbing or poking at the eye(s);
- emotional or behavioral changes;
- decreasing abilities to perform daily functions or walk as the result of impaired vision.

People who have cataracts should visit an ophthalmologist regularly. The ophthalmologist will monitor the growth of the cataract and check whether it is affecting vision. If a cataract is small and not obstructing vision, it is usually just observed.

The treatment of cataracts involves surgically removing the cloudy lens from the eye. An implant may be placed at the time of the surgery. This may reduce the need for glasses after surgery, although contacts or glasses may still be necessary, with or without an implant. Ordinarily, the operation is done under little or no sedation. Instead, local anesthesia is used to numb the eye while the patient remains awake. Some people with DS may need to have the operation done under general anesthesia, however. Following the operation, prescription eye drops need to be administered for a period of time. There are no medications that can remove cataracts.

BLEPHARITIS

A common eye problem for people with DS of all ages is blepharitis, inflammation or infection of the eyelids. This causes redness of the eyelids and mattering (sticky secretions) of the eyelids and eyelashes. It is also sometimes associated with conjunctivitis, or pink eye—an inflammation or infection of the conjunctive (the outer clear membrane that covers the eye).

Blepharitis can be caused by:

- bacterial infection,
- acne rosacea, or
- seborrhea (a chronic inflammatory skin disorder of the sebaceous glands that causes red and flaking skin, as well as dandruff on the scalp).

Prevention and treatment consists of:

- instructing (and reinforcing) the individual to keep her hands away from her eyes;
- warm compresses on the eyes to loosen crusting/mattering;

- ◆ light scrubbing with a mixture of half water and half baby shampoo using a washcloth or cotton swab;
- ◆ treating scalp dandruff/seborrheic dermatitis or acne rosacea when present (see Chapter 6);
- ◆ if necessary, using antibiotic eye drops, particularly if conjunctivitis occurs.

It is usually necessary to treat blepharitis on an ongoing basis. That is, people who are prone to blepharitis usually get the condition over and over again. If the person develops a bacterial infection, she could transfer the bacteria to others. Therefore, she needs to be encouraged to keep her hands away from her eyes and wash her hands regularly to prevent spreading the bacteria to others.

STRABISMUS

Strabismus, abnormal alignment of the eyes, also occurs more frequently in people with DS. One or both eyes can point inwards toward the nose (esotropia), point out toward the sides (exotropia), or point up (hypertropia) or down (hypotropia). This misalignment is usually caused by eye muscle imbalance.

Strabismus is generally present from early childhood. Vision in the eye that is misaligned is often impaired and the normally aligned eye is the predominant source of vision. That is, the person primarily sees with one (good) eye. In this situation, the person's depth perception (or ability to see in 3-D) is significantly reduced. This makes it difficult to walk up stairs or up and down curbs, to do fine motor tasks such as threading a needle or catching a ball, to drive, and to do other tasks requiring binocular vision.

Strabismus requires treatment in childhood. Otherwise, the misaligned eye will lose its ability to see adequately due to lack of use. Early intervention helps improve or even restore the vision in the misaligned eye. Treatment may include using eyeglasses, patching, or surgery to force the person to use her weaker eye. However, if the intervention is not done by adolescence, treatment is unlikely to improve vision. At that point, treatment usually focuses on using eyeglasses to optimize vision.

IMPAIRED DEPTH PERCEPTION

Interestingly, many people with DS have impaired depth perception even if they do not have strabismus. Many family members and caregivers have described how an adult with DS has trouble with activities that require depth perception. These observations have been supported by our observations of a large number of patients carefully climbing onto the exam table. We suspect there is an impairment in the vision centers of the brain. Whether or not an adult has a history of strabismus, if she has difficulties seeing in 3-D, this should be considered when evaluating appropriate jobs for her. For example, before pursuing a job that involves working around moving machines, evaluate whether the person can maneuver safely in that environment. Likewise, carefully consider difficulties with depth perception when determining whether the person should learn to drive.

RETINAL DETACHMENT

As previously noted, the retina is the back portion of the eye where visual images are focused and signals are sent on to the brain. With age, everyone has a slight chance that their retina might become detached (separated from the structure of the eye), leading to buckling and folding of the retina. The risk of detachment is higher if you have a significant degree of nearsightedness.

In general, adults with DS have the same slight risk of retinal detachment as adults without DS. Although this is a less common problem than the other problems discussed in this chapter, we are discussing it here as a precaution for the small number of adults with DS who have self-injurious or aggressive behavior. The person may be particularly at risk of a detached retina if she strikes her head or hits her head against hard objects. It is very important to get an eye exam after a head injury, especially if vision impairment is suspected.

Signs of a detached retina are typically the same as those for other causes of impaired vision. The difference is that these changes tend to occur abruptly with the detachment. The person might also complain of spots, shapes, or lights floating in front of her eyes.

If a retinal detachment is suspected, the person should be immediately seen by an ophthalmologist. The sooner it is treated, the better the chances that vision will not be lost. If the retina has become detached, the ophthalmologist may choose to observe the eye if only a small area is involved. However, for larger areas or areas affecting central vision, surgery or another procedure may be needed to reattach the retina.

MACULAR DEGENERATION

Macular degeneration is a cause of vision impairment seen in older individuals. In people without Down syndrome, it is more common in adults over 50 years of age. The condition occurs as the macula, the center of the retina responsible for central vision, deteriorates over time. A blind spot develops in the area of central vision, which makes reading, driving, recognizing faces, and doing detail work difficult.

Fortunately, macular degeneration seems to be less common in people with Down syndrome. It has been hypothesized that this is due to extra copies of genes that suppress angiogenesis, or blood vessel growth. Increased angiogenesis is part of macular degeneration. Similarly, cancer is less common in people with Down syndrome (see Chapter 14). In cancer, increased angiogenesis is essential to provide nutrients to feed growing tumors. Reduced angiogenesis may reduce the incidence of both cancer and macular degeneration.

GLAUCOMA

Glaucoma is caused by several conditions that cause an elevation in the pressure inside the eye. This increased pressure results in optic nerve damage. Recently, researchers found that glaucoma occurs much more frequently in adults with Down syndrome (Yokoyama et al., 2006).

Glaucoma is the second leading cause of blindness. There are usually no symptoms except the gradual loss of vision. Often the loss of vision is so gradual that the person doesn't notice it until the disease is quite advanced. Less commonly, glaucoma may cause discomfort and redness of the eyes.

Early diagnosis and treatment can minimize or prevent optic nerve damage and limit glaucoma-related vision loss. Just as for other people, it is important for a person with Down syndrome to have her eyes examined regularly, and make sure that the eye doctor measures her intraocular pressure.

Treatment usually consists of eye drops used to lower the pressure in the eye. Oral medications and surgery are also sometimes options.

PREVENTATIVE CARE

Impaired vision is a significant problem for many adults with Down syndrome. Therefore, it is important to take steps to optimize good eye health. To maintain eye health, we recommend that you:

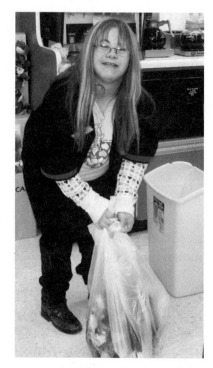

- ◆ Ensure that the person has regular eye exams by a vision specialist. We recommend every two years. If you rely on the adult with DS to report changes in her vision, you may miss significant changes. Many adults with DS don't notice or can't report a change in vision or a significant eye problem.
- ◆ Gently wash the eyelids and eyelashes daily to prevent infections.
- ◆ Teach the adult to avoid rubbing her eyes.
- ◆ Ensure that the adult uses protective eyewear when doing tasks or jobs that could result in eye injuries.

Chapter 9

Cardiac

· · · · · · ·

Concerns

◆ · ◆ · ◆ · ◆ · ◆ · ◆ · ◆ · ◆

As he approached his fortieth birthday, John and his parents wanted to discuss his risk for heart disease at his annual exam. He had had no heart problems when he was born and had never had any symptoms suggestive of heart problems. We discussed other risk factors for heart attack (myocardial infarction). John did not smoke, there was no family history of heart attacks, he did not have diabetes mellitus, he exercised regularly, his blood pressure was normal, and he was not overweight. His cholesterol, however, was moderately elevated at 256. We discussed the low incidence of coronary artery disease (blockages of the arteries supplying oxygen to the heart) in people with Down syndrome. John and his family decided against using medications to lower his cholesterol due to this low incidence.

The following year at John's annual exam, his family asked if we could be sure that John wasn't building plaques in his arteries despite the low incidence of coronary artery disease in people with Down syndrome. We suggested a rapid CT scan (computerized tomography) of the coronary arteries, a test that is often used to assess for coronary artery disease in people without Down syndrome. John and his family decided to proceed with a CT. John had a calcium score of zero, which indicated no evidence of the development of plaque. With this information, John and his family again decided against cholesterol-lowering medications. John did, however, stay on a diet low in saturated fats.

CONCERNS FOR ADULTS WITH CONGENITAL HEART DISEASE

◆ ◆

Down syndrome (DS) and heart disease are two conditions that are commonly considered together. Forty to sixty percent of children with DS are born with heart disease. The congenital heart conditions are usually structural problems of the inner walls of the heart or the heart valves. Common problems include:

- ventricular septal defect (VSD)—a hole in the wall between the two ventricles or large chambers of the heart;
- atrial septal defect (ASD)—a hole between the two atria or smaller heart chambers);
- atrioventricular canal defect—defects in both walls of the heart that effectively result in one large chamber;
- abnormalities of the mitral and/or aortic valves.

Most people with DS now have these conditions surgically corrected early in childhood. However, issues that require special attention in adulthood may remain. Adults with unrepaired heart disease are at added risk of complications, as discussed below.

TREATMENT FOR ADULTS WITH REPAIRED HEART DEFECTS

Adolescents and adults who have had congenital heart defects surgically corrected need ongoing cardiac evaluations and sometimes additional treatment. This is because after a heart defect has been repaired, there are still two potential causes of problems: structural and rhythm. In some individuals, the surgically corrected area or adjacent area may deteriorate over time. This could lead to a decline in the heart's ability to function. It could also leave the heart more vulnerable to infection. Rhythm disturbances can also occur. The beat of the heart can become irregular, too fast, or too slow.

For these reasons, we recommend that adults with repaired heart defects see a cardiologist who is familiar with the care of adults with congenital heart disease at least every five years. In addition, these adults may need to get a preoperative assessment from a cardiologist before undergoing anesthesia for surgery. Also, they may need to take antibiotics before certain medical or dental procedures, as described in the section on "Antibiotic Prophylaxis," below.

TREATMENT FOR ADULTS WITH UNREPAIRED HEART DEFECTS

For individuals who did not have their congenital heart disease corrected in childhood, ongoing cardiac care is extremely important. Fortunately, far fewer people with Down syndrome now go without surgical correction. However, cardiac surgery was not available to *anyone* born before the mid 1960s or so, and then for a period of time it was sometimes not available to children with DS.

In some cases, the heart condition may not have required surgical correction because it was less complicated and the cardiologist may have felt the heart function would stay stable over time. Or there may have been holes or defects that closed on their own. However, for some types of heart disease, if cardiac surgery is not performed, the heart will deteriorate over time.

Parents and caregivers of adults with uncorrected heart defects should watch for the following symptoms that can indicate heart dysfunction:

- ◆ increased fatigue,
- ◆ less ability to tolerate exercise or physical activity,
- ◆ shortness of breath,
- ◆ agitation, irritability, or other psychological changes that could be signs that the person feels ill,
- ◆ chest pain, and
- ◆ dizziness.

POSSIBLE COMPLICATIONS FOR ADULTS WITH UNREPAIRED HEART DISEASE

CYANOTIC HEART DISEASE

Some people with DS with congenital heart disease who did not have correction (or did not have correction early enough) will develop cyanotic heart disease. "Cyanotic" in general means blue. In the context of heart disease, it refers to blood with inadequate oxygen, which will make the person's skin appear blue. This color will be visible not only in the hands and feet but also the lips, and often more extensively.

The cyanosis develops due to a hole or defect in the heart that interferes with oxygenation of the blood. In a person without the hole or defect, what normally occurs is that blood flows from the body, to the right side of the heart (right atrium, then to right ventricle), to the lungs, back to the left side of the heart (left atrium to left ventricle), and then back out to the body. Blood returns to the heart from other parts of the body after dropping off oxygen and picking up carbon dioxide.

What typically occurs in an individual with cyanotic heart disease is that some of the blood is circulated to the body without going through the lungs to pick up oxygen. Instead, when the blood reaches the heart, some of it crosses a hole in the heart from the right side of the heart to the left and then out to the body. When blood flows directly from the right to the left side through the hole, it goes back to the body without picking up more oxygen and dropping off the carbon dioxide in the lungs. The low oxygen in the blood and tissues of the body causes the person to look blue or cyanotic.

Obviously, there are much more significant implications for the person than just appearing to be blue. The decreased oxygen in the blood impairs the function of all the organs of the body. Over time, the function of the heart and all other organs of the body gradually deteriorates.

It can take years for cyanotic heart disease to develop in someone with an unrepaired heart defect. When a child is born with a heart defect such as an atrioventricular defect, a ventricular septal defect, or an atrial septal defect, the blood does not initially flow from the right side through the hole to the left side of the heart, bypassing the lungs. At first, the blood enters the right side normally from the body, goes to the lungs, and then enters the left side of the heart. Normally, the pressure is higher in the left side of the heart than the right. Therefore, some of the blood flows through the hole from the left side to the right side of the heart. Due to blood entering the right side from both the body and the left side (through the hole), there is a greater blood flow through the lungs. The greater blood flow through the lungs causes the blood vessels in the lungs to thicken and the pressure increases.

Because the blood flows from the right side of the heart to the lungs, as the pressure increases in the lungs, it also increases in the right side of the heart. At some point, the pressure in the right side of the heart will exceed that in the left side. Then some of the blood will begin to flow from the right side to the left through the hole, bypassing the lungs. This is when cyanosis occurs.

Cyanosis may appear in infancy, but may not develop until late into adulthood. Some adults with these types of heart problems never develop cyanosis. People who do develop cyanosis may need to limit exercise to less strenuous activities. Even when cyanosis develops, the person often lives several to many more years. Unfortunately, however, the development of cyanosis typically decreases a person's life expectancy.

Assessment: If cyanosis develops, a cardiologist will assess the person via a history and physical exam. He may also order an EKG, blood work, and echocardiogram to decide on the best course of treatment.

If surgery is being considered, a cardiac catheterization may be needed. During a cardiac catheterization, a catheter (a thin tube through which pressures can be measured and dye can be injected) is inserted into a vein in the groin or arm. The catheter is then threaded up to the heart to assess heart function.

Cardiac catheterization is usually done with local anesthetic. The patient has to lie still for a significant amount of time (the time varies depending on the problem, the heart structure, etc.). When the dye is injected, the person may experience a warm sensation in the chest. People with Down syndrome may need to have this procedure done under general anesthesia if they cannot lie still, are likely to become frightened by the machines, or become agitated by the number of people in the room assisting with the procedure.

Treatment Options: Treatment options for both cyanotic heart disease and mitral regurgitation (see below) may include medication, oxygen, or surgery. Diuretics such as furosemide (Lasix) may be used to reduce retention of excess fluid in the lungs, the extremities, and other parts of the body. Furosemide causes the kidneys to excrete urine, salt, and water. Digoxin (lanoxin) is sometimes used to improve heart function. Medications such as captopril (Capoten) or lisinopril (Prinivil or Zestril) are sometimes used to reduce the blood pressure in the arteries in the body so that the heart does not have to work so hard to pump blood forward.

Bosentan (Tracleer) or sildenafil (Viagra) are sometimes used for those who have elevated blood pressure in the blood vessels in their lungs related to cyanotic heart disease. These medications can reduce the blood pressure in these vessels. They may also improve blood flow through the lungs and increase the amount of oxygen in the blood. Bosentan's use is restricted in the United States to certain practitioners (usually to cardiologists who are prescribing it for elevated blood pressure in the lungs due to heart disease). This is because of the need to monitor the patient's heart and side effects and because of the risk of birth defects if taken by a pregnant woman.

Supplemental oxygen may help people with cyanotic heart disease by increasing the amount of oxygen the lungs can deliver to the blood. It also may help people who have non-cyanotic heart disease as their heart function declines. We have found that adults with DS generally tolerate oxygen therapy pretty well. The oxygen is delivered through a canula in the nose or via a mask. A hose from the canula or mask is attached to one of a variety of oxygen supplies:

- ◆ a large metal bottle that contains oxygen gas;
- ◆ a large container with liquid oxygen (smaller containers can be connected to it so a smaller amount of liquid oxygen can be made portable);
- ◆ a concentrator that pulls oxygen out of the air and "concentrates" it to the needed concentration.

Especially as heart function declines, most people with DS realize that they feel better when they are breathing the supplemental oxygen and are more willing to use it.

Surgery may benefit people with cyanotic heart disease if it is done before the blood flows from the left side of the heart to the right, and it may also help those with non-cyanotic heart disease. Generally speaking, surgery involves repairing the holes in the heart that were not repaired when the person was younger.

Unfortunately, as the pressure in the blood vessels in the lungs increases and the blood begins to flow from the left side to the right, surgical correction is no longer beneficial and can actually decrease heart function. Due to damage to the heart and the blood vessels in the lungs, the surgery that is required in that situation is a heart and lung transplant. Unfortunately, this procedure can cause severe complications and a significant number of people still die quite prematurely. Also, some people die waiting for a compatible heart and lung to become available. Some hospitals, doctors, or transplant organizations have also been reluctant to approve transplants for people with Down syndrome for one reason or another.

Comfort Care: If the person's health continues to decline despite treatment, comfort care needs to be provided. This may include oxygen, morphine to decrease pain and to reduce discomfort related to breathing difficulties, use of hospital beds or wheelchairs, and hospice care. The issues of advance directives and end-of-life care are addressed more extensively in Chapter 22.

Acrocyanosis: Another Cause of Blue Hands or Feet

Blue hands and feet are actually quite common in people with Down syndrome. Sometimes the blueness is due to cyanotic congenital heart disease or to pulmonary hypertension (high blood pressure), poor peripheral blood circulation, or Raynaud's phenomenon. Often, however, the cause is acrocyanosis—a benign, painless disorder caused by constriction or narrowing of small blood vessels in the skin. The spasm of the blood vessels decreases the amount of blood that passes through them, resulting in less blood being delivered to the hands and feet. The affected areas turn blue.

Anxiety, pain, and cold temperatures can worsen the symptoms of acrocyanosis, while warmth can decrease symptoms. We also find that it tends to be more pronounced in our patients with DS who have developed Alzheimer disease. Acrocyanosis is generally not uncomfortable and usually does not cause any other problems.

The increased incidence of acrocyanosis in people with DS may be related to differences in the autonomic nervous system. The autonomic nervous system controls the function of the small blood vessels in response to a variety of stimuli and does seem to work differently in people with DS.

Sometimes an adult with DS and cyanosis may become anxious if he feels ill or realizes he is going to die soon. Careful use of medications to reduce anxiety may play a role in treatment in these situations.

VALVULAR HEART DISEASE

Valvular heart disease refers to damage to the valves in the heart that play an important role in directing and controlling blood flow. Some people with DS are born with valvular heart disease, although this occurs less commonly than the defects noted above. Others who weren't born with valvular heart disease may develop these problems later in life. This is true for all adults, but may be more common for adults with Down syndrome. Some of the defects that may develop include:

- ◆ mitral regurgitation—blood flowing backward from the left ventricle to the left atrium through an abnormal mitral valve (see above);
- ◆ aortic regurgitation—blood flowing backward from the aorta, the large artery coming out of the heart, back into the left ventricle;
- ◆ aortic stenosis—an abnormally small opening in the aortic valve that restricts normal blood flow out of the left ventricle;
- ◆ pulmonic stenosis—an abnormally small opening in the pulmonic valve that restricts normal blood flow out of the right ventricle.

Symptoms of valvular heart disease are the same as those previously described for heart dysfunction. These conditions may require no treatment, but sometimes require medications. Generally, they can be treated successfully and the person can continue to do all or most of his usual activities. If the valvular heart disease progresses, sometimes the valve must be surgically replaced.

MITRAL VALVE PROLAPSE

Another condition that deserves mention is mitral valve prolapse (MVP). In MVP, the mitral valves, between the left atrium and left ventricle, bulge backwards into the left atrium. Most commonly, this condition does not cause symptoms and does not become worse over time. A small subset of people with MVP may have symptoms, including:

◆ dizziness or syncope (passing out),
◆ fatigue,
◆ chest pain,
◆ abnormal heart rhythm, and
◆ sudden death (rare).

Occasionally, the mitral valve degenerates over time. This causes mitral regurgitation (see the section above). Most of the time, MVP requires no treatment. However, if someone has a tendency toward dizziness, encouraging adequate salt and fluid consumption may reduce the symptoms. Beta blocker medications such as propranolol (Inderal) may help with abnormal heart rhythms. Surgery to replace the valve may be necessary in a few adults later in life if the valve deteriorates. The surgical success rate for this procedure is high.

PRECAUTIONS FOR ADULTS WITH REPAIRED AND UNREPAIRED DEFECTS

ENDOCARDITIS

Some people born with heart disease and some with acquired heart problems, whether or not they have been repaired, are at higher risk of endocarditis, or an infection of the heart. This is because one complication of an abnormal heart structure is an increased tendency for infectious agents, especially bacteria, to attach to the inner lining of the heart. It is unlikely to "stick" to a normal heart. Once the infectious agent has attached, it is difficult to eradicate and it can cause significant, even life-threatening damage to the heart.

Any infectious agent that enters the body and gets into the bloodstream will pass through the heart. Bacteria, fungi, or other infectious agents may enter through diseased gums, breaks in the skin, or other sources. For people with congenital heart disease, it is very import to try to prevent such infections through good oral hygiene and skin care. If the person does get an infection, it should be treated promptly. A fever that lasts longer than expected may warrant blood tests including blood cultures to assess for organisms in the blood stream.

If there is a possibility of endocarditis, it may be wise to do an echocardiogram. The echocardiogram can look for "vegetations," which are the infective organisms mixed in blood clots that are adhering to the inside of the heart.

ANTIBIOTIC PROPHYLAXIS

Antibiotic prophylaxis—taking antibiotics to prevent bacterial endocarditis—is recommended in some circumstances for people who have structural abnormalities of the heart or who have had a heart defect surgically repaired. In the past, the American Heart Association recommended that antibiotics be taken before a wide range of medical and dental procedures in order to prevent bacterial infection of the valves or inner wall of the heart. In 2007, the American Heart Association (AHA) made significant changes to the recommendations, eliminating the recommendations for antibiotics for many congenital heart conditions.

Currently, the AHA recommends that antibiotics be taken only before:

- dental procedures involving manipulation of the gums or procedures involving a risk of perforation of the mouth tissue;
- invasive procedures involving incision (cutting) or biopsy of respiratory tissue (e.g., trachea or lungs).

(The previous recommendations that antibiotics be taken before gastroenterologic or urologic procedures were eliminated.)

The AHA recommends that anyone who falls into the categories below receive antibiotics before dental procedures:

- artificial heart valve,
- previous history of infective endocarditis,
- cardiac transplant with valve repair,
- unrepaired cyanotic congestive heart disease,
- repaired congenital heart disease within six months of repair or with a residual defect at the site of, or adjacent to, the repair.

The following are the antibiotics recommended (to be taken 30 to 60 minutes before the procedure):

- amoxicillin; 2000 mg orally;
    if not able to take orally, then:
    - ampicillin 2000 mg IM (intramuscular injection) or IV (intravenous),
    - cefazolin 1000 mg IM or IV,
    - ceftriaxone 1000 mg IM or IV,
- for those with an allergy to penicillin:
    - cephalexin 2000 mg (do not use if the person has a history of severe reaction to penicillin),
    - clindamycin 600 mg,
    - azithromycin 500 mg,
    - clarithromycin 500 mg,
- for those with a penicillin allergy who are not able to take medications orally:
    - cefazolin 1000 mg IM or IV (see warning above regarding cephalexin),

> ➤ ceftriaxone 1000 mg IM or IV (see warning above regard-
> ing cephalexin),
> ➤ clindamycin 600 mg IM or IV.

There are additional regimens recommended (but not discussed here) if the individual has bacterial resistance to penicillin.

POSSIBLE CARDIAC ISSUES FOR ALL PEOPLE WITH DOWN SYNDROME

CORONARY ARTERY DISEASE

The coronary arteries are the blood vessels that supply blood to the heart muscle.
Coronary artery disease (CAD) occurs when these arteries become narrowed, typically
by fatty plaques. (This condition is also known as atherosclerosis—"hardening of the
arteries.") CAD can lead to myocardial infarctions ("heart attacks"), congestive heart
failure (reduced ability of the heart to pump blood), and abnormal heart rhythms.

CAD is the leading cause of death in adults without DS. Adults with DS, however, seem to have a much lower rate of CAD, even though they have a much higher
incidence of congenital heart disease. CAD actually seems to be quite uncommon in
people with DS.

It is not clear at this time why people with DS have a lower incidence of CAD. One
theory is that because people with DS have an extra 21st chromosome, they produce
more of some proteins. One (or more) of these proteins may somehow lead to a reduced incidence of CAD. Further research is needed to understand this situation.

The risk factors for CAD among adults in general are:

- a family history of CAD, especially if it begins at age 50 or younger,
- cigarette smoking,
- diabetes mellitus,
- obesity,
- inactive life style,
- hypertension (high blood pressure),
- abnormal levels of lipids in the blood; specifically: elevated low density lipoproteins (LDL—so-called "bad cholesterol"), decreased high
density lipoproteins (HDL—so-called "good cholesterol"), and elevated triglycerides,
- male sex,
- increasing age,
- stress.

Among adults with DS, some of the risk factors are more common, less common, or about the same:

- ◆ More Common:
    - ➤ diabetes mellitus
    - ➤ obesity
    - ➤ sedentary lifestyle (although this may be improving)
- ◆ Less Common:
    - ➤ hypertension (high blood pressure)
    - ➤ cigarette smoking
    - ➤ increased age (life expectancy for people with DS is lower than for those without DS, but it is increasing)
- ◆ Probably of Equal Incidence:
    - ➤ male sex
    - ➤ family history of CAD
    - ➤ lipid abnormalities (e.g., high cholesterol levels)

As far as stress is concerned, we don't think we truly understand this issue in adults with Down syndrome. At the Adult Down Syndrome Center, we have often heard that "people with DS don't have stress" in their lives. And it's true, many adults with DS do not worry about some of the financial and other issues that cause stress for other adults. However, in our experience, people with Down syndrome do seem to experience stress about other issues. In fact, as we discussed in *Mental Wellness for Adults with Down Syndrome*, sometimes they are very sensitive to events going on around them. This "emotional radar" can help a person with DS be more sensitive to others, but may also cause him to internalize or experience stress from events that don't actually concern him. Therefore, at this time, we would only conclude that more research is needed on the amount of stress that people with DS experience and the effect of stress on their physical health.

ADDRESSING RISK FACTORS FOR CAD

As illustrated by the case example of John at the beginning of the chapter, the jury is still out as to whether addressing risk factors for heart disease in people with DS actually reduces the incidence of CAD. Lifestyle modifications (such as regular exercise and diets lower in saturated fat) are recommended because even if these strategies do little to prevent heart disease, there are likely other benefits and the risks and side effects are limited. Therefore, we recommend the following strategies for all adults with Down syndrome, regardless of whether they test as having high cholesterol:

- ◆ get regular exercise,
- ◆ eliminate smoking,
- ◆ reduce salt consumption if blood pressure is high,
- ◆ lose weight if overweight (through healthy eating and regular exercise),
- ◆ limit saturated fats in the diet (to a similar level as recommended for people without DS).

We also recommend:

- appropriate, but not "too tight" control of diabetes (see Chapter 15),
- appropriate control of hypertension (but not "too tight," so as to avoid low blood pressure).

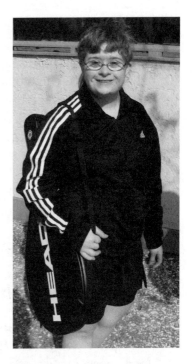

Periodic blood testing of cholesterol levels (every one to five years depending on risk factors and previous cholesterol levels) can help guide treatment.

We are less likely to recommend cholesterol-lowering medications for our adult patients with Down syndrome. We regularly discuss other risk factors (including family history), the level of the cholesterol, the individual's ability to follow lifestyle changes and their effects on cholesterol and health, and the patient's and family's desires regarding treatment. Coronary CT Angiography is a possible method to further assess the coronary arteries. It has not been studied in people with Down syndrome. However, in those without Down syndrome, it has been used as a noninvasive method to view the coronary arteries and screen for atherosclerotic disease. Some of our patients and their families have used this procedure to screen for coronary artery disease when the individual had risk factors for atherosclerosis.

In general, given the lower incidence of CAD, the benefit of prescribing cholesterol medications is less clear for people with DS. Also, we have concerns about the side effects in people with DS. For the statins (e.g., atorvastatin, or Lipitor), pravastatin (Pravachol), we worry that some people with DS may not be able to report whether they are experiencing the muscle pain that is occasionally caused by these medications. Also, concerns have recently been raised, based on anecdotal evidence, that some cholesterol-lowering drugs may be associated with cognitive impairment in people without DS. It is not clear whether this also occurs in people with DS. However, we have had a number of patients who experienced memory or other cognitive impairments after starting statin medications. These impairments improved after the medications were stopped.

Especially given the decline in skills and Alzheimer disease that can occur in adults with DS (see Chapter 19), there may be good reason for caution in prescribing cholesterol-lowing medications for people with Down syndrome.

HIGH OR LOW BLOOD PRESSURE

Blood pressure (BP) is a measurement of the pressure in the arteries in the body. Blood pressure is recorded as two numbers. The upper number is the systolic pressure and the lower number is the diastolic number. The blood pressure rises during the time the heart contracts (systole) and falls when the heart relaxes to refill with blood (diastole). This fluctuation occurs with each heart beat.

Hypertension (high blood pressure) is defined as a sustained elevation of blood pressure. In adults, high blood pressure is diagnosed if the systolic blood pressure is 140 mm Hg or greater and/or the diastolic blood pressure is 90 mm Hg or greater. The pressure must be elevated on at least two separate days to make the diagnosis.

BP is lower for children, so the diagnosis is made at lower levels for children and varies according to age.

The blood pressure (BP) of people with DS tends to be lower than that of people without DS, and hypertension (high BP) is less common.

Autonomic Nervous System Function and Relaxation of Smooth Muscle

The autonomic nervous system directs the functioning of the body systems that we don't have to think about controlling, including our heart rate, blood pressure, the opening or constricting of the airway in our lungs, and function of our gastrointestinal tract and urinary bladder. Part of our control over these systems is through the relaxation or contraction of our smooth muscles. (There are three types of muscle in the body: 1) skeletal muscles, like the biceps that move in response to a conscious signal from the brain; 2) cardiac (heart) muscle; and 3) smooth muscle that is involved in functions of the body that don't require active thoughts to direct—e.g., functions of the stomach.)

One possible theory regarding the differences in frequency of certain conditions in DS is that these differences are related to the autonomic nervous system and smooth muscles. Sometimes when smooth muscles are "too relaxed," as in people with DS, it can lead to problems. For example, constipation or retention of urine may occur due to reduced contraction of the muscles. These problems are more common in people with DS. On the other hand, sometimes relaxation of smooth muscles is beneficial. For example, when the muscles in the airway are more relaxed, a person is less likely to have the increased airway resistance that is part of the problem in asthma. Asthma seems to be less common in adults with DS. Similarly, this relaxation of smooth muscles may contribute to reduced blood pressure.

In addition, although the heart is not a smooth muscle, heart rate is controlled by the autonomic nervous system and heart rate (HR) tends to be lower in people with DS. A normal HR for adults is 60 to 100. Our patients most commonly have a HR around 60 and some even lower. As with low blood pressure, a lower HR is generally a concern if it is significantly lower than usual or it is causing symptoms (usually low blood pressure and dizziness).

HYPERTENSION (HIGH BP)

High blood pressure or hypertension seems to be much less common in people with DS. The cause for this is not clear, but one proposed explanation may be a difference in the autonomic nervous system (see box on page 114).

In people without DS, hypertension can be classified as either: 1) essential hypertension (hypertension without a definable cause), or 2) secondary hypertension (hypertension related to a definable cause). Secondary hypertension has several possible causes, including:

- abnormal endocrine function such as hyperthyroidism (overactive thyroid) and Cushing's disease (excess cortisol production);
- stenosis (narrowing) of the renal arteries (arteries supplying the kidneys);
- kidney disease;
- medication side effects (e.g., prednisone or certain medications used for "colds"—upper respiratory infections).

Hypertension is a risk factor for coronary artery disease and peripheral vascular disease (narrowing of the arteries outside of the heart or brain—e.g., in the legs). It also can cause kidney disease and strokes. Because of these serious health risks, hypertension is important to treat.

Because hypertension is relatively rare in people with DS, it is important to look for secondary causes if high blood pressure is present. Likely causes of secondary hypertension in a person with DS include:

- kidney disease,
- medication side effects,
- hyperthyroidism, and
- severe obesity.

Treatment of hypertension includes:

- weight loss (the goal being to get down to the ideal body weight, but if a person is overweight, any weight loss may be beneficial),
- regular exercise,
- limiting salt intake (table salt is sodium chloride and the goal is to reduce sodium intake),
- treating any secondary causes that have been identified,
- medications (such as hydrochlorothiazide, tenormin (Atenolol), lisinopril (Zestril), and many others.

HYPOTENSION (LOW BP)

As mentioned above, people with DS are more likely to have low blood pressure than high blood pressure. Many adults with have a blood pressure between 85-110 systolic and 50-70 diastolic, although there is certainly individual variation.

Clearly, it is a good thing not to be at risk for the health problems that can accompany high blood pressure. But there are also some disadvantages to having low blood pressure.

The first concern comes when a person with DS is evaluated by a practitioner not familiar with the individual or with people with DS in general. If this health care professional is not aware of the individual's usual BP, he or she may express concern that the person with DS has developed hypotension. Hypotension, in contrast to just lower-than-usual blood pressure, refers to 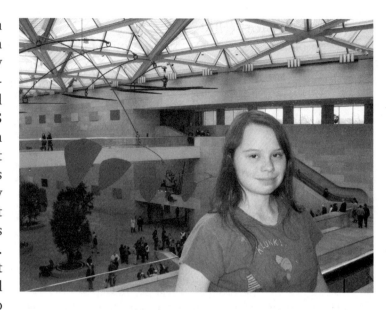 an abnormally low blood pressure that has many possible causes and is associated with insufficient blood flow to the organs of the body. Therefore, knowledge of the individual's typical BP and a careful assessment for effects of hypotension can prevent over diagnosis and treatment of hypotension. Certainly, if the person's BP has changed significantly from past readings, he should be evaluated.

On the other hand, at times, people with Down syndrome do have symptoms of hypotension. These can include:

- ◆ *Orthostatic hypotension* (a lowering of blood pressure with a change in position)—ordinarily, when a person goes from lying down to sitting or standing or from sitting to standing, the body prevents low blood pressure to the brain by constricting blood vessels, increasing heart rate, and/or increasing the pumping of the heart. As previously discussed, possibly due to autonomic nervous system function and/or smooth muscle function, these systems seem to function differently in people with DS. Therefore, some people with DS are more susceptible to dizziness when sitting or standing up. This is not unique to people with DS, but does appear to be more common.

- ◆ In frightening or painful situations, the human body may respond with a drop in heart rate and/or blood pressure. This is the same reason that some people faint when having blood taken. This response is exaggerated in some people with Down syndrome and may lead to dizziness or fainting in these situations. This is called a *vasovagal event* or reaction.

- ◆ When a person is drinking insufficient fluids and becomes dehydrated, blood pressure may drop. People with DS may be more susceptible to symptoms in this situation for the reasons noted above. Also, we have found that many people with DS regularly drink insufficient fluids. Given this chronic dehydration, they are susceptible to more serious dehydration in situations in which they are not able to drink fluids or have increased loss of fluid (e.g., diarrhea). Therefore, dehydration may contribute to low BP and may make people with DS more susceptible to symptoms of low BP when they change position or are in frightening or painful situations.

Steps to prevent and treat abnormally low blood pressure include:
- ◆ Maintain good fluid balance at all times by drinking adequate fluids (see Addendum 1: Drinking More Fluids).
- ◆ Avoid or appropriately treat situations that cause a drop in blood pressure. For example, a woman might experience cramping each month with her period, and the pain then leads to a vasovagal event that causes low heart rate and dizziness. If so, treat the menstrual discomfort more aggressively. Or, if someone feels lightheaded when he watches gory movies, recommend that he watch a different type of movie.
- ◆ Increase salt consumption. For example, periodically eating saltine crackers during the day can be beneficial. Sometimes it helps to eat a few crackers and drink a large glass of water before getting out of bed in the morning.
- ◆ Some people require medications to raise their blood pressure. Midodrine (Proamatine) is approved for use in people with orthostatic hypotension. Fludrocortisone is also approved for orthostatic hypoten-

Helping People with DS Tolerate the Blood Pressure Cuff

Some people with DS don't tolerate having their BP checked. They may find the squeezing of the blood pressure cuff painful or not understand that the cuff is not going to keep squeezing their arm tighter and tighter.

There are several ways to help someone learn to tolerate BP testing.

First, you can ask the healthcare professional to gradually accustom the individual to the BP cuff and its sensation. First, the practitioner might just put the cuff on loosely, without pumping it up. Later, he or she might only pump it a small amount, and over time increase the pressure in the cuff. This may take several visits. It may also be helpful to practice at home with a toy cuff or one available in a drug store or grocery store slowly increasing the amount the cuff is inflated.

Second, a parent, sibling, or other trusted person can demonstrate that BP testing is not so bad. While the person with DS observes, the parent can cheerfully get his BP tested. Afterwards he can comment on what it felt like: "That cuff got pretty tight, but I knew it was going to get looser soon."

sion. It is also used for adrenal insufficiency (insufficient function of the adrenal gland). Consider evaluation of adrenal function through a blood test prior to use of this medication.

VARICOSE VEINS

Varicose veins (varicosities) are enlarged superficial veins (veins close to the surface of the skin). Varicose veins often run in families and occur most often in the legs. They do seem to be a little bit more common in adults with Down syndrome.

Varicose veins may have no symptoms, but sometimes they ache. They may also lead to:

- swelling of the feet and legs,
- brownish discoloration of the skin, and
- leg ulcers that are difficult to heal.

If there are no symptoms, treatment is not needed. Otherwise, we advise:

- Avoid prolonged standing in one spot. If it is necessary to stand in one spot, it is helpful to shift weight from one foot to the other, lift one foot and flex and extend the foot, or walk around for a few minutes every hour or so.
- Avoid prolonged sitting with the feet down below the waist. As with prolonged standing, it can help to move the feet or get up and walk for about 5 minutes every hour. Also periodically elevate the legs to at least the level of the hips.
- Limit salt intake to help reduce swelling.
- Wear support stockings to reduce discomfort and swelling. A surgical supply house or some pharmacies can measure the person for custom-fit support stockings, which have greater compression than most over-the-counter products. However, many people will decline to wear the stockings in hot, humid weather, which is when they are most needed, because of the discomfort associated with these stockings.

Chapter 10

Asthma, Coughs, and Other Pulmonary Problems

Olivia, age 19, came to the Adult Down Syndrome Center complaining of a persistent cough. She had been treated for pneumonia twice in the past year. Both times after recovering from pneumonia, she had continued to cough intermittently. She would often cough during or after meals. Olivia's symptoms had increased in the last several weeks. There was no reported wheezing and her history and physical exams showed no other problems, specifically no neurological decline

Olivia was referred for a video swallow evaluation. The speech-language pathologist (SLP) who evaluated Olivia found that she had no swallowing problems when she ate slowly, but when she rushed, she did not chew well and she would aspirate (breathe in) some fluids and solids into her upper airway. Olivia was referred to an Ear, Nose, and Throat (ENT) physician so she could be evaluated for structural problems, but none were found. The SLP then recommended that Olivia eat more slowly. To help her pace herself, the SLP advised Olivia to put down her fork or spoon after each bite and take a sip of liquid. She was also encouraged to be more conscious of chewing each bite thoroughly.

Within a few weeks, Olivia's cough had markedly improved. For the next year, she had no episodes of pneumonia.

Pulmonary (lung) problems are relatively common in adolescents and adults with Down syndrome (DS). People with Down syndrome are more prone to develop a number of lung infections and other lung conditions. But they are also less likely to develop certain other pulmonary problems such as asthma and lung cancer. With thorough assessment and treatment, the lung problems that people with DS do develop can usually be reversed.

PNEUMONIA

People with DS seem to be more likely to develop pneumonia—an infection of the lungs in which fluid fills the small air sacs of the lungs. There are two major reasons for this increased incidence. First, swallowing problems are fairly common in people with DS. This makes it more likely that the person will aspirate (breathe in) foods, liquids, and saliva, which can bring infectious agents into the lungs. Second, immune dysfunction is more common in DS and this can limit the person's ability to fight off infections anywhere in the body, including in the lungs.

Symptoms of pneumonia may include:

◆ cough,
◆ fever,
◆ shortness of breath,
◆ chest discomfort,
◆ coughing up blood, and
◆ weakness.

If pneumonia worsens, it can cause:
◆ mental confusion,
◆ difficulty breathing, and even
◆ death.

Pneumonia can be caused by many different infectious agents, including bacteria, viruses, fungi, and parasites. Often (but not always) a person will first develop a cold or the flu—a viral infection of the upper airway and lungs. These infections may weaken the individual and impair the normal function of the respiratory system. Symptoms that suggest that the illness has progressed beyond a cold or the flu include:

◆ persistent fever (lasting more than 3-4 days),
◆ shortness of breath,
◆ low oxygen level (which may be observed as blue lips or fingertips),

- ◆ a worsening cough, usually producing thick, colored sputum (sometimes blood-tinged),
- ◆ progressive weakness,
- ◆ decrease in blood pressure.

Some people with DS become agitated or irritable as they feel increasingly ill.

Pneumonia is usually diagnosed based on the history of the illness, physical exam, and possibly additional testing. When pneumonia is suspected, additional testing may include:

- ◆ checking the oxygen level in the person's blood (most commonly done with a pulse oximeter—a small device that clips onto a finger or ear and measures oxygen without having to penetrate the skin),
- ◆ chest x-ray,
- ◆ blood tests (to check for evidence the body is fighting off infection).

Often people who have bacterial pneumonia can be treated with oral antibiotics (pills or liquid) without being hospitalized. Viral infections generally only require supportive care and do not require antibiotics. However, sometimes hospitalization is required for either type of pneumonia if:

- ◆ The person's blood pressure drops to a concerning level.
- ◆ She is significantly short of breath.
- ◆ The oxygen level drops to a concerning level.
- ◆ The person is too ill to take oral medication (and needs IV medication).
- ◆ She is too weak to care for herself or to be cared for at home.
- ◆ She doesn't respond to treatment at home.

In the hospital, additional testing may be done to assist with the diagnosis. A bronchoscopy (a tube placed through the mouth into the lungs) may be ordered to help clarify the organism causing the pneumonia. For example, parasites and fungi are sometimes harder to diagnose and may require a bronchoscopy. The bronchoscopy may need to be done under anesthesia, especially if the person is already having trouble breathing.

In the hospital, additional evaluations and treatments may include:

- ◆ close monitoring of the person's oxygen level,
- ◆ intravenous fluids,
- ◆ intravenous antibiotics,
- ◆ oxygen therapy,
- ◆ ventilator therapy, if breathing becomes more labored or impaired,
- ◆ respiratory therapy to provide nebulizer treatments if there is any wheezing, and
- ◆ physical or occupational therapy to help the person regain her strength.

SWALLOWING DYSFUNCTION AND PNEUMONIA

Swallowing is a complex function that requires a number of steps that must each occur in the proper order. While some of the steps require more conscious activity (such as chewing), much of swallowing occurs without conscious input. The movement of the muscles of the throat, the epiglottis covering the airway, and other steps occur automatically. However, some people have neurological impairments related to DS that affect the steps of swallowing that should occur automatically.

There are also other causes of swallowing dysfunction:

- Many people with DS have missing teeth or unusually shaped or positioned teeth, leading to difficulties chewing.
- As with Olivia, above, the problem can be more behavioral: eating too rapidly, not chewing food well, talking while swallowing, taking bites that are too large, etc. More careful attention to chewing and swallowing can generally solve these problems.
- Less often, a mass or other structural change can cause swallowing problems. Rarely, severe atlantoaxial subluxation can cause a bulge into the back of the throat that impairs swallowing (see Chapter 13). A foreign body can also cause swallowing dysfunction if it becomes lodged in the throat
- Additional neurological impairment (beyond impairment related to DS alone) sometimes occurs, as discussed below.

Many neurological problems can cause swallowing dysfunction, particularly if the person already has difficulties with swallowing. As discussed in Chapter 19, Alzheimer disease causes swallowing dysfunction in some older people with DS. Strokes and multiple sclerosis (MS) can also cause weakness of the swallowing muscles or impaired coordination of swallowing. (Note, however, that strokes and MS are not more common in people with DS.) In addition, seizures—which *are* more common in people with DS—can lead to aspiration of saliva and other secretions (for example, of vomited stomach contents if the seizures are associated with vomiting). In fact, anything that causes a change in consciousness can contribute to aspiration.

If swallowing dysfunction is suspected, evaluation should include:

- an assessment of the person's generalized debility (weakness) since any cause of generalized weakness may contribute to swallowing dysfunction, especially in someone who already has a tendency to impaired swallowing;
- a careful history and physical exam, especially to evaluate whether the person has lost any neurological function (loss of thinking/cognitive skills, or new movement problems such as weakness of the arms and/or legs);
- Some or all of the following tests:
  - ➤ blood sugar—to assess for diabetes,

> ➤ blood urea nitrogen and creatinine—to assess for kidney dysfunction,
> ➤ thyroid stimulating hormone (TSH)—to assess for thyroid dysfunction,
> ➤ complete blood count (CBC)—to assess for anemia,
> ➤ vitamin B12 level—to assess for B12 deficiency,
> ➤ other blood tests as indicated by the person's history and physical,
> ➤ a swallowing evaluation by speech-language pathologist (SLP), which may include video (x-ray) evaluation done with a SLP and a radiologist),
> ➤ CT scan or MRI of brain—to assess for abnormalities in the brain (e.g., brain tumor, strokes, evidence of Alzheimer disease),
> ➤ lateral cervical spine (neck) x-ray—to assess for atlanto-axial instability,
> ➤ evaluation by an ENT physician—to assess for structural or anatomical abnormalities of the upper airway.

Note: If someone with DS has recurrent pneumonia, particularly if she has had other infections as well, it may be a good idea to get an immune function evaluation from an infectious disease specialist. Immune dysfunction is thought to be more common in people with DS and may involve a number of the parts of the immune system.

PREVENTING PNEUMONIA

If the tests above show that pneumonia is related to swallowing dysfunction or another medical problem, prevention will be focused on treating the underlying problem or swallowing dysfunction.

If no other cause for pneumonia is found, monitoring and modifying eating habits or the texture of foods may help prevent repeat episodes. Parents and caregivers can encourage:

- ◆ a slower rate of eating,
- ◆ more thorough chewing of food,
- ◆ putting the fork or spoon down between bites,
- ◆ taking a sip of liquid between bites,
- ◆ cutting food into smaller bites, and
- ◆ eating softer foods.

Those with more difficulties swallowing may benefit from:

- ◆ thickening the consistency of liquids if there are problems swallowing thin liquids (the consistency of water);
- ◆ swallowing therapy under the guidance of a speech therapist aimed at learning and practicing proper swallowing techniques;

◆ electrical stimulation—a nonpainful electrical stimulation therapy of the swallowing muscles that is performed by a speech therapist.

In addition, people who are having ongoing difficulties with swallowing and as-piration may benefit from seeing a dietitian for advice about changing the textures of foods or finding palatable foods that can be more easily swallowed.

ASTHMA

Asthma is a chronic condition that makes it harder to breathe during "attacks." When an attack is triggered, two physical changes occur in the body, restricting airflow:
1. broncho-constriction (contraction of the muscles of the airways of the lungs, causing narrowing of the airways), and
2. inflammation of the airways, resulting in swelling of the airways and mucous production that further contributes to the narrowing of the airways.

Symptoms of asthma may include:
◆ wheezing (a high-pitched, musical sound made particularly when breathing out),
◆ cough,
◆ chest tightness or chest pain,
◆ shortness of breath,
◆ symptoms that come and go (are intermittent).
These symptoms can occur or worsen with exercise or certain conditions like bad air quality.
In those who have asthma, an attack can be triggered by a variety of factors, including:
◆ a respiratory infection,
◆ smoke or other airborne pollutants,
◆ exercise, and
◆ allergies.
The risk factors for asthma include:
◆ family history (other family members have asthma);
◆ viral lower respiratory infection during infancy (bronchiolitis, a lung infection caused by Respiratory Synctial Virus, is associated with wheezing—it has been suggested but not proven that it contributes to the later onset of asthma);
◆ exposure to tobacco smoke;
◆ living in the inner city (if exposed to higher levels of pollens, molds, and air pollution).

Down syndrome is *not* a risk factor for asthma. In fact, the condition seems to be less common in adults with DS than in others. Asthma is more common in children with DS than in adults with DS, so it appears that some people with the condition do "outgrow" it.

Treatment includes taking medications to relax the airways and to reduce the inflammation and mucous. The use of inhalers, nebulizer machines, and other devices can direct the medication directly to the lungs. Some people with DS find the use of an inhaler challenging because it takes a coordinated effort to release the medication from the inhaler followed rapidly by a deep inhalation. A spacer device that attaches to the inhaler may improve the benefit of the inhaler because the same level of coordination is not required to get the medication to the lungs. Oral or intravenous medications are also sometimes needed if the severity of the condition warrants or if the person is unable to use inhalers or other devices that direct the medication directly to the lungs.

If the symptoms occur frequently, an individual may require daily medications to prevent symptoms. Whether the person requires daily medications or not, when an asthma episode occurs, the person needs to take her medications as soon as possible. This means that people with asthma should keep a supply of their medication with them at all times.

Not being able to manage one's own asthma can interfere with a person's ability to live independently or with minimal supervision. Untreated or improperly treated asthma episodes can be hazardous to the person's health and/or frightening. The person may have to be hospitalized if she has:

- persistent wheezing that does not respond to medications,
- progressive shortness of breath,
- low oxygen level,
- an inability to take medications via an inhaler, nebulizer, or by mouth.

To avoid hospitalization for treatment, it is important to help the person learn to recognize symptoms and treat herself to the extent possible.

CHRONIC COUGH

A cough that lasts more than three weeks is called a chronic cough. In our experience, adults with DS are more likely to have persistent coughs. The underlying cause for a chronic cough may include:

- postnasal drip (nasal, pharynx, and/or sinus mucous dripping down the back of the throat),
- asthma,
- gastroesophageal reflux disease (a condition in which acid or other stomach contents come back up into the esophagus),
- chronic bronchitis,

- smoking,
- medication side effect,
- cancer, and
- chronic infections (e.g., tuberculosis).

In adults with DS, the most common causes seem to be:
- postnasal drip, and
- gastroesophageal reflux disease.

These are discussed in the sections below.

CHRONIC COUGH CAUSED BY POSTNASAL DRIP

Postnasal drip involves the drainage of mucous from the nose, pharynx, or the sinuses into the upper airway (the throat) and sometimes the lungs. Postnasal drip may occur as the result of:

- allergies
- chronic vasomotor rhinitis—that is, increased chronic nasal drainage that isn't associated with allergies; often the cause is not clear, but may be made worse by irritants such as smoke, pollution, etc.
- sinusitis—an infection of the sinuses that is usually caused by a virus or bacteria but that sometimes has other causes such as fungi
- medication side effects—most commonly from nasal (spray) decongestants such as phenylephrine (Neo Synephrine) or oxymetazoline nasal (Afrin). Use of these medications for more than three to five days can cause rebound congestion—a condition in which the congestion is worse after a dose wears off than it was prior to the dose. Rebound congestion can result in a vicious cycle of using the medication more frequently and for longer periods of time to reduce the side effect of congestion. Also, medications (such as captopril) from the ACE inhibitor category that are used for heart disease or hypertension can cause chronic cough
- less often, a foreign body in the nose may cause chronic nasal drainage and postnasal drip

After a medical practitioner takes a good history and performs a thorough physical exam to determine the cause of a chronic cough, he or she may request additional tests, including:

- a chest x-ray,
- a screening CT scan of the sinuses,
- passing a scope through the nose, upper airway, and sinuses to look for blockage, drainage, infection, foreign body, and other causes,
- allergy testing.

However, if the cause appears to be postnasal drip, treatment may be begun without further investigation. Treatment may include:

- cough suppressants,
- irrigating the nose and sinuses with saline solutions, a Neti pot, or nasal irrigation,
- antihistamine pills—e.g., diphenhydramine (Benadryl) or loratadine (Claritin),
- steroid nasal sprays—e.g., fluticasone (Flonase) or mometasone (Nasonex),
- other medications for allergies—e.g., montelukast (Singulair),
- medications to "thin" the secretions—e.g., guafenisin (Mucinex).

Chronic Cough Caused by Reflux

Gastroesophageal reflux disease (GERD) is more common in people with DS and can cause a chronic cough. The condition results when acid or stomach contents reflux (flow back) out of the stomach into the esophagus. They may go higher into the upper airway and even be aspirated into the lungs. In addition to a cough, other symptoms may include:

- heartburn,
- sore throat (often recurrently in the morning),
- difficulty swallowing,
- regurgitation,
- worsening of symptoms when lying down (gravity helps keep acid and stomach contents from refluxing when standing or sitting).

As with postnasal drip, the diagnosis of GERD may be suspected based on the person's history and physical exam. If so, the physician may recommend treatment designed to minimize reflux. Treatment is discussed in Chapter 11.

Other Causes of Chronic Cough

If neither postnasal drip nor gastroesophageal reflux is suspected as the cause of the cough, or if the symptoms persist despite treatment, it is necessary to take a systematic approach to assess for other causes and treatments. Just a few of the many possible causes were described above. In general, the cause is more likely to be something common, such as bronchitis, rather than less common, such as lung cancer. Furthermore, as discussed in Chapter 14, cancers, in general, are rarer among people with DS than in other people.

Careful review of the person's history, as well as a physical exam and additional testing and treatments can often help healthcare professionals eliminate potential causes or find the cause(s). However, in some individuals, the cause and correct treatment for a chronic cough can be elusive, and a painstaking evaluation may be necessary. Occasionally, an adult with DS develops a "habitual cough"—a cough that is be-havioral or tic-like. Repetitive movements and sounds are relatively common in people with DS, and are covered in detail in our previous book, *Mental Wellness in Adults with Down Syndrome* (Woodbine House, 2006).

Influenza

Influenza ("the flu") is a respiratory infection caused by influenza virus types A and B. Although vomiting and diarrhea are often called "the flu," these are not symptoms of true influenza. The symptoms of influenza include sudden onset of:

- fever,
- body aches,
- sore throat,
- nonproductive cough—meaning it doesn't produce phlegm (mucous),
- headache,
- chills,
- nasal congestion, and
- fatigue and malaise.

People with Down syndrome seem to be more likely to get the flu due to immune system dysfunction. They are also more likely to develop complications such as bacterial pneumonia once they have the flu.

The diagnosis of influenza is usually suspected on the basis of the individual's history and physical exam. Rapid influenza testing is available in the office but has been found to be quite inaccurate. The testing available in labs is far more accurate. These tests require a swab of the back of the nose (nasopharynx) and take a few days to process. Generally, this testing is only done on the sickest individuals who require hospitalization. Particularly if the diagnosis is not clear or pneumonia is suspected, additional tests such as a chest x-ray and blood tests may be needed.

Treatment of influenza includes:

- drinking more fluids, since fever causes a person to become dehydrated more quickly,
- medications to reduce fever and decrease body aches—e.g., acetaminophen (Tylenol), ibuprofen (Advil), etc.,
- getting more rest,
- staying home from school or work, not only to allow for more rest and healing but also to prevent spreading the infection (the virus can be transmitted by touch and through the air),
- strict hand washing,
- using a cool-mist vaporizer (especially when sleeping),

Viral Infections

Like influenza, most upper respiratory infections ("colds") are caused by viruses. Viruses do not respond to treatment with antibiotics. While antiviral agents can speed recovery in influenza, there are no antiviral agents to treat the common cold. Symptomatic treatments (such as discussed earlier for postnasal drip) may help reduce symptoms, but don't speed up recovery.

- ◆ medications (antiviral agents) that must be started within 48 hours of the onset of symptoms to effectively reduce the duration of the illness:
  - ➤ rimantadine (Flumadine) and amantadine (Symmatrel), which are only effective against Influenza A
  - ➤ zanamivir (Rilenza) and oseltamivir (Tamiflu), which are effective against types A and B
- ◆ hospitalization may be necessary to treat complications such as dehydration, hypoxemia (low oxygen in the blood), pneumonia, or other serious complications.

Note that antibiotics are not used to treat influenza. Sometimes, however, the flu can lead to bacterial pneumonia, which requires treatment with antibiotics. Note also that which strains of the flu are resistant to which antiviral medications changes on an ongoing basis and may vary by area, so updated data for your particular area is important. Worsening of the illness, as well as development of the symptoms outlined above for pneumonia, warrant an evaluation to assess for pneumonia.

PREVENTING THE FLU

We strongly advise taking precautions to prevent people with DS from getting the flu. As discussed in Chapter 3, the influenza vaccine reduces the incidence of the infection. Influenza vaccination is given once between October and March. In addition, the antiviral agents listed above may be used as a preventative measure within 48 hours of exposure to someone who has the flu. Handwashing and prevention of spread through the air by coughing or sneezing into your sleeve are recommended.

Here are a few common situations where it makes sense to consider giving the person an antiviral agent:
- ◆ The person exposed to influenza has not yet had the influenza vaccine this season (October—March).
- ◆ The person lives in a setting such as a residential facility in which someone who lives or works there has developed influenza. Taking the medication may be a good idea even for those who have had the vaccine because

there are always strains of flu that the vaccine does not protect against. Often the person who developed influenza has had the vaccine.

The flu vaccine does not prevent all people from developing influenza. In a setting where a number of people live and the infection could quickly spread, antiviral agents are an effective additional preventative measure.

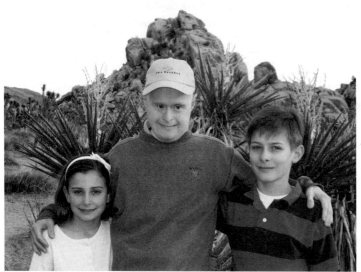

It is especially important to try to prevent the flu or other lung infections in teens and adults with untreated congenital heart disease. People with untreated congenital heart disease are more at risk for developing lung infections and tend to have more serious infections when they do have a lung infection. This is because the impaired blood flow in the lungs reduces the lungs' ability to resist infection. Since lung infections put an increased stress on the heart, preventing lung infections to begin with is strongly recommended for people with untreated congenital heart disease. Assessment and treatment (if indicated) should be done within the first 48 hours of illness to see if antiviral medications should be given as a preventative measure, or whether additional infections (e.g., pneumonia) have occurred.

Chapter 11

Gastrointestinal

· · · · · · · · · · · ·

and

· · · · · · · ·

Liver Concerns

· · · · · · · · · · · · · · ·

Sara, age 21, was brought to the Adult Down Syndrome Center because her parents were concerned about recent changes in her mood and behavior. For several months, she had been irritable and less tolerant of her family members. She was nearing high school graduation and her family initially assumed that this was the cause. Her sleep and her appetite both remained good, although her parents said she was becoming more easily fatigued. She had no abdominal pain, constipation, or diarrhea, and there were no changes in her skin. Her primary physician had drawn thyroid blood tests that were normal. She had assessed Sara as having depression and recommended an evaluation at the Center.

At the Center, we noted that Sara had lost six pounds over three months. Then, when we did blood work, we found that her anti-tissue transglutaminase antibody was elevated consistent with celiac disease. Sara underwent an esophagogastroduodenoscopy (EGD)—a test in which a scope is passed through the mouth into the esophagus, stomach, and small intestine. A biopsy of her small intestine confirmed the diagnosis of celiac disease. Sara then started on a gluten-free diet, the treatment for

*celiac disease. Her mood improved, she regained the six pounds she had
lost, and her energy level returned to normal.*

A number of gastrointestinal conditions are more common in people with
Down syndrome (DS). Some of these conditions have symptoms such as
diarrhea that point immediately to a possible medical problem with the gastrointestinal system—the stomach, intestines, liver, gall bladder, and pancreas. Others have
more subtle symptoms, and may be mistaken for behavioral or psychological problems, as was the case with Sara.

There are, therefore, several good reasons to consider the possibility of a gastrointestinal problem whenever an adolescent or adult with DS is being evaluated for
a change in health or behavior. First, many of the gastrointestinal conditions have
symptoms, and assessing for them and treating them will reduce the person's pain and
suffering. Secondly, for the conditions that have subtle symptoms in the beginning,
finding the condition early can avoid additional complications.

Furthermore, as discussed in Chapter 5, psychological and behavioral changes are often the first sign of a physical health condition in a person with DS. Gastrointestinal conditions appear to be a frequent cause of these symptoms. One
reason may be that some of these conditions cause few other outward signs. The
symptoms are often just subjective discomfort that only the person with the symptoms is aware of. If the person with DS has difficulty verbally communicating his
symptoms, he may communicate them through a behavioral change. Therefore, an
awareness of the gastrointestinal conditions that occur more frequently in people
with DS is important when considering behavioral or psychological changes, as
well as when assessing symptoms that seem to be more obviously connected to a
gastrointestinal problem.

CELIAC DISEASE

Since the 1990s, the Down Syndrome Medical Interest Group has recommended
that all children with DS be screened for celiac disease between two and three years
of age. As a result, many teenagers and young adults with DS have had this screening
blood test at some point in their lives, and older adults may also have had the test if
their doctor is knowledgeable about health conditions associated with DS. However,
even if a teenager or adult with DS has had one negative screening test for celiac disease, that does not mean that celiac disease should not be considered as one possible
cause of gastrointestinal problems. Celiac disease can develop at any age, even in
people who have previously experienced no symptoms or who previously had a negative evaluation.

Celiac disease is related to sensitivity to gluten. Gluten is a protein in wheat,
barley, and rye. Exposure to gluten in foods causes an inflammation in the intestine

that, in turn, causes the villi (microscopic fingers in the small intestine) to slough off. This reduces the surface area of the small intestine, decreasing its ability to absorb vitamins, minerals, and calories. Over time, celiac disease results in malabsorption of nutrients in food.

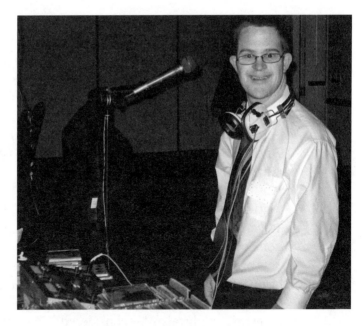

People who have celiac disease have a genetic predisposition to the disease. That is, it tends to run in families, and there are groups of people (such as those of Northern European ancestry) who are more likely to develop the disorder. When individuals who have the genetic predisposition are exposed to some environmental stimuli (thought to probably be an unknown virus), an immune reaction is set off and celiac disease becomes active. The immune system attacks the villi.

DS increases a person's susceptibility to celiac disease. Celiac disease is more common in people with DS than in the general population. It is estimated that 7 to 15 percent of people with DS may have the disorder.

The most commonly recognized symptoms of celiac disease are diarrhea and weight loss because of poor absorption. However, celiac disease can be associated with many additional symptoms, including:

- ◆ constipation,
- ◆ abdominal discomfort,
- ◆ bloating,
- ◆ muscle cramps,
- ◆ dizziness,
- ◆ nervousness,
- ◆ weakness,
- ◆ fatigue,
- ◆ a sense of lack of energy or motivation,
- ◆ increased appetite,
- ◆ large amount of flatulence,
- ◆ seizures,
- ◆ poor absorption of several nutrients.

Longstanding untreated celiac disease is associated with intestinal lymphoma (a type of cancer) and other gastrointestinal malignancies.

DIAGNOSIS OF CELIAC DISEASE

The diagnosis of celiac disease usually starts with an assessment of the person's symptoms and a physical exam. It is not necessary to see a gastroenterology specialist at this stage. A primary practitioner can do this assessment and order the blood tests needed for further assessment. These include tests of:

◆ Anti-tissue transglutaminase antibody (IgA) (TTGA),
◆ Anti-tissue transglutaminase antibody (IgG),
◆ Anti-endomysial antibody (IgA),
◆ Anti-gliadin IgA,
◆ Anti-gliadin IgG (the least specific test),
◆ It is generally recommended to also draw a total IgA (theoretically, if someone has a deficiency of total IgA, the above tests— which are subsets of IgA—would also be low even if the person had celiac disease.

At the Adult Down Syndrome Center, we generally order the TTGA and the total IgA.

Genetic testing might also be considered. The genes DQ2 and DQ8 on chromosome 6 are associated with celiac disease. If the genes are present, the person is susceptible to developing celiac disease, but it does not mean the person has celiac disease. Many people with the genetic predisposition don't develop celiac disease. As noted above, some other factor, possibly a viral infection, may need to occur before the disease is triggered. At this time no other genes are known to be associated with celiac disease. Therefore, if the testing is negative for the celiac genes, the person cannot go on to develop celiac disease. Unfortunately, presently the genetic tests are expensive, only available at a few labs, and are often not covered by insurance.

Interestingly, we have seen an elevated globulin (blood test) in many of our patients. (This is addressed under autoimmune conditions in Chapter 13.) Recently, we have begun to find that many of our patients with an elevated globulin have celiac disease. So if we find an elevated globulin, we do further blood testing for celiac disease.

The definitive test for celiac disease is a small bowel biopsy. This test is performed by a gastroenterologist—a medical doctor who specializes in disorders of intestines, liver, and liver. The gastroenterologist does the test by passing an endoscope—a flexible tube equipped with video capabilities—through the mouth and down to the small bowel, where a small sample of intestinal tissue is taken (biopsied). This procedure is called an esophagogastroduodenoscopy. It usually requires sedation and may require general anesthesia for some people with DS.

Some families opt not to put their son or daughter with DS through an endoscope procedure. They choose to proceed with the gluten-free diet based on the symptoms and the results of blood tests. Other families want to know for sure that the diagnosis is correct before changing the person's diet. The biopsy is the only way to be certain that the person does, in fact, have celiac disease. In either approach, the diagnosis is confirmed if the symptoms respond to appropriate treatment (discussed below).

TREATMENT OF CELIAC DISEASE

Treatment consists of completely eliminating gluten from the person's diet, since even a small amount of gluten can cause symptoms. This requires avoiding wheat, barley, and rye in all foods. Since these grains are included in many processed foods as well as in other prepared products such as medicines, following the diet can be quite challenging. It can be especially difficult to switch to a gluten-free diet if the person has a relatively limited diet, resists changes, cannot read labels to determine whether the product contains gluten, and/or does not understand the connection between eating "forbidden" foods and experiencing unpleasant symptoms as a result.

We recommend consulting with a registered dietitian or nutritionist to help the adult with DS and his family or caregivers understand the gluten-free diet. A dietitian can provide information on foods containing gluten, on reading labels, and on sources of additional information such as organizations and websites. If the person with DS does not prepare his own meals, whoever is involved in meal preparation should also consult with a dietitian.

For an individual to successfully follow the gluten-free diet, he needs to understand and avoid the large number of foods and other substances that contain gluten. We have found that it can help to use visual supports, since people with DS are often visual learners. Suggestions for helping someone with DS stay gluten-free include: 1) making a picture guide of acceptable foods, and 2) saving food labels from acceptable foods (or making color copies of the labels) and categorizing the foods as snacks and main dishes. Be sure to include pictures of restaurant foods.

Getting to know other families who have a family member with celiac disease is very helpful. Others who are living with the disease can give tips on foods and recipes that are palatable but gluten-free. In addition, they can share information about how to avoid gluten at parties, when going out to eat, and at other times or places in which the person must deviate from his usual diet. The Celiac Foundation (www.celiac.org) is a good resource and can be a link to a local support group.

> Ben, a 29-year-old man with DS, was very embarrassed by his diarrhea and occasional incontinence of stool caused by his celiac disease. He became increasingly resistant to leaving his house because he feared having an accident.
>
> With treatment of his celiac disease, Ben's diarrhea and incontinence improved. However, Ben continued to fear having accidents if he left the house. With guidance from the Adult Down Syndrome Center, his staff developed a successful strategy for getting him comfortable with traveling away from home again. To encourage Ben to leave the house, they offered him incentives such as trips to favorite stores or restaurants located nearby. Staff members were careful to map out all possible bathrooms that Ben could use on the way, if needed. Staff gradually increased the distance Ben went from home. Over a period of time, as Ben became used to more normal

bowel elimination and the strategy developed by staff, he was able to leave his home without fear and without need of any additional incentives.

DIARRHEA AND FOOD SENSITIVITIES

Even in the absence of celiac disease, many people with DS have problems with diarrhea and food sensitivities. There is not one type of food or a subset of foods that are particularly problematic for people with DS. The two exceptions to this would be foods containing gluten, as noted above, and foods containing lactose (lactose intolerance, milk intolerance), discussed below. Often when someone has symptoms of food sensitivities, it takes some investigation to discover what food(s) may be a problem for the individual.

LACTOSE INTOLERANCE

Lactose intolerance is caused by the inability to digest lactose, the primary sugar in cow's milk. People who are lactose intolerant produce insufficient amounts of lactase, the enzyme that breaks down lactose. Lactose intolerance most often develops in the teenage and adult years. It appears to be more common in people with DS.

Symptoms of lactose intolerance typically experienced after consuming dairy products are:

- ◆ bloating,
- ◆ cramping,
- ◆ abdominal discomfort,
- ◆ diarrhea,
- ◆ flatulence,
- ◆ rumbling in the abdomen.

Symptoms usually occur thirty minutes to two hours after consuming foods that contain lactose. Many people can consume some lactose-containing foods, but consuming larger amounts causes symptoms.

The diagnosis can be made by a primary care physician or gastroenterology (GI) specialist by doing a lactose breath hydrogen test (which involves breathing into a device). If the person is unable to cooperate with the test, then the doctor might recommend trying the treatments below and then monitoring the person to see if symptoms improve.

Treatment consists of avoiding foods that contain lactose, consuming lactase-treated foods, or taking lactase supplements.

Foods to avoid include:

- ◆ milk,
- ◆ cheese,
- ◆ ice cream, and
- ◆ prepared products such as cereal that contain milk or lactose.

Many people cannot consume these products even when they are cooked or used as ingredients in baking. However, yogurt and fermented dairy products such as hard cheeses are usually better tolerated.

In addition to avoiding foods containing lactose, the following steps can also be helpful:

- Drink lactaid milk—milk that is pretreated with lactase.
- Take lactase tablets (e.g., Lactaid or Lactrase brands) before eating lactose-containing foods.
- Take a calcium and vitamin D supplement to make up for the calcium that is not being consumed by avoiding dairy products.

Some people have lactose intolerance together with celiac disease. Particularly if the person is strictly following a gluten-free diet but symptoms persist, consider lactose intolerance.

INTOLERANCE OF OTHER FOODS

Our patients with DS have also described a wide variety of other foods that lead to gastrointestinal symptoms such as diarrhea, bloating, or cramping. We have not identified any particular foods or patterns of foods that are more likely to cause these problems.

If other causes of gastrointestinal symptoms have been ruled out and there is no clear offending food or drink, keeping a food diary can help in making the diagnosis. The individual records everything that he eats or drinks throughout the day and also records any symptoms following consumption of foods. Particularly if the times and amounts of the types of food are recorded, it may be possible to find a pattern and then discover the problematic food or drink. It may also be helpful to see a dietitian for help in pinpointing the problematic food.

IRRITABLE BOWEL SYNDROME

Irritable bowel syndrome (IBS) is usually associated with many of the same symptoms as celiac disease and lactose intolerance—namely, abdominal pain, diarrhea, and/or constipation. These symptoms are often worse when the person is under more psychological stress.

The diagnosis of IBS is usually not given unless testing has ruled out other causes, as there are no tests that can be done to diagnose IBS. The cause is unknown. A consult with a GI specialist is often helpful to assess for other causes of the symptoms.

People with IBS have intestinal motility abnormalities. That is, food and waste products don't move through the intestines in the normal way. People with IBS often seem to have increased but abnormal motility with spasms of the intestines. For some people food moves faster through the intestines, for some slower, and for some, the food may sometimes move slowly and sometimes move rapidly through the intestines. There also may be an increased perception of the pain associated with motility. Sometimes IBS is associated with constipation, sometimes with diarrhea, and some people have diarrhea and constipation at different times.

IBS is probably more common in adults with DS. The motility of the gut is commonly abnormal in people with DS. In addition, many people with DS seem to physically react to stress with a change in their gastrointestinal system.

Treatment includes:

- ◆ If other causes for the symptoms have been ruled out, reassure the person that there is no other underlying condition. IBS does not progress to cancer or inflammatory conditions such as ulcerative colitis or Crohn's disease.
- ◆ Increase fiber in the diet or take fiber supplements (increase fiber slowly to avoid increased intestinal gas). A dietitian can advise you how to do this.
- ◆ Avoid large meals, fatty foods, and caffeine.
- ◆ Sometimes medications to reduce anxiety can help. We have had particular success with paroxetine (Paxil), a selective serotonin reuptake inhibitor.

GASTROESOPHAGEAL REFLUX DISEASE (GERD)

Gastroesophageal reflux is the backward flow of stomach acid into the esophagus (the tube running between the mouth and the stomach). GERD is more common in people with DS of all ages. Obesity, sleep apnea, and overeating are all reasons we see an increased frequency in adolescents and adults.

The most common symptom of GERD is heartburn, which is a burning or pain in the chest that can occur after meals. Other symptoms include:

- ◆ sore throat,
- ◆ regurgitation of digested food,
- ◆ abdominal pain,
- ◆ hoarseness,
- ◆ bronchospasm (asthma),
- ◆ difficulty swallowing,
- ◆ aspiration (breathing food into the lungs),
- ◆ chronic cough,
- ◆ loss of enamel on the teeth.

Untreated, persistent GERD can lead to:

- ◆ Barrett's esophagitis (changes in the tissue of the esophagus that predispose the person to cancer of the esophagus), and

◆ scarring of the esophagus, which can cause narrowing and make it harder for food to pass through it to the stomach.

An endoscopy can diagnose these complications (see below).

Treatment of GERD includes:
- ◆ not overeating,
- ◆ reaching/maintaining ideal body weight (obesity contributes to reflux),
- ◆ limiting caffeine,
- ◆ not lying down for an hour (or more, if needed) after a meal (e.g., not eating right before going to bed),
- ◆ avoiding clothing that constricts the abdomen (which can increase pressure in the abdomen, pushing stomach contents into the esophagus),
- ◆ putting the legs at the head of the bed up on blocks to allow gravity to help keep stomach contents in the stomach. (Propping the head and chest on more pillows usually doesn't help and often makes reflux worse by causing flexion at the waist and increasing the pressure in the abdomen, similar to the problem with wearing constricting clothing),
- ◆ taking medications such as:
  - ➤ antacids to reduce acid in the stomach—e.g., aluminum hydroxide/magnesium hydroxide (Maalox),
  - ➤ H_2 receptor blockers that reduce acid in the stomach—e.g., cimetidine (Tagamet), ranitidine (Zantac), or famotidine (Pepcid),
  - ➤ proton pump inhibitors that reduce acid in the stomach—e.g., omeprazole (Prilosec), lansoprazole (Prevacid), pantoprazole (Protonix), rabeprazole (Aciphex), or esomeprazole (Nexium),
  - ➤ metoclopramide (Reglan), usually along with a medication to reduce acid (Metoclopramide stimulates the upper gastrointestinal tract and apparently helps push stomach contents forward to the small intestine, thereby reducing reflux).

If the heartburn persists or the person develops recurrent vomiting, testing to evaluate for Barrett's esophagitis or a stricture (narrowing) of the esophagus should be done. Tests may include:
- ◆ An endoscope (EGD) exam: a scope passed by a gastroenterologist through the mouth into the esophagus, stomach, and duodenum (first part of the small intestine). This can be challenging for some people—both with and without DS—to tolerate. Heavier sedation or even general anesthesia may be required for these people.
- ◆ An x-ray test: A special kind of x-ray called an esophogram can detect a narrowing. The patient must drink liquid barium and then have

x-rays. Liquid barium is a thick, chalky liquid that some people may balk at swallowing.

Neither test is pleasant to undergo. However, one advantage of the EGD is that if a narrowing is found during the test, the doctor can treat the narrowing on the spot. He or she can insert a balloon through the endoscope and into the esophagus to dilate (widen) the esophagus and make it easier for food to pass through.

PEPTIC ULCER DISEASE

In general, an ulcer is a place where normal body tissue has been worn away or disrupted. For example, a deep burn with an acid can cause an ulcer of the skin. Similarly, the acid in the stomach can damage the tissue and cause an ulcer. When one or more ulcers develops in the stomach, the condition is known as peptic ulcer disease.

Ulcers don't seem to be more common in people with Down syndrome, but sometimes the symptoms can be missed. In addition, possibly due to the increased pain tolerance of (some) people with DS, the problem may not be diagnosed until symptoms have gotten more serious.

Symptoms may include:
- ◆ abdominal pain (especially an hour or so after eating),
- ◆ resistance to eating,
- ◆ vomiting,
- ◆ symptoms associated with blood loss:
  - ➤ dark stools,
  - ➤ blood in the stool,
  - ➤ vomiting blood,
  - ➤ fatigue,
  - ➤ syncope (passing out—due to the loss of a large amount of blood).

In the past, certain foods (such as spicy foods) were blamed for ulcers. However, it is now known that a bacterial infection (with Helicobacter pylori) is a common cause for ulcers. The use of anti-inflammatory medications such as ibuprofen (Advil, Motrin) or naproxen (Naprosyn) can also contribute to ulcers.

If an ulcer is suspected, the doctor may order blood tests and stool tests. Treatment can often be prescribed based on the symptoms, the physical findings, and the lab results. Sometimes, however, an endoscopic exam or EGD (see section above) is needed to make the diagnosis or to assess for complications.

Treatment most often consists of:
- ◆ avoiding foods that may contribute to symptoms (for example, acidic foods such as orange juice);

- H2 blockers to reduce acid—e.g., ranitidine (Zantac) or famotodine (Pepcid);
- proton pump inhibitors (medications that reduce acid in the stomach)—e.g., omeprazole (Prilosec), lansoprazole (Prevacid), pantoprazole (Protonix), rabeprazole (Aciphex), and esomeprozole (Nexium).

If Helicobacter pylori is diagnosed or suspected, antibiotics are prescribed to kill the bacteria. There are a number of different regimens, each with a combination of antibiotics and other medication, usually taken for two weeks.

Occasionally, if an ulcer is not responding to medications, surgery may be recommended. Surgery usually involves removing the ulcer and cutting the nerve that stimulates the stomach to make acid.

CONSTIPATION

Constipation is a change in the frequency, size, consistency, and ease of bowel movements that leads to an overall decrease in the volume of bowel movements. Constipation is common in people with DS of all ages. This may be because of the lower muscle tone or the apparent dysfunction of the autonomic nervous system (discussed in Chapter 9). In the gastrointestinal system, these differences result in decreased motility (movement) through the gut. Constipation is one of the ways this is manifested.

Constipation sometimes develops in young adults who are living independently or semi-independently for the first time. When they were younger, their parents probably made sure they ate food with fiber, drank enough water, and got some exercise. Once they're on their own, however, they may eat unhealthier foods, avoid fruits and vegetables, get less exercise, etc.

For a person to have "normal" bowel movements, it is not necessary to have a daily bowel movement. Having between three bowel movements a week and three a day is considered normal. However, a change in bowel movement frequency for an individual can be abnormal for that individual. Constipation may present in lots of ways and symptoms and signs of constipation may include:

- decreased frequency of bowel movements,
- increased size of infrequent bowel movements,
- small, hard bowel movements,
- occasional formed stool with intermittent diarrhea,
- bloating of the abdomen,
- abdominal discomfort,
- decreased appetite.

In extreme cases of constipation, fecal impaction occurs. This involves large, hard stool that the person is not able to pass. Fecal impaction can develop into a serious medical condition requiring hospitalization.

It can be challenging for parents or caregivers to recognize constipation in a person with DS who is independent in the bathroom without intruding on his privacy. In those situations, it may be helpful to have the individual record his bowel movements on a chart. Particularly if constipation has been a serious problem in the past, a regular discreet review of the chart with his parents or caregivers can help assure he is having regular bowel movements.

A health care practitioner generally diagnoses constipation on the basis of a good history and physical—in which he looks for complaints as noted above. In more severe cases of constipation, the doctor may note physical findings during the abdominal exam, such as hardness of the abdomen, palpable stool in the abdomen, bloating, or discomfort.

When constipation is more severe, additional testing for constipation may include plain x-ray (without barium), barium x-ray (barium enema), and/or colonoscopy (a scope passed into the rectum to view the large intestine). Colonoscopies are generally performed with no anesthesia or under "conscious sedation," in which the person becomes very relaxed and may fall lightly asleep but can be easily awakened. This test usually requires heavier sedation or general anesthesia in people with DS.

PREVENTING OR REDUCING CONSTIPATION

The following are ways to improve motility and reduce constipation:
- ◆ Increase fiber in the diet or add fiber supplements. This would include eating more whole grain foods, more fruits and vegetables, and/or taking a supplement such as Metamucil or Benefiber.
- ◆ Increase fluid consumption. Dehydration contributes to constipation. Many people with DS resist drinking water. Beverages the person might drink if he dislikes water include:
  - ➤ one or two diet sodas per day (one or two will provide some of the daily fluid needed, usually without the bloating that can occur if the person drinks more)
  - ➤ noncaloric flavored water
  - ➤ diluted juices
- ◆ Exercise regularly.

Over-the-counter laxatives are not usually recommended because they can foster a dependency. That is, over time the body may need the laxative to continue to have bowel movements. However, in some individuals, regular use of medications is the only solution. Medications that may help include:
- ◆ fiber supplements such as psyllium (Metamucil) or wheat dextrin (Benefiber)
- ◆ docusate sodium (Colace)—a stool softener that draws water into the colon to reduce dryness of the bowel movements

- polyethylene glycol (Miralax)—which causes water retention in the colon
- bisacodyl (Dulcolax), a stimulant that can be taken as a pill, a suppository, or an enema (Fleets)
- tap water enemas

Symptoms and signs that can indicate more serious constipation include:
- bloating,
- abdominal pain,
- bleeding from the rectum.

These symptoms usually require additional evaluation. If the pain is increasing, especially if associated with vomiting, the person should see a doctor immediately or even go to the emergency room. These can be signs of a fecal impaction.

LONG-TERM, PAINFUL CONSTIPATION

Sometimes long-term constipation can lead to a cycle in which the person has painful bowel movements, so he tries to hold them back, and then becomes even more constipated as a result. In this situation, the symptoms usually include diarrhea (as liquid stool leaks around a large amount of constipated stool) or even a complete lack of stools. An aggressive management plan is needed to eliminate the stool that is causing discomfort. This usually requires some of the medications listed above. Once the large amount of stool has been removed, the person will need a maintenance plan to prevent accumulation of stool, as well as treatment to limit the anxiety about having bowel movements.

In designing a means to reduce anxiety and avoidance, it may help to know that people with DS have characteristics which may make them a little more susceptible to this type of problem. They often have excellent visual memories and they tend to replay past events over and over, especially negative experiences (see Chapter 5 in *Mental Wellness in Adults with Down Syndrome*). Consequently, each time they approach a toilet, they may re-experience the pain and discomfort. This then triggers their anxiety and a pattern of avoidance. In addition, people with DS tend to be creatures of habit and to keep patterns going even if these patterns are not productive (see the information on grooves in Chapter 9 in *Mental Wellness*).

The good news is that the characteristics that get people in trouble may also help to solve problems. For example, we have found that people with DS are not only responsive to visual memories but to visual cues as well (see Chapter 2 of this book for more on this). Visual cues are surprisingly effective in helping people to reset patterns of behavior they have gotten stuck in. The form and type of visual cue depends on the age, cognitive level, and interests of the person. For instance, some people may respond positively to using a picture schedule showing the steps of the process of elimination in more positive terms. Others may simply need a positive notation on a calendar after each positive elimination experience to reduce anxiety, or may respond favorably to positive rewards, such as earning points toward a desired object.

The goal of these procedures is to reduce the association of anxiety with elimination and allow a more normal pattern of elimination to occur. Finally, once this pattern is established, the person's tendency to repeat patterns or grooves becomes an asset and not a liability, as the pattern of normal bowel elimination continues and is reinforced in day-to-day life.

GALLSTONES

The gall bladder is an organ that sits below the liver and stores bile from the liver. When we eat, the gall bladder contracts and releases bile down a tube (the common bile duct) into the small intestine. Bile helps us digest food, but can also harden into gall stones (cholelithiasis), which are more common in people with DS.

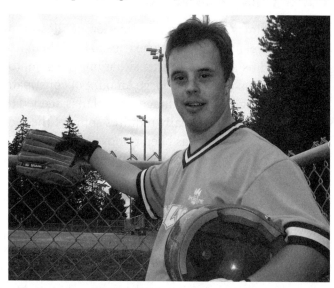

Liquid bile contains cholesterol, bile salts, and bilirubin (a break-down product of red blood cells). If the bile contains too much of these substances, it may harden into pieces of stone-like material called gall stones. In addition, if the bile is not readily expelled from the gall bladder, the stasis (nonpassage) of the bile may lead to stone formation.

One theory is that decreased motility and subsequent stasis of bile may be the cause of increased gall stones in people with DS. In addition, people with DS may have greater turnover of red blood cells, which could lead to higher levels of bilirubin.

Gallstones may not result in any symptoms, or they may cause significant problems. People can live with gallstones for many years if they are not causing symptoms. No treatment is necessary in this situation. In the general population, less than half of people with gallstones ever develop symptoms. However, about 5 to 10 percent of people with gallstones do develop symptoms each year.

Symptoms include:
♦ episodic abdominal pain, usually in the right upper quadrant or epigastric areas (the upper abdomen in the middle where the stomach sits), with the pain often radiating to the back,

♦ nausea,
♦ vomiting,
♦ diarrhea,
♦ indigestion or bloating,
♦ intolerance of fatty food (getting the symptoms above after eating a fatty meal).

Some people with DS may not be able to report their symptoms, and may therefore have behavioral changes in response to the symptoms. We have seen several individuals who reacted to gallstones with periodic aggressive or agitated behavior. Their behavior improved after treatment of the gallstones.

Lab findings and imaging tests that help make the diagnosis include:
♦ blood tests of liver function (an elevation of some liver tests suggests gallstones)
♦ an ultrasound of the gall bladder to look for gallstones
♦ a computed tomography (CT) scan of the abdomen, which can show gallstones
♦ a HIDA scan (cholescintigraphy) to evaluate gallbladder function and help determine if the gallstones that are present (usually seen on an ultrasound) are the cause of the symptoms. (As noted, gallstones are often asymptomatic. Even if gallstones are present and the person has symptoms suggestive of gallstones, a HIDA scan may be ordered to help confirm that the gallstones are in fact causing the symptoms.)
♦ Additional testing may include an MRCP (magnetic resonance cholangiopancreatography) or an ERCP (endoscopic retrograde cholangiopancreatography). An MRCP is an MRI test. An ERCP is done through an endoscope passed through the stomach to the small intestine. Both tests further assess the bile duct that flows out of the gallbladder to evaluate for stones that may be "stuck" in the duct and blocking the flow of bile from the gallbladder to the small intestine. (See box on the next page.)

Eating a low-fat diet may help reduce symptoms of gallstones. However, the ultimate treatment is surgically removing the gallbladder (which contains the stones) and removing any stones that may be in the common bile duct. Gallbladder surgery is now usually done through a laparoscope (a scope passed through small incisions in the abdomen). This surgery is done under general anesthesia in the operating room and people with DS generally tolerate the procedure well. Occasionally an open procedure is required. This is the older approach to gall bladder surgery, and requires a larger incision and more recovery time.

Even after the gall bladder is removed, some people will continue to need to eat a diet lower in fats to avoid symptoms. Consultation with a dietitian may be necessary.

GI Tests

CT scan: A computed tomography test. The person must lie still on a table that enters a large doughnut-shaped machine. The test is painless, but takes several minutes. Most people with DS tolerate the scanning well, but some need sedation or even anesthesia.

HIDA scan: This is a nuclear medicine scan. A radioactive solution is given in an IV, so the person must have a needle inserted into a vein. The person must also lie still on a table, sometimes for an hour or two. Many people with DS tolerate the procedure well, but occasionally a person with DS will require sedation.

MRCP: The MRCP is a magnetic resonance imaging (MRI) test that focuses specifically on the gall bladder and bile duct. Some people—with and without DS—have trouble tolerating MRI-testing because an MRI is done with the body in a small tube (closed MRI) or between two large plates (open MRI). The closeness of the machine and the loud banging/clanking noises can be disturbing. Sometimes heavy sedation or general anesthesia is needed for a person with DS to be able to remain still long enough for the test to be completed.

ERCP: For the ERCP, an endoscope is inserted into the mouth and threaded down through the stomach and into the small intestine. Placing the tube in the mouth and throat can be uncomfortable and cause gagging. There may be some cramping as the tube is passed through the stomach and small intestine. As with a regular endoscopy, EGD (as discussed in celiac disease and ulcers), an ERCP will likely require heavy sedation or general anesthesia.

LIVER PROBLEMS

The liver is the large organ in our right upper abdomen. It has many functions including:

- helping to detoxify the blood;
- storage of glycogen (the form of glucose/sugar used for energy stored by our body);
- decomposition of red blood cells;
- production of biochemicals necessary for digestion;
- synthesis of cholesterol.

The majority of liver problems seen in people with DS tend to be due to environmental or infectious causes.

FATTY LIVER

Fatty liver is a condition in which fat deposits build up in the liver. Inflammation and fibrosis (like scarring) can also occur. Infrequently, fatty liver can lead to cirrhosis, a condition that can result in liver failure.

People usually have no symptoms when fat builds up in the liver. The condition is most often detected when a liver function test (blood test) finds elevated levels of fat, or, inadvertently, when the person has an ultrasound, CT scan, or MRI of the abdomen.

Causes of fatty liver include:

- ◆ excessive alcohol consumption,
- ◆ metabolic abnormalities, including:
  - ➤ excess body weight,
  - ➤ insulin resistance (such as occurs in diabetes),
  - ➤ high levels of triglycerides in the blood,
- ◆ medications, including:
  - ➤ aspirin,
  - ➤ corticosteroids,
  - ➤ tetracycline,
- ◆ pregnancy,
- ◆ some viruses.

Treatment of fatty liver consists of addressing the cause. In people with DS, the most common causes appear to be metabolic abnormalities. Treatment icludes

- ◆ assessing for and treating diabetes, if present;
- ◆ losing weight (down to the ideal body weight);
- ◆ reducing consumption of simple sugars (such as found in cookies, candy, soda pop);
- ◆ reducing consumption of saturated fats.

If an adult with DS has diabetes, is overweight or obese, or eats excessive amounts of sugary or fatty foods, it may be advisable to have periodic (perhaps annual) liver blood tests to check for the development of fatty liver. Dieting and other weight loss efforts can be challenging for many people with Down syndrome. Techniques to help a person with DS with these goals are addressed in Chapter 2.

HEPATITIS

Hepatitis is an inflammation of the liver. The inflammation can be either acute—sudden, but relatively short lived—or chronic—persisting over a long period of time.

When the inflammation is acute, the person can be ill with diarrhea, vomiting, and jaundice (the eyes and skin turn yellow due to liver dysfunction). Infrequently, the liver may fail in acute hepatitis. Some types of hepatitis can develop into a chronic infection that can cause liver failure or increase the risk of liver cancer. In people with DS, hepatitis is most commonly caused by viral infections.

The three most common types of hepatitis are:
- ◆ hepatitis A,
- ◆ hepatitis B,
- ◆ hepatitis C.

The differences among these types are explained below.

The most common symptoms of hepatitis are:
- ◆ fever,
- ◆ malaise,
- ◆ nausea and vomiting,
- ◆ decreased appetite,
- ◆ jaundice (skin and eyes turn yellow),
- ◆ enlarged liver,
- ◆ dark urine,
- ◆ pale stools,
- ◆ abdominal pain,
- ◆ fatigue, and
- ◆ joint discomfort.

The vast majority of people who develop hepatitis have few or no symptoms and the condition may only be recognized later with blood testing.

Hepatitis is diagnosed on the basis of information gathered through:
- ◆ the person's history,
- ◆ physical exam,
- ◆ liver function blood tests, and
- ◆ specific blood tests for the type of hepatitis the individual is suspected to have.

If hepatitis B or C is suspected, tests may also include:
- ◆ imaging studies (ultrasound, CT scan)
- ◆ a liver biopsy in which a bit of the liver is surgically removed (often with a needle passed through the skin) and examined microscopically.

HEPATITIS A

Hepatitis A is most commonly passed by the fecal-oral route. That is, someone with hepatitis A sheds the virus in his stools and can transmit it to others if they ingest the virus. For example, someone might accidentally get stool from an infected person on his hand by changing a diaper, touching a toilet seat, or touching the individual and then casually touching his hand to his mouth or to something he is eating. Or an infected person might fail to wash his hands after using the bathroom and then accidentally contaminate food that others eat.

Symptoms of hepatitis A include diarrhea, fatigue, fever, jaundice, and others. Treatment is generally supportive in nature. For example, if the person develops a significant problem with diarrhea, treatment would include monitoring the status of his electrolytes (e.g., sodium and potassium) and his hydration status and treating him with oral or intravenous fluids, as needed.

Generally, the illness lasts several days to a few weeks, and, with supportive care, the person fully recovers. Much less often, the individual will develop fulminant hepatitis A. This complication can lead to *liver failure.* Liver failure can cause severe jaundice, ascites (fluid in the abdomen), hemorrhages in the GI tract, coma, and death. It requires hospitalization and much more aggressive treatment.

Good sanitation, hygiene, and hand washing (especially for food handlers, health care workers, and day care workers) are important measures to prevent the spread of hepatitis A. People who are known to have hepatitis A should not return to work until they are no longer contagious. Due to the infectious nature of the illness, the potential for spread to many others, and the availability of these preventative measures, a case of hepatitis A generally must be reported by law to the local health department.

The hepatitis A vaccine and hepatitis A globulin are recommended for people who have been exposed to hepatitis A. Hepatitis A globulin consists of antibodies against hepatitis A that are given to help eliminate the virus. Hepatitis A vaccine is also recommended for individuals more likely to be exposed to hepatitis A at work, including day care workers, sewage workers, and those traveling to places where hepatitis A is common.

HEPATITIS B

Hepatitis B has historically been viewed as an illness that is transmitted by blood transfusion or other exposure to infected blood in a health care setting, through sharing needles (for example, between persons who use illegal IV drugs), or through having multiple sexual partners, particularly homosexual males. However, donated blood is now routinely checked for hepatitis B, so blood transfusions are rarely a cause. It is also uncommon for people with DS to use illegal IV drugs or have multiple sexual partners. And yet, hepatitis B is fairly common in people with DS. The reason is that hepatitis B can be transmitted through *any* body fluid, including blood, semen, tears, urine, stool, saliva, etc. If an individual has close contact with someone with hepatitis B, particularly in a situation where hygiene guidelines may not be carefully followed, he can become infected. Adults with DS are most likely to be exposed to hepatitis B in group residential facilities or day programs (like workshops).

Acute hepatitis B can make individuals quite ill (see symptoms above) and can sometimes cause acute *liver failure.* Unlike hepatitis A, which usually only causes short-lived infections, hepatitis B can become a chronic illness. This puts the individual at greater risk for *cancer of the liver* and can eventually cause liver failure. In addition, people with chronic hepatitis B are potentially infectious to those around them. In the general population, about 1 percent of individuals who contract acute hepatitis B go on to develop chronic hepatitis B. In people with DS, however, the figure is 10 percent.

Some individuals who have had acute hepatitis B don't develop chronic active hepatitis B, but do become chronic carriers of the disease. Although they don't have chronic inflammation of the liver with the potential complications, they are still potentially contagious to those around them.

As with hepatitis A, prevention is important. "Universal precautions" are recommended. For example, a care provider who helps a person with DS with hygiene should wear gloves when touching potentially infectious substances (e.g., urine and stool). Using good hand washing techniques is always a wise precaution. If taken with every individual—even those who are not known to have hepatitis B—these precautions can prevent accidental exposure. A case of hepatitis B must also be reported to the local health department.

Hepatitis B vaccine is recommended for everyone who lives in a residential facility. We also recommend the vaccine for everyone who works in a workshop-type setting where there is contact with many people with intellectual disabilities (who may have had contact with hepatitis B in residential or other settings). Family members of people who have hepatitis B (acute or chronic) should also be immunized. They may also need to take immune globulin to prevent hepatitis B, preferably given within 48 hours of initial exposure.

Medications are not prescribed to treat acute hepatitis B except as needed to support the individual. For example, a medication to reduce vomiting might be prescribed for someone with that particular symptom. For chronic hepatitis B, however, there are a variety of medications that can specifically treat the virus. They include:

◆ adefovir (Hepsera),
◆ entecavir (Baraclude),
◆ lamivudine (Epivir),
◆ interferons (see the box below).

If a person with DS has chronic hepatitis B, we recommend consultation with a gastroenterologist who treats liver disease. These medications require careful monitoring for effectiveness and side effects.

Liver Failure

Liver failure occurs when the liver shuts down and stops doing its usual functions.

A person with liver failure requires medical support until the liver recovers. Unfortunately, sometimes the liver does not recover and the liver is irreversibly damaged. In that situation, the only treatment is liver transplant, which involves a complicated operation and recovery period. In addition, the anti-rejection medications that must be taken after a transplant require careful attention and extensive monitoring. We have had no transplant experience in our practice. There is limited documentation of liver transplants for people with DS in the literature.

HEPATITIS C

Hepatitis C is most commonly transmitted through infected blood or its products, but in about 40 percent of cases, the mode of transmission is unknown. Now that blood is tested before transfusion, the incidence of infection from a blood transfusion is rare. Sharing syringes for illegal IV drug use, sexual activity with an infected individual (especially homosexual males), and exposure to household contacts are all potential sources of infection. For our patients, the most common cause we have found is from blood transfusions received prior to 1992 (when testing blood for hepatitis C became available). Most often, we see hepatitis C in adults who required blood transfusions as part of heart surgery.

Like hepatitis B, hepatitis C can cause both acute and chronic infections. Chronic hepatitis C can cause *liver failure.* It is now the most common cause of chronic liver disease and the most frequent reason for liver transplantation in the United States.

The same prevention and avoidance measures recommended for hepatitis B are also recommended for hepatitis C. Unfortunately, at this time, there is no available vaccination for hepatitis C.

Interferon Therapy

Interferon therapy can be effective in treating chronic hepatitis B and acute and chronic hepatitis C. This medication can be challenging to take, however. It is given by injection multiple times a week and the treatment course may last as long as 48 weeks. In addition, there are many potential side effects, including suppression of the bone marrow's ability to make red blood cells, white blood cells, and platelets.

In addition to the potential physical side effects, there are very serious potential psychological side effects. These include:

- psychosis ("losing touch with reality"—hallucinations, delusions, and disorganized speech),
- aggressive behavior,
- depression, and
- suicidality.

In addition, one research study has suggested that interferon may not be effective against hepatitis C in children with DS (Miyoshi et al., 2008). In this particular study, interferon was effective in half of the children without DS and none of the children with DS.

None of our adolescent and adult patients have received interferon to date. Therefore, we have no recommendations based on experience. We recommend consulting with a specialist in liver disease if interferon is recommended for someone with DS.

Unlike with hepatitis A and B, if the diagnosis of acute hepatitis C is made, specific medications to destroy the virus are recommended. Treatment is with interferon (see box below). Ribavirin is added for some patients. For chronic hepatitis C, both medications are generally recommended.

PRECAUTIONS FOR ALL PATIENTS WITH HEPATITIS A, B, OR C

In addition to the treatments discussed above, everyone with liver disease from hepatitis should avoid consuming alcohol or other potential liver toxins. This includes medications that can affect the liver, such as acetaminophen (Tylenol), erythromycin, statin medications (e.g., Lipitor), and others. For individuals with hepatitis B or C who have not had hepatitis A, we recommend getting the hepatitis A vaccine. For individuals with hepatitis C, we also recommend hepatitis B vaccine if they have not had the vaccine and don't demonstrate immunity to hepatitis B.

HERNIAS

◆ ◆ ◆ ◆ ◆ ◆ ◆ ◆ ◆ ◆ ◆ ◆ ◆ ◆ ◆ ◆ ◆ ◆

Hernias are formed when there is a defect in the abdominal wall and the tissue within the abdominal cavity pushes through the area. It usually causes a noticeable lump in that area. Hernias may be uncomfortable, but many do not have symptoms.

Hernias are more common in people with DS. The common areas for hernias in people with DS are:

- ◆ inguinal (in the groin; seen more commonly in men),
- ◆ umbilical (at the umbilicus or belly button),
- ◆ epigastric (in the abdominal area above the umbilicus), and
- ◆ at the site of a previous abdominal surgery.

The diagnosis is usually based on the physical exam. Sometimes, however, an imaging study (usually a CT scan) may be necessary to determine whether a bulge is really a hernia (rather than a mass in the abdominal wall, for example).

If the hernia causes any discomfort, then treatment should be considered. In addition, sometimes a large hernia may limit function because it is "in the way," even though it may not be uncomfortable *per se*. If lifting heavy objects causes discomfort or increases the bulge, this activity should be avoided. If a hernia is not causing any symptoms, studies have shown that it can be monitored.

Treatment is generally surgical repair of the defect. Binders—special girdle-like devices—can sometimes help keep tissue from protruding through the defect. However, this is usually either a temporary solution or one used for people for whom surgery is very risky due to other health problems. If there are any questions about the appropriate treatment, ask for a consultation with a general surgeon.

There are multiple surgical approaches. Depending on the location, size, previous surgical history, the person's tolerance of the surgery, and the person's other health problems, some surgical options include:

- same-day surgery (go home the same day vs. spending one to several days in the hospital);
- laparoscopic surgery vs. an open procedure;
- use of mesh to prevent the hernia from recurring.

After surgery, the person generally needs to limit work and other activities for several days to several weeks.

Although it is not a common complication, the most significant concern with a hernia is if the tissue from within the abdomen protrudes through the hernia and gets stuck in the defect. The hernia is then referred to as "incarcerated." When this occurs, the site usually gets red and swollen, and is generally tender. This is a surgical emergency because the tissue that is protruding through the defect gets pinched, often swells, and the blood supply to the tissue can be impeded. This can cause that tissue to die, which can lead to multiple complications. Sometimes the tissue can be reduced (or pushed back in). If not, emergency surgery is needed for incarcerated hernias.

As noted above, a hernia can just be monitored if there are no symptoms. However, if the physician notices that protruding tissue cannot easily be pushed back through the hernia, it may indicate that the hernia is more likely to become incarcerated. In this case, it's a good idea to get a surgical consultation to discuss whether surgery is advisable.

IF IN DOUBT, CHECK IT OUT!

There are numerous possible gastrointestinal conditions. Many of them can produce similar symptoms, and some of the symptoms can be quite subtle. For people with Down syndrome, the main sign that something is wrong may be a behavioral change.

The following symptoms should always be investigated—particularly if they are persistent, and even if mild:

- abdominal pain,
- vomiting blood (requires urgent evaluation),
- blood in the stool,
- unexplained weight loss,
- heartburn.

Even if the symptoms have been a chronic concern, if there is a change, they should be evaluated.

Diagnosing gastrointestinal problems in people with DS can be a challenge. As noted, the symptoms may be subtle. In addition, people with DS often have a high pain tolerance. Therefore, if the diagnosis is not clear from the evaluation, consider a referral to a gastroenterologist. We often find ourselves referring people to a gastroenterologist even when we might not have referred someone else (without DS). The challenge of diagnosis in people with DS sometimes makes additional GI testing necessary to make the diagnosis.

Chapter 12

Urology

. . . .

Matthew, age 25, was having intermittent episodes of agitation and conflict with his siblings and parents. Most of the time he was his usual pleasant self, but over the preceding few months, these episodes had developed. Matthew's limited verbal skills hampered efforts to figure out what was bothering him.

Then, in what appeared to be an unrelated event, Matthew became ill with influenza and needed to be hospitalized for pneumonia. While he was in the hospital, the nursing staff noticed that he seemed to have difficulty urinating. He was using his hands to push on his lower abdomen. A catheter was placed into his bladder and an abnormally large amount of urine was obtained. Subsequent testing showed that Matthew had an overly large, distended bladder with decreased muscle tone. There was no obstruction preventing the urine from passing out of his bladder, but the bladder could not adequately contract to eliminate his urine. Matthew was treated with medication and his bladder function improved.

Later, at an appointment at the Adult Down Syndrome Center, Matthew's parents shared several observations. They hadn't really given it much thought before, but Matthew had been intermittently pushing on his abdomen prior to the hospitalization and now he was no longer doing it. They now believed that he had been trying to initiate his urinary stream by pushing on his abdomen. They also noted that Matthew's agitation had significantly diminished since he was treated for the bladder condition. In retrospect, it appeared he had been uncomfortable from a very distended bladder and had not been able to tell his parents what the problem was.

Problems involving the urological system (bladder, kidneys, ureters, prostate, penis, and testes) are fairly common in people with Down syndrome (DS). Some of these problems are related to physical and behavioral characteristics that many people with DS share. For example, as in Matthew's case, difficulties emptying the bladder or initiating the urinary stream can occur due to low muscle tone and longstanding habits such as holding the urine in. Likewise, kidney dysfunction due to dehydration can occur if the person routinely drinks insufficient fluids, as many people with DS do. In addition, problems related to difficulties with hygiene can occur. Of course, adolescents and adults with DS can also develop some of the same problems that other adults may have.

PROBLEMS RELATED TO DIFFICULTIES EMPTYING THE BLADDER

Most people with DS have some degree of low muscle tone. That is, the amount of elasticity in the muscles is looser or "floppier" when at rest. Low muscle tone can be found in skeletal muscle such as the muscles of the arms or legs. This improves with time for many people with DS. Low muscle tone can also be found in smooth muscle— that is, in organs such as the colon or the urinary bladder. In the colon, low muscle tone appears to contribute to constipation. Similarly, in the bladder, low muscle tone may result in incomplete emptying of the bladder or difficulty initiating the urinary stream.

Another apparent cause of lowered muscle tone in the bladder of some people with DS is a functional or behavioral one. Many people with DS urinate infrequently. This may be related to decreased muscle tone, a decreased perception of the sensation of the need to urinate, or a conscious decision to hold the urine in. With infrequent urination, the urinary bladder may get very stretched out. Similar to over-stretching a rubber band, the stretching of the bladder may, over time, reduce the elasticity of the bladder, reducing the bladder's ability to completely contract and empty.

When the bladder is not contracting well and tends to be full of urine, it can cause a number of problems:

- **Increased likelihood of urinary tract infections:** Urine is generally sterile (without organisms). If bacteria do enter the bladder, they are usually flushed out through regular, complete emptying of the bladder. However, if the bladder does not empty, the urine will, in effect, stagnate in the bladder. As a result, bacteria are more likely to flourish in the bladder, which can lead to a urinary tract infection.
- **Urinary incontinence:** As additional urine is made in the kidneys and passed into the bladder through the ureters, an overly distended bladder may reach a point where the urine overflows out of the bladder. The person may not be able to control the flow of urine in this situation and incontinence is the result. In addition, when the bladder is very distended and has low tone, the person may have little sense of

the need to urinate. However, with the addition of more urine in the bladder, the person may rapidly reach the threshold for the need to urinate. This can cause a sudden sense of urgency, and also, with such a full bladder, a reduced ability to hold back the urine.

- ◆ **Discomfort:** As in Matthew's case, a large, distended bladder, coupled with a reduced ability to initiate the urinary stream, can cause significant discomfort.
- ◆ **Kidney problems:** Over time, an overly large volume of urine in the bladder may result in pressure in the urinary system that eventually affects the kidneys. Chronic "back pressure" from the bladder can damage the kidneys. This may also result in urine flowing backwards toward the kidney, which can lead to kidney infections if the urine contains bacteria.

There are a variety of tests that may be done to evaluate someone who is having problems emptying the bladder. They include:

- ◆ An ultrasound of the bladder before and after urination. The person is instructed to drink a significant amount of fluids and not to urinate. The ultrasound is then performed. The person is then asked to urinate completely and the ultrasound is repeated. The volume of urine in the bladder before and after urination is recorded and compared. A large amount of urine remaining in the bladder after urination is consistent with retention of urine. It may also indicate, however, that the person did not try to empty her bladder. Therefore, it is important that the person with DS understands and follows the instructions.
- ◆ Placing a catheter in the bladder. The person is instructed to urinate and completely empty her bladder. After she urinates, a catheter is introduced through the urethra into the bladder and the volume of urine is recorded. As with the ultrasound, retained urine can indicate the inability to empty the bladder. While this test can be done in an office that doesn't have an ultrasound machine, it obviously can be challenging for people with DS to tolerate. Therefore, we usually order an ultrasound to be done at an imaging center rather than attempting to place a catheter in the bladder.
- ◆ A voiding cystometrogram. This test requires placing a catheter in the bladder, filling the bladder with fluid, and then asking the patient to report when she feels the sensation of bladder fullness. For multiple reasons, this can be challenging for people with DS (and we don't usually order the test).
- ◆ A urinalysis (and possibly urine culture) to check for a urinary tract (bladder) infection.
- ◆ A cystoscopy (passing a scope through the urethra into the bladder) to visualize the urethra and bladder. The cystoscopy can be used to

look for any obstruction. An enlarged prostate (in men), a narrowing or stricture in the urethra, a mass or tumor of the bladder obstructing the urethra, and other causes can be assessed. If there is an obstruction, usually there is higher pressure in the bladder as the muscle contracts harder to push out the urine. However, over time, the bladder may become very stretched and the bladder may not contract as well. Theoretically, this test can be done in the office of a urologist's office—a physician who specializes in conditions of the urinary tracts of males and females, and on the reproductive system of males. However, for people with DS, the test must often be done in the operating room with anesthesia.

TREATMENTS FOR PROBLEMS EMPTYING THE BLADDER

OBSTRUCTIONS

If an obstruction is found that is not due to an enlarged prostate, it may need to be surgically removed. This can often be done under anesthesia in the operating room via the cystoscope—a form of endoscope used to examine the ureter and the bladder. It is passed through the urethra into the bladder. Occasionally, obstructions can be removed via the cystoscope in the urologist's office or in the operating room. Less frequently, obstructions must be removed via an open procedure in the operating room under anesthesia.

If an enlarged prostate is blocking the flow of urine, medications may be used either to improve urinary flow or to reduce prostate size. Medications that can improve urinary flow include:

- doxazosin (Cardura),
- tamsulosin (Flomax),
- terazosin (Hytrin),
- alfuzosin (Uroxatral).

One side effect of these medications that must be monitored for is lowered blood pressure. This can be especially evident with the first dose. Sometimes lowered blood pressure occurs only when a person stands up. The lowered blood pressure could cause dizziness or a fall. Taking the medication just before bed can reduce this problem for some individuals. It is recommended that alfuzosin and tamsulosin be taken with food in the stomach.

Medications that can reduce prostate size include: dutasteride (Avodart) and finasteride (Proscar).

Similar to other obstructions, an obstruction due to prostate enlargement can also be surgically removed using a variety of techniques. Many procedures can be done through or with cystoscopy. Some of the modalities used with these procedures include scalpel, laser, microwaves, electric current, and radio waves. Much less frequently, the prostate is surgically removed. Surgical removal is usually reserved for treating prostate cancer.

"FLOPPY" BLADDER

Sometimes no obstruction is found. For a large, floppy bladder without obstruction, we have found the following treatments helpful:

- ◆ Sometimes leaving a catheter in the bladder for a few weeks will help the bladder to regain elasticity by preventing the bladder from getting stretched beyond normal. The urine is collected in a leg bag connected to the catheter. The bag is frequently emptied. Most of our patients who have needed this treatment have not required hospitalization. A few have required short hospital stays.
- ◆ Encouraging frequent (every two to three hours during the day) urination can prevent the bladder from getting overly stretched.
- ◆ Using medications prescribed to improve urinary flow in prostate enlargement can be quite helpful. Although the medications are not FDA approved for this use without prostate enlargement, we have found that for many people with DS who have large, "floppy" bladders, these medications improve bladder emptying and reduce the amount of urine left in their bladder after urination. We have found benefits for both men and women.

Problematic Bathroom Habits Linked to Difficulties Emptying the Bladder

In our experience, people with DS sometimes develop problematic routines when they have bowel or bladder elimination problems. For example, as described above, a large bladder with limited muscle tone can lead to difficulty emptying the bladder or retention of urine. Some adults with this difficulty sit on the toilet for an extended period of time attempting to urinate. A number of our patients with DS have developed a compulsive behavior of sitting in the bathroom, which can interfere with their ability to work, take part in recreational activities, or do anything outside of the home.

The treatment for people with these types of difficulties is not only focused on the compulsive behavior but also on the underlying physical health issue. Without addressing the person's difficulty with urinating, the behavior will be more difficult to treat. However, the compulsion to sit on the toilet may continue even after the health condition is treated successfully. This type of compulsive behavior may respond to redirection. For example, a timer may help the person learn to reduce the time spent in the bathroom. Sometimes medication can also help to decrease the compulsive behavior. More information on treating obsessions and compulsions is included in our previous book, *Mental Wellness in Adults with Down Syndrome.*

◆ Prescribing bethanecol (Urecholine) can improve bladder contraction and emptying of the bladder. This medication works by stimulating the part of the nervous system that causes bladder contraction.

SMALL BLADDER CAPACITY

Sometimes ultrasound testing of the bladder finds that the person has the opposite of a large, floppy bladder. The ultrasound may show a bladder with a small capacity that contracts even with a small amount of urine and is overactive or "spasmodic." This can cause incontinence because the person frequently has sudden urges to urinate and may not be able to hold the flow back or get to the bathroom quickly enough. This condition is treated with anti-spasmodic medications:

◆ tolterodine (Detrol, Detrol LA),
◆ oxybutynin (Ditropan, Ditropan XL),
◆ darifenacin (Enablex),
◆ trospium (Sanctura, Sanctura XR),
◆ solifenacin (Vesicare).

Urinary Incontinence: A Symptom with Many Possible Causes

There are many possible reasons that an adolescent or adult with DS may become incontinent—or unable to control urination. Some of them are directly related to the urologic system and some are related to problems affecting other body systems. Causes include:

◆ urinary tract infections,
◆ overflow incontinence (large volume of urine in the bladder),
◆ urinary obstruction,
◆ spasmodic (hyper-reflexic) bladder,
◆ diabetes mellitus (see Chapter 15),
◆ medication side effects,
◆ any condition that makes it more difficult to get to the bathroom in time (e.g., osteoarthritis),
◆ atlanto-axial instability (AAI) or spinal cord impingement at any level (see Chapter 13),
◆ seizures (see Chapter 17),
◆ Alzheimer disease (see Chapter 20),
◆ behavioral issues.

If an individual with DS develops incontinence (assuming she was continent and not having accidents previously), the first step is to get an assessment from the primary care provider. He or she will do a good history and

In our experience, all of these medications seem to work equally well for adults with DS. Most people need to take the medication for life, but occasionally an adult with DS is able to stop the medication without recurrence of symptoms.

URINARY TRACT AND BLADDER INFECTIONS (UTIs)

Urinary tract and bladder infections are more common in adults with DS of both genders, but especially so in women. For both men and women, holding in the urine for any of the reasons described above can lead to bacteria in the bladder and subsequent infections. Regular, more frequent urination helps to flush out any bacteria that have entered the bladder. A large, full bladder may also cause reduced blood flow to the bladder, which can contribute to infections.

Women may have hygiene issues that can further contribute to UTIs. All women are more prone to UTIs than men because of the closer proximity of the urethra (the tube that carries the urine from the bladder outside of the body) to the anus (the opening from which stool/poop is expelled from the body). As a result, it is fairly easy for bacteria in the stool to contaminate the urethra. This risk is increased in

physical exam to check for the problems noted above (and perhaps others as well). Based on the history and physical, additional testing may include:

- urinalysis and urine culture (to assess for infection, blood in the urine, and other abnormalities);
- blood testing (to assess kidney function, diabetes, and other abnormalities);
- ultrasound of the bladder, pre- and post-void (to assess how the bladder fills with urine and empties; also to look for abnormal anatomical changes of the bladder);
- lateral cervical spine (neck) x-ray (to assess for AAI);
- a cystoscopy, discussed above, to assess for obstruction or other abnormalities (this test would be done by a urologist);
- CT or MRI of the spine and/or brain to check whether anything is impinging on the spine, and to assess for a brain mass or other neurologic abnormalities (these tests might be ordered by the primary provider or a urologist or neurologist);
- EEG (electroencephalogram) to assess for seizures (see Chapter 17).

If all of these problems are ruled out, the next step would be a psychological evaluation performed by the primary provider, a psychologist, clinical social worker, or psychiatrist. An adult with DS might become incontinent due to psychological issues—e.g., as a reaction to stress, as a way of getting out of a situation she can't tolerate, or due to fear that she can't leave her work area to use the toilet.

women who wipe from back (near the anus) to front (toward the urethra). Women with DS should be instructed on appropriate (front to back) wiping technique. Premoistened wipes may also be helpful.

Symptoms of a urinary tract (or bladder) infection include:

- ◆ incontinence of urine—people with UTIs often feel a sense of urgency to urinate and may not be able to hold their urine,
- ◆ a burning sensation with urination,
- ◆ urinating frequently,
- ◆ blood in the urine.

UTIs are primarily treated with antibiotics. Often a short course (three days) is adequate. However, if the infection comes back or spreads up to the ureter(s) and kidney(s), it will require longer treatment. The symptoms of an infection that has spread may include back pain and fever.

Antibiotics commonly used to treat UTIs include:

- ◆ amoxicillin,
- ◆ trimethoprim-sulfa (Bactrim), and
- ◆ ciprofloxacin (Cipro).

The antibiotic prescribed depends on what type of bacteria is found when the urine is cultured. Other antibiotics than those listed above may be used based on the results of the culture and the determination of which antibiotics the bacteria are sensitive to. Phenazopyridine (Pyridium) may also be prescribed to reduce discomfort during urination. It is used temporarily to "numb" the painful bladder and urethra sensation while the antibiotic is eliminating the bacteria. This medication can turn the urine orange.

Anyone who has a UTI will also be advised to drink more water to flush out the kidneys and bladder. If the person with Down syndrome resists drinking water, other fluids may be used such as diet soda, flavored waters, and juices. Diluting the juice will help limit the excess calories.

KIDNEY PROBLEMS

◆ ◆ ◆ ◆ ◆ ◆ ◆ ◆ ◆ ◆ ◆ ◆ ◆ ◆ ◆ ◆ ◆ ◆

The kidneys are a pair of organs in the abdomen. The kidneys filter excess sodium, water, and waste products from the blood and make urine. Urine passes from the kidneys to the ureters to the bladder, and then from the bladder out of the body through the urethra. The kidneys also produce hormones that:

- ◆ stimulate red blood cell production in the bone marrow,
- ◆ control blood pressure, and
- ◆ maintain calcium in the bones.

There are many causes for kidney dysfunction ("renal insufficiency"). These causes can be broken down into three basic categories:

- **renal**—dysfunction whose cause primarily affects the kidney;
- **pre-renal**—dysfunction whose primary cause occurs before the blood reaches the kidney to be filtered;
- **post-renal**—dysfunction whose primary cause occurs after the blood is filtered in the kidney and the urine is made.

Ultimately, all three causes have an impact on the function of the kidneys themselves. Both pre-renal and post-renal causes of kidney dysfunction seem to be more common in people with DS.

PRE-RENAL CONDITIONS

Kidney dysfunction due to pre-renal conditions is frequently seen in adults with DS. When it is mild, there are usually no symptoms and the problem is only found during the course of a physical exam and blood tests. The most common cause appears to be dehydration. We have found through completing histories, physical exams, and lab work that many people with DS don't drink enough fluids and are continuously at least mildly dehydrated. One of the effects of dehydration is inadequate blood flow to the kidneys. As a consequence, the kidneys don't appropriately clear the blood of waste.

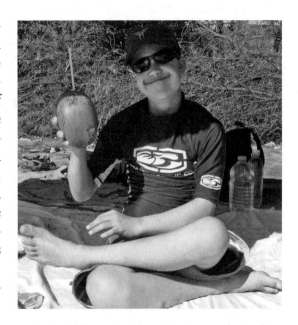

The Consequences of Dehydration

Inadequate fluid intake can cause dehydration. In addition, losing excess fluids, such as through diarrhea, can also cause dehydration. In people with DS, dehydration can contribute to the following problems:

- ◆ renal insufficiency,
- ◆ dizziness,
- ◆ dry skin,
- ◆ periodontal (gum) disease, if saliva is decreased,
- ◆ a sense of weakness,
- ◆ constipation.

If someone is mildly dehydrated, encouraging her to increase her fluid consumption can often resolve mild renal insufficiency. We recommend at least 6 to 8 glasses of fluid (preferably water) per day. Many people with DS decline to drink enough water, but can get enough fluids if they drink flavored water, flavored drinks (e.g., Crystal Light®), juice, and soda (preferably low-calorie, caffeine-free). See Addendum 1 at the back of the book for more suggestions for encouraging adequate fluid intake.

POST-RENAL CONDITIONS

Post-renal dysfunction is also fairly common in people with DS. Any condition that prevents urine from flowing out of the kidneys can lead to increased pressure in the kidneys. This can cause kidney dysfunction and eventually kidney damage. Some children with DS are born with obstructions of the ureter (the tube between the kidneys and the bladder). If the obstructions are not treated in childhood or scarring later occurs and narrows the ureters, kidney dysfunction can occur. (Scarring can be caused by a urinary tract infection or previous surgery.)

Kidney stones are another reason for obstruction of the ureter, but these don't appear to be more common in people with DS. A kidney stone occurs when substances in the urine (such as calcium or uric acid) are present in abnormally high concentrations and collect into a stone-like mass. Genetics plays a role in the formation of kidney stones.

A mass either outside the ureter or inside the ureter or bladder can also obstruct urine flow. For example, a large ovarian cyst, enlarged uterus, or large lymph nodes could obstruct the ureters. Again, these don't appear to be more common in people with DS. Severe constipation may also put pressure on the ureters, obstructing flow. This may occur more often in some people with DS.

Another place where urine may be obstructed is as it passes out of the bladder through the urethra. The flow of urine may be obstructed if the urethra is narrowed—due either to a congenital problem or to scarring caused by injuries, surgery, or catheters. As discussed elsewhere in this chapter, an enlarged prostate or a bladder that doesn't contract well may also cause urinary pressure to build, causing kidney dysfunction.

There may be no symptoms that the kidneys are being damaged. However, sometimes an obstruction will cause warning symptoms that lead to an evaluation. Symptoms of obstruction can include:

- ◆ difficulty urinating,
- ◆ urinating frequently, usually small amounts,
- ◆ discomfort in the lower abdomen, sometimes associated with a sensation of needing to urinate,
- ◆ back discomfort,
- ◆ blood in the urine (this can be caused, for example, by kidney stones).

If the pressure persists for a prolonged time, permanent kidney damage can occur.

DIAGNOSIS OF KIDNEY PROBLEMS

There are two blood tests that indirectly measure kidney function and may be done as part of a complete physical—blood urea nitrogen (BUN) and creatinine. Urea nitrogen and creatinine are waste products that kidneys ordinarily remove from the blood. If the results of these tests are elevated, it can indicate that the person's kidneys are not functioning adequately. We don't recommend routine screening, but do order these tests if the history and/or physical exam suggest kidney disease or inadequate fluid consumption.

An ultrasound of the kidneys can assess for signs of increased urinary pressure within the kidneys. An ultrasound of the bladder before and after the person urinates can assess the ability of the bladder to adequately empty. These ultrasounds are painless, but require the person to drink a lot of water, which can be uncomfortable.

TREATMENT OF KIDNEY PROBLEMS

Treatment of kidney problems depends on the condition. Generally, the primary care provider will manage the problems as appropriate and will consult a urologist and/or a nephrologist when needed, depending on the underlying problem. (Nephrology is a branch of internal medicine and pediatrics dealing with the study of the function and diseases of the kidney).

If the problem worsens, the person may need dialysis—a process in which a machine takes over the function of the kidneys and removes waste products and excess water from the body. Dialysis can be challenging due to the frequent (usually three times a week) treatments that can each take several hours and require the individual to lie still. The patient must also allow herself to be connected to the dialysis machine. We have had very limited experience with dialysis for adults with DS, but with coaching and encouragement, some people with DS are able to tolerate dialysis.

The other treatment for serious kidney dysfunction is kidney transplantation. Although we have had no experience with kidney transplantation, some people with DS have successfully undergone transplantation. Before proceeding with a transplant, a thorough discussion is needed to review the procedures, the need for medication and follow-up care, and other aspects of care needed to make the transplant successful.

CIRCUMCISION
◆ ◆ ◆ ◆ ◆ ◆ ◆ ◆ ◆ ◆ ◆ ◆ ◆ ◆ ◆ ◆ ◆ ◆ ◆

Many men, including men with DS, are circumcised (have the foreskin on the penis removed) in the first few days of life. On the other hand, many men are not circumcised.

If a man with DS has *not* been circumcised, it is important that he be taught proper hygiene. This includes pulling the foreskin back at least daily and washing the head of the penis. If not regularly cleaned, a white substance, smegma, tends to build up under the foreskin and can lead to bacterial or fungal infections. Specifically, ***balanitis*** (infection of the glans/head of the penis) and **posthitis** (inflammation of the foreskin) can occur. Symptoms include swelling, redness, pain, ulceration, and discharge. The condition can be infectious, if caused by bacteria or fungus, but there are other causes of inflammation that are not infectious.

Phimosis—tightness of the foreskin that prevents it from being drawn back—is another condition that can be caused by poor hygiene. It can also be caused by recurrent infections. If a man cannot retract the foreskin due to phimosis, the chance of recurrent infections increases. In addition, sometimes the phimosis is so tight that it can obstruct the meatus (opening) of the urethra and make urination difficult. In advanced situations, the person may not be able to urinate due to obstruction.

When balanitis, posthitis, or phimosis is caused by infection, they are treated with topical antifungal or antibacterial creams or ointments or oral antifungal or antibacterial tablets. Pain medications may be needed as well. Soaking in a bathtub may also be helpful. Gentle cleaning with soap and water is recommended.

If a man has recurrent infections, difficulty urinating, or there is concern about future problems (perhaps due to the person not being able to perform appropriate hygiene), the only additional treatment is surgical. That is, circumcision, or removal of the foreskin, should be considered. This is performed in the operating room under anesthesia and the man will require pain medication after the surgery.

These problems can be uncomfortable and can cause serious problems if left unrecognized and untreated. However, it can be challenging to balance an adolescent's or adult's right to privacy with the need to assess for a problem. If the person showers and uses the bathroom independently, it would be an inappropriate invasion of his privacy for family members or caregivers to check for proper hygiene or signs of infections. However, it is important that the man have someone in his life who can be confided in, in confidence, if there is a concern about any private area of the body. This might be a parent, a trusted male in his life, a doctor, etc. (We recommend consulting Terri Couwenhoven's book, *Teaching Children with Down Syndrome about Their Bodies, Boundaries, and Sexuality,* for strategies in teaching the individual how to communicate about sensitive issues.) If the person does not have the speech skills to describe medical problems, consider providing him with a picture or communication device to indicate the need to see a doctor.

As with other health problems, in some cases caregivers will have to follow-up on behavioral clues that the person is experiencing discomfort or an infection. For example, he may walk differently, spend more time in the bathroom, be more quiet, be louder and more agitated, or touch his genitals more.

CONCLUSION

Problems involving the urological system (bladder, kidneys, ureters, prostate, penis, and testes) are fairly common in teens and adults with DS. However, many of these problems can be prevented or minimized through educating the person about good hygiene and toileting habits, as well as the need to drink adequate amounts of fluids. If parents or caregivers are unwilling or unable to educate the adult with DS about these issues, they can ask the adult's doctor or nurse for help educating him or her. If need be, a dietitian can also help the person figure out ways to include more fluid in her diet.

Chapter 13

Orthopedic

. . . .

Problems

. . . .

Jason, age 18, had been doing very well in high school. A senior who was fully included in his classes, he was planning on attending a college program about 600 miles from his home the following fall. Unfortunately, about half way through the school year, his teachers became concerned that he seemed bored with school and was not paying attention in class. He was putting his head on his desk during class and his grades were falling. He had also begun falling in physical education class and appeared less coordinated.

At his evaluation at the Adult Down Syndrome Center, Jason denied any neck pain, but he indicated that it was hard to hold his head up and that was why he was laying his head on the desk at school. Results of his physical exam included:

- ◆ *an unsteadiness with walking,*
- ◆ *mild decreased strength in his arms and legs, and*
- ◆ *increased reflexes in his arms and legs.*

His blood work was all normal, including his thyroid blood tests. A lateral cervical spine (neck) x-ray done in flexion, extension, and neutral demonstrated atlantoaxial subluxation (slippage of the first vertebrae in the neck with respect to the second vertebrae), with measurement of 10 mm between the dens of C2 and the arch of C1. An MRI of his neck was ordered, and this showed compression of the spinal cord at the first cervical vertebrae.

Jason was diagnosed with atlantoaxial instability and was referred to an orthopedic surgeon who specializes in spinal surgery. Jason underwent surgery to decompress the spinal cord and stabilize his cervical spine. After a recovery period that included physical and occupational therapy, Jason was able to return to school. With the aid of a tutor during his recovery period, he graduated with his class and was able to start college in the fall.

People with Down syndrome (DS) are more likely to develop two broad types of orthopedic problems—that is, problems with the bones, joints, ligaments, or tendons. These include:
1. Problems that are caused by ligamentous laxity of the joint (explained below), including:
   ◆ atlantoaxial instability,
   ◆ hallux valgus (bunions),
   ◆ overpronation of the ankles, and
   ◆ subluxation of the patella (knee cap slipping out of place).
2. Problems that may be associated with early aging, including:
   ◆ osteoarthritis at a young age,
   ◆ spinal stenosis, and
   ◆ osteoporosis.

PROBLEMS ASSOCIATED WITH LIGAMENTOUS LAXITY

◆ ◆ ◆ ◆ ◆ ◆ ◆ ◆ ◆ ◆ ◆ ◆ ◆ ◆ ◆ ◆ ◆ ◆ ◆ ◆

Ligaments are connective tissues that connect one bone to another bone, holding the joint together. In people with DS, the ligaments are abnormal (more "stretchy"). This contributes to a number of problems. In joints, it tends to make them looser. The upside is increased flexibility. The downside is that joints may be unstable. If the joints are too loose, the bones will move too far apart from each other or slip partially or completely out of the socket or away from the adjacent bone.

VERTEBRAL SUBLUXATION (INCLUDING ATLANTOAXIAL INSTABILITY)

The vertebrae are the stack of bones that surround and protect the spinal cord and run from the base of the skull to the tailbone. They are numbered starting at the top and are categorized according to their location, either:
   ◆ cervical (in the neck),
   ◆ thoracic (in the thorax; attached to the ribs),
   ◆ lumbar (in the lower back), or
   ◆ sacral (a wedge-shaped fusion of five bones that is attached to the pelvis).

Due to lax ligaments connecting the vertebrae, people with DS are considerably more likely to experience vertebral subluxation—slippage of one vertebra in reference to the one next to it. If the vertebra slips far enough, it can cause compression of the spinal cord. The most common site for this to occur is at the first and second vertebrae of the neck (C1-2 subluxation) This is called atlantoaxial instability (the atlas is the first vertebrae in the cervical spine and the axis is the second). Subluxation, however, can occur at any level of the vertebral column.

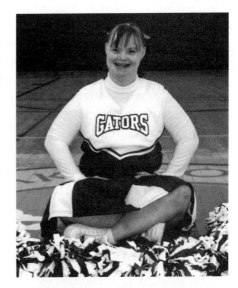

SYMPTOMS OF VERTEBRAL SUBLUXATION

Although subluxation can occur at any level of the vertebral column, it occurs less often in the thoracic part (the vertebrae in the back of the chest) of the vertebral column. (The ribs attached to the thoracic vertebrae increase stability in this part of the vertebral column.) In our practice, the cervical (neck) and lumbar (lower back) parts of the spine are more commonly affected and are more likely to cause symptoms.

Our experience has been that in the lumbar spine, the most common symptom is pain. In the cervical spine, neurological changes that occur when the spinal cord is damaged are the most common.

Symptoms of vertebral subluxation include:

- holding the head in unusual positions (cervical);
- pain (all levels);
- weakness of the arms (cervical);
- weakness of the legs (all levels);
- incontinence of urine and/or stool (all levels);
- abnormal breathing as a result of pinching of the nerves that stimulate the diaphragm to contract and cause breathing movements (cervical).

In our practice, approximately 1 percent of our patients have significant, symptomatic vertebral subluxation. Approximately 2 to 3 percent have asymptomatic vertebral subluxation—that is, x-rays have shown that the individuals' vertebrae are slipping, but they are not experiencing any of the symptoms listed above.

THE RISKS OF VERTEBRAL SUBLUXATION

If vertebral subluxation is left untreated, progressive compression of the spinal cord can occur and cause:

- permanent paralysis,
- decreased neurological drive to breath,
- death.

When symptoms occur, weakness (or paralysis) is a pretty common feature of cervical subluxation (including atlantoaxial subluxation). Sometimes the paralysis is reversible with surgery. However, once weakness has occurred, there is likely to be some permanent paralysis, even though further damage can usually be prevented and sometimes some strength can be regained. Although these symptoms are not common, we have unfortunately seen a few people with DS who did not undergo surgery lose the drive to breathe and then die.

PREVENTION OF VERTEBRAL SUBLUXATION

Many doctors believe that it is important to screen people with DS for the presence of AAI (or cervical subluxation at other levels) so that those who have the vertebral instability can avoid activities that might lead to vertebral subluxation. Others

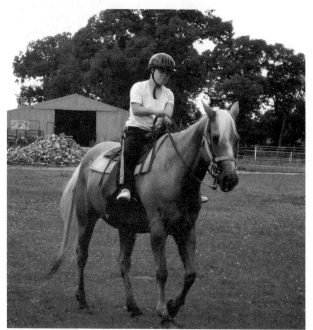

do not think screening is worthwhile. For years, medical professionals have debated whether screening x-rays should be done in people with DS who do not have symptoms.

To date, there is no clear answer based on scientific study. However, the Down Syndrome Medical Interest Group Health Screening guidelines recommend that all children with DS have a lateral cervical spine x-ray between ages two and three. That is, they should have an x-ray of the neck done from the side with the head held in its usual upright position; flexed forward; and extended backwards. Less than 5 mm of movement of C1 in reference to C2 is considered normal. Five mm or more is diagnostic for atlantoaxial instability. There isn't clear data as to when and if additional x-rays should be done.

Our approach has been to obtain a lateral cervical spine x-ray for a teen or adult with DS if the person:

- ◆ has not had a previous set;
- ◆ has any of the symptoms consistent with cervical subluxation (see below);
- ◆ is being examined as a part of a preoperative evaluation and has not had a cervical spine x-ray for a number of years.

We also consider repeating the x-rays every ten years for all of our patients for screening purposes. For patients who have had a previous borderline or mildly abnormal set of x-rays, we repeat the x-rays every one to two years. This is in addition to taking a good history and performing a neurological exam at least annually to assess for changes consistent with cervical subluxation.

Adolescents and adults with DS may also be required to have neck x-rays done before participating in sports or activities that have the potential to lead to neck injury. For example, for liability reasons, horseback riding or gymnastics programs or school physical education departments may require medical documentation that your child does not have AAI. For years, Special Olympics has required that people with DS get a pre-participation neck x-ray. The concern is that if someone has instability in the neck, then participation in certain sports could lead to a sudden, serious injury. Generally, if a person has AAI, then it is recommended that they not play contact sports, dive, tumble, or do the butterfly stroke in swimming.

The other situation in which screening is important is in a preoperative evaluation. A person who has AAI (or cervical subluxation at other levels) may develop spinal cord compression in the operating room because of positioning of the head during intubation (placing of the breathing tube). A neck x-ray is advised before surgery for those who have not previously had one. If a person does have AAI (or subluxation at other levels), the anesthesiologist will take special care by using direct visualization of the intubation with a laryngoscope.

Obviously, even if screening is carefully done and a person with AAI (or cervical subluxation at other levels) tries to avoid all activities that could cause a sudden blow to the head or movement of the neck, unforeseen injuries can occur—for instance, as the result of an automobile accident or a fall. Because of these risks, some doctors recommend treating even people with AAI who have no symptoms—to minimize chances that the spinal cord will be compressed in an accident. However, there are no data to indicate what amount of subluxation should be present in an asymptomatic individual before the possible advantage of preventing an injury outweighs the risks of surgery.

TREATMENT

When the spinal cord is being compressed, the only treatment is surgery. The vertebrae must be adjusted away from the spinal cord and then stabilized so the corrected position is maintained. The spine is stabilized with rods or screws and/or a bone graft (often from the hip). The individual may have to wear a halo for several months after the surgery. A halo is a device that is screwed into the skull with 4 screws and holds the neck stable while it heals. Several weeks to months of physical and occupational therapy may also be needed to help the person regain strength or lost skills. People who had neurologic impairment before the surgery tend to need physical therapy for several months.

If surgery is being recommended, you should have a thorough discussion with the orthopedic surgeon or neurosurgeon. Topics to be discussed include:

- ◆ What are the indications for surgery? (What symptoms or neurological findings justify proceeding with an operation?)
- ◆ What are the risks of surgery? (see below)

> ◆ How might the individual's health status affect treatment?
>> ➤ Can he physically tolerate surgery?
>> ➤ Are there other serious underlying health issues that are likely to significantly shorten his life before the benefits of surgery could be experienced?
>> ➤ Will the person be able to participate in the rehabilitation process after surgery? This question should be asked particularly for someone who does not have evidence of spinal cord compression or neurological injury but does have significant subluxation. If the person cannot participate in the recovery and rehabilitation process, the surgery and the period of time being incapacitated after the surgery can lead to a temporary loss of skills or function that can become permanent. In a sense, sometimes these individuals have the problem corrected, but don't recover from the process of having the problem corrected.

In the past, surgeons have reported a very high rate of complications during and after neck surgery. One study even quoted a 40 percent mortality rate for people with DS. However, at Advocate Lutheran General Hospital (the hospital the ADSC is associated with), we have been fortunate to have a very fine surgical team, as well as superb teams in the surgical intensive care unit and on the orthopedic unit. While there have been some complications, the rate of complications is much lower than previously described. We have developed an improved understanding of the potential problems. Complications include:

- difficulty weaning the person off the ventilator,
- swallowing problems,
- pneumonia,
- infections,
- worsening of neurologic functions (for example, weakness, gait unsteadiness),
- pulmonary embolism (blood clot to the lung),
- persistent pain, and, rarely,
- death.

When a person has developed neurologic symptoms due to spinal cord compression, surgical correction may improve function. However, often the best result obtained is prevention of further loss of neurologic function. It seems that the longer the spinal cord is compressed and the more damage the spinal cord suffers, the less likely the person's neurologic function will be completely restored.

To help optimize the results of the surgery, we sometimes recommend additional preoperative exams and testing, over and above the usual ones (which include a recent thyroid blood test for people with DS). We consider having the following assessments done before the operation, based on the individual's health history and physical exam:

- an echocardiogram or cardiac clearance by a cardiologist for anyone with a history of heart problems;
- a swallowing evaluation (to anticipate swallowing problems after the operation);
- a sleep study (to assess for sleep apnea, which is more common in people with DS and can cause significant problems post-operatively, especially if undiagnosed);
- a consult with a neurologist to assess for other neurologic problems that may be contributing to the symptoms.

SCOLIOSIS

Due to lax ligaments, scoliosis (abnormal curvature of the spine) is more common in people with DS. This is generally a bigger concern in childhood and early adolescence than in adulthood. If the curvature is diagnosed before the person stops growing, it can often be minimized by having the individual wear a brace.

Although scoliosis is more common in people with DS, we have seen few patients with untreated significant abnormal curvature. Untreated, severe scoliosis can cause breathing difficulty if the curve makes it harder to expand the lungs. It can also cause pressure on the spinal cord.

If scoliosis is severe enough to cause these problems, the spine can be surgically straightened. This surgery carries some of the same risks as operating on the spine for AAI (discussed above). However, surgery for scoliosis is more often done in the thoracic and lumbar region of the spine and not the upper cervical region, so it is less likely that the nerves that drive breathing would be affected. The recovery period is long, so if surgery is suggested, parents and caregivers should ask similar questions about the indications and risks of surgery as described above for AAI.

BUNIONS

The joint where the big toe is attached to the foot is subjected to great pressure during the course of normal walking. Over time, the big toe can turn so that the tip of the toe points toward the second toe. The big toe then bears weight at an unusual angle. The joint degenerates and a bulge appears on the inside (medial part) of the foot. This condition is known as a bunion (hallux valgus).

Bunions appear to be more common in people with DS, probably because of laxity of the joint. Bunions can cause discomfort and make it harder to walk. Interestingly, despite significant deformity, many people with DS who have bunions complain of little or no pain and appear to have minimal loss of function.

Treatment includes:

- wearing wider shoes;

  ◆ avoiding high heels (because they put increased stress on the joint);
  ◆ soaking the feet in warm water to reduce pain;
  ◆ using anti-inflammatory medications or acetaminophen (see below, under treatment for osteoarthritis);
  ◆ using pads or inserts to reduce or relieve discomfort at pressure points.

If symptoms persist despite these measures, we recommend a consultation with a podiatrist or orthopedic surgeon who provides foot care. Surgery can correct the deformity, relieve the symptoms, and improve function.

There are many different surgical approaches. Usually, however, surgery involves some cutting and repositioning of the bones. Pins or screws are usually used to hold the bones in place. It can take several weeks to months for recovery. A wheelchair, walker or crutches, or a cane may be necessary during recovery. If both feet have bunions, some surgeons recommend doing one foot at a time so walking will be less affected. Others recommend doing both feet at the same time because walking will be affected either way and the person will only have to have to go through surgery once.

Sometimes bunions recur following surgery. This does appear to occur more often in people with DS, probably due to laxity of the joint.

Because of the possibility of recurrence, we recommend beginning with conservative therapy for treating bunions (wider shoes, ibuprofen, foot soak). We recommend surgery if these other measures are inadequate and there are significant symptoms or loss of function that would justify the discomfort of surgery.

PROBLEMS WITH THE KNEECAP

Another joint that can have increased laxity and cause problems for people with DS is the patella (knee cap). The patella acts as a fulcrum. It is attached to muscles in the upper and lower leg and helps transmit the power of the large muscles in the front of our thighs to extend our lower legs. The patella should track nicely through the groove formed by two large protrusions (medial and lateral epicondyle) at the bottom end of the femur (the large thigh bone where it connects with the knee). For visualization purposes, make a fist with your left hand. Look at the knuckles of the index and middle finger. The two knuckles can be compared to the medial and lateral condyles of the femur. Sending the index finger of your right hand through the groove between the two knuckles of your left hand is how the patella should glide between the two condyles.

Unfortunately, it is more common in people with DS for the patella to track a little bit out of the groove; usually toward the outside of the knee. In the hand analogy, if you move your index finger a little bit to one side, and then try to glide it, it bumps into your knuckle. Similarly, the patella bumps into the condyle. This can be uncomfortable in itself, put additional stress on the knee (and hip), and can eventually cause wear on the backside of the patella. Knee pain that results from the patella tracking poorly is called *patella-femoral syndrome.* When the posterior part (back side) of the patella becomes damaged, it is called *chondromalacia* of the patella.

Steps in prevention and treatment of patella-femoral syndrome include:
- ◆ wearing a good supportive shoe (one with appropriate arch support that fits snugly with laces or Velcro straps, rather than a slip-on or flip flops);
- ◆ strengthening the muscles of the thigh, especially the muscles of the inner thigh near the knee, using exercises such as:
  - ➤ ball squeezing: Put a slightly deflated volleyball, soccer ball, or basketball between the knees and squeeze.
  - ➤ terminal extension exercises: Sit in a chair with one foot off the floor a few inches. Lift the foot, bring the foot upwards, and straighten the lower leg so the knee is straight. Slowly return the foot to a few inches off the floor. Repeat. Once the individual can do 2 or 3 repetitions of about 20 lifts each, add light weights to the ankle.

Sometimes the kneecap will move far to the side of the knee and become stuck out of position. This is usually due to sudden trauma or force on the knee, such as a fall or a forceful blow to the knee. This is called *dislocation of the patella.* It can be quite painful. The kneecap needs to be pushed back into place. The person or his parent or caregiver may be able to gently push it back into place but this may need to be done by a doctor. Sometimes a muscle relaxant needs to be injected to relax the thigh muscles so the patella can be put back into place.

If someone is prone to dislocated kneecaps, he can try wearing a knee brace and/or try physical therapy (PT) to help prevent recurrences. If the patella becomes dislocated repeatedly despite a brace and physical therapy, surgery can be done to prevent recurrences. Consult with an orthopedic surgeon if this surgery is recommended to find out about risks and recovery times. PT will probably be needed after the surgery.

OVERPRONATION OF THE ANKLE

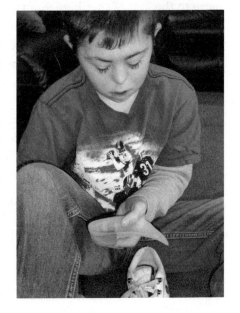

In normal walking, our foot lands on the outside of the heel, then the rest of the foot strikes the ground, and we roll the foot inward so the push-off for the next step comes primarily from the big toe. Some people roll their feet too far inward. This is called overpronation. It is often associated with flat feet. Significant overpronation can cause foot, ankle, knee, hip, and even back pain.

Overpronation seems to be more common in people with DS. A physical exam is usually enough to make the diagnosis.

Treatment involves preventing the foot from rolling too far. Ways to achieve this include:

♦ Wear shoes designed for overpronators. Running shoes come in many varieties and some are made with a sturdier medial (near the arch) part. Consult a knowledgeable person at your local running shoe store or you local shoe store.

♦ Use an insert (inserted in the shoe) that supports the arch and limits overpronation. These can be purchased at a shoe or sports store.

♦ Use a custom orthotic that fits inside the shoe. These are usually obtained from a podiatrist. He or she will make a cast (mold) of the foot and have an orthotic made specifically for the person's foot.

ORTHOPEDIC PROBLEMS ASSOCIATED WITH AGING

As discussed in Chapter 4, the aging process seems to be speeded up in adults with DS. That is, adults with DS are subject to the usual health problems associated with aging, but tend to develop these problems twenty or even thirty years earlier than other people do. In aging people in general, there are many health problems related to deterioration of joints that can result in orthopedic problems; adults with DS can develop any or all of these, sometimes long before they would be considered "elderly."

OSTEOARTHRITIS/OSTEOARTHROSES

Arthritis in general means inflammation of the joint. Osteoarthritis, the type of arthritis commonly associated with aging, occurs when the cartilage lining the end of the bone is damaged. It is more correctly called osteoarthroses because it is related more to the loss of cartilage, but there may be some inflammation as well.

Osteoarthritis is more common in people with DS. Even in their twenties and thirties, many people with DS have x-rays that demonstrate arthritic changes such as bony changes and narrowing of the joint. These changes may be related to the early aging associated with DS.

Interestingly, even when their x-rays show significant signs of arthritis, many adults with DS don't complain of pain. As previously discussed, people with DS often have a greater pain tolerance (or decreased pain perception). This may be the reason that pain is not a complaint despite the x-ray findings.

Some adults with DS do complain of pain. Others don't complain of pain but change the way they use the affected joint. For example, someone with arthritis in the hip may be noted to be limping. This may mean that the person feels pain, even though he is not complaining about it. It may also mean that the arthritis has progressed far enough to actually affect the function of the joint. For example, the person may be limping because the arthritis has damaged the joint to a point where it no longer works properly.

Osteoarthritis tends to run in families, so there is probably a genetic component to it. Having DS also puts people at greater risk of developing osteoarthritis. This may be for a number of reasons:

- If the person is obese, increased weight puts more stress on, and causes more trauma to, joints.
- Loose joints are more at risk for injury. In turn, a joint that has been injured is at greater risk for developing arthritis.
- There may be other factors genetically coded on the 21st chromosome that increase risk.

The diagnosis is made based on the person's history and physical exam. X-rays may also be done to look for changes of the joint and the bones. Sometimes an MRI is done to look for other (nonarthritic) changes in the joint. For example, sometimes a *torn meniscus*—the fibrous cushion in the knee—will cause pain and changes in function that mimic the symptoms of arthritis.

TREATMENT OF OSTEOARTHRITIS

Treatment can reduce discomfort and improve function. Treatment can also help individuals who have decreased function of a joint due to osteoarthritis but who don't complain of discomfort. Treatment includes:

- Anti-inflammatory medications such as ibuprofen (Advil, Motrin) and naproxen (Naprosyn, Aleve). These can be given "prn" (as needed for symptoms) or can be given on a regular schedule. Scheduled dosing eliminates the person having to regularly ask for the medication. A trial of scheduled dosing of anti-inflammatory medicine can be particularly helpful when the person does not complain of pain but only has a functional change. A scheduled dosing eliminates the need to figure out when to give the medication and allows a period of time to figure out if it does provide benefit. These medications should be given with food to reduce possible stomach upset. They can also be given with medications to reduce acid in the stomach, including H_2 blockers such as ranitidine or famotidine or proton pump inhibitors such as omeprazole (see Chapter 11) or misoprostol (Cytotec). These can be considered if the person has a history of gastroesophageal reflux (GERD) or ulcers or develops upset stomach with the anti-inflammatory medication.
- Acetaminophen (Tylenol). Acetaminophen can also provide symptom relief. It can be used as needed or scheduled just as with the anti-inflammatory medications.
- Avoidance of activity that increases stress to the problematic joints.
- Physical activity and physical therapy. Good general fitness, improving the strength of muscles around an affected joint, and maintaining or reaching ideal body weight can all help improve symptoms

and function of arthritic joints. If an arthritic joint limits activity, a person's overall general fitness level will progressively worsen. Consultation with a physical therapist may also be helpful. Often times the person "favors" the affected joint, causing the muscles around it to weaken. This can lead to even greater disability. A physical therapist can help evaluate the problem and recommend a plan to maximize function, strength, and mobility of the joint.

◆ Occupational therapy. An occupational therapist can recommend modifications in ways of performing tasks, adaptive equipment that can improve function, safety precautions to prevent further injury, and can provide other advice to limit the disability caused by the arthritis.

If these treatments are not sufficient, additional considerations for diagnoses and treatment include:

◆ further imaging tests, such as MRI to assess for other damage within the joint which might require a different treatment;

◆ consultation with a rheumatologist—a medical doctor who specializes in diagnosis and treatment of arthritis—or with an orthopedic surgeon or sports medicine physician;

◆ narcotic pain medication (such as Vicodin);

◆ injections of corticosteroids into the joint (it is recommended to limit these injections to perhaps no more than 3 injections per year up to a maximum of 12 injections per joint);

◆ injection of hyaluronic acid (which is thought to temporarily restore normal properties of fluid in the joint);

◆ chiropractic treatment (some individuals report reduced discomfort with manipulation).

SPINAL STENOSIS

Subluxation is not the only reason the spinal cord can become compressed. One of the changes associated with arthritis is the development of bony outgrowths, called osteophytes. In the spine, as these outgrowths develop, they can cause the spinal canal to narrow, even to the point of putting pressure on the spinal cord. This can cause the same symptoms seen with cervical subluxation, described above.

As with subluxation of the vertebrae, spinal stenosis can occur at any level of the vertebral column. Again, the cervical and lumbar areas tend to be more common sites for problems in people with DS.

Although the risk of sudden compression of the spinal cord seems to be less of a concern with spinal stenosis than with atlanoaxial instability (AAI), the stenosis can get progressively worse (albeit usually slowly) and cause damage to the spinal cord.

Similar to AAI, the diagnosis is made through history, physical, and neck x-rays. The neck x-rays won't show subluxation (unless the person has both spinal stenosis and subluxation). If the history and physical exam suggest spinal cord injury, an MRI of the spinal cord should be done (even if the x-rays don't show concerning findings).

Treatment for spinal stenosis includes:

- anti-inflammatory medications such as ibuprofen and narcotic pain medications to reduce discomfort;
- epidural spinal injections (injections of steroids next to the covering around the spinal column) to reduce inflammation and symptoms;
- physical therapy.

If the problem progresses, does not respond to the above measures, or causes significant neurological impairment, surgery may be needed. Surgical intervention is similar to that for subluxation. There are some differences in the surgical procedures, but the potential complications and challenges are similar.

OSTEOPOROSIS

Osteoporosis, or "thinning of the bones," is a problem that we all experience to one degree or another as we age. The concern about osteoporosis lies in the fractures that

Changes in Gait

When an adolescent or adult with DS begins walking differently (more slowly, more awkwardly, with a limp), it is important to look for the reasons for this change in gait. As previously mentioned, there are several orthopedic problems that can lead to changes in gait: subluxation or stenosis in the vertebral columns, bunions, overpronation, and osteoarthritis If an orthopedic problem is suspected, the focus should be on the joint or joints that are causing discomfort. Further investigation is needed, possibly including x-rays of any joint that doesn't seem to be functioning normally or that the person appears to favor.

If no orthopedic problem is discovered, there are other conditions that are fairly common in DS that should be investigated. These include:

- an inner ear problem, leading to balance problems;
- painfully cracked skin on the soles of the feet;
- boils in the groin area;
- balanitis (inflammation of the glans of the penis) or posthitis (inflammation of the foreskin of the penis) (see Chapter 12);
- worsening vision due to cataracts or other causes;
- dizziness due to celiac disease, low blood pressure, or medication side effects;
- sexual abuse.

Especially if the individual is not usually able to tell others verbally when he is experiencing pain or is experiencing a change in functioning, a change of gait should always be regarded as an indication that something is wrong.

may occur because of the weaker bones. More than one-third of adult women in the general population will sustain a fracture in their lifetime as a result of having osteoporosis. Men are also susceptible to osteoporosis but not as much as women are. In particular, the decrease in estrogen after menopause increases the rate of osteoporosis in women.

There is some evidence that suggests that adults with DS of both sexes are more at risk for osteoporosis. In addition, osteoporosis runs in families. Osteoporosis is more common in:

- ◆ whites and Asians (less common in African Americans and Latinos),
- ◆ women than in men,
- ◆ people with lean body type, especially low body weight,
- ◆ individuals who consume inadequate calcium or vitamin D,
- ◆ individuals who consume too much phosphate or protein,
- ◆ people who are physically inactive,
- ◆ people who smoke, drink more than two alcoholic beverages per day, or have a high caffeine intake,
- ◆ people with certain medical conditions, including celiac disease (see Chapter 11),
- ◆ individuals taking certain medications, including corticosteroids such as prednisone (for greater than 3 months), medroxyprogesterone (Depoprovera), chronic heparin, seizure medications (dilantin, Phenobarbital), chemotherapy, tamoxifen, and lithium,
- ◆ those receiving radiation therapy.

PREVENTION OF OSTEOPOROSIS

Although all of us will get some degree of osteoporosis if we live long enough, there are several relatively simple steps that can be taken to build up bone strength and slow down the loss of bone. These include getting enough of the right kinds of exercise and including adequate amounts of calcium and vitamin D in the diet

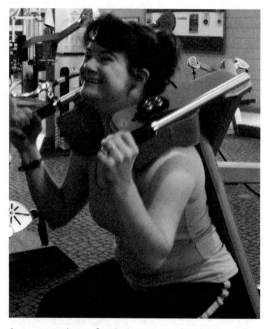

Exercise: Regular exercise is important. Weight-bearing activities, such as walking, jogging, dancing, and aerobics improve skeletal (bone) health. Non-weight-bearing activities, such as swimming, improve well-being and increase confidence and coordination. Although non-weight-bearing exercises don't improve bone density, they may help the individual be more fit so he can participate in weight-bearing exercises and also improve balance to help prevent falls that can lead to fractures.

It is important to exercise starting at a young age. It is much more difficult to improve bone density at an older age than it is to improve/maintain bone density throughout life. In addition to participating in exercises like walking, some weight lifting can help improve bone density. Adding some light hand weights to aerobics, dancing, or walking can benefit the entire body.

Nutritional Advice: Adequate amounts of vitamin D and calcium are crucial to bone health and to slowing or preventing osteoporosis.

The Recommended Daily Allowance for vitamin D ranges from 200 International Units (IU) for children to 600 IU for older adults. Some regular exposure to sunlight also helps. Exposure of our skin to sunlight (UV rays) triggers the body to synthesize Vitamin D. Unfortunately, it is difficult to get adequate sun exposure (especially in colder climates) to make enough vitamin D. Therefore, it is usually necessary to take in additional vitamin D through diet and supplementation. However, very few foods in nature contain vitamin D. Good sources are fish, such as salmon, tuna, and mackerel, as well as fish liver oils. Smaller amounts are found in cheese, egg yolks, and beef liver. Foods that are fortified with vitamin D are also good sources.

Some foods that are fortified with Vitamin D include:
- milk,
- cheese,
- yogurt,
- juices, and
- cereals.

It is important to review nutrition labels to check whether a particular food is vitamin D fortified. We have found many people with DS to be vitamin D deficient. You may want to discuss blood testing for vitamin D level with your physician. (The test to order is 25-hydroxy Vitamin D.) Additional supplementation may be appropriate if the person is deficient.

Adequate calcium intake is also important. For men and pre-menopausal women, a daily intake of 1000 mg of calcium is recommended. For menopausal woman, 1500 mg of calcium is recommended. As with vitamin D, it can also be difficult to get enough calcium in the diet. Foods that are a good source of calcium include:
- dairy (milk, yogurt, cheese),
- leafy green vegetables (broccoli, kale, spinach),
- fruits (oranges, tangerines, blackberries, dried fruit such as raisins),
- beans and peas (tofu, peanuts, peas, black beans, baked beans),
- fish (salmon, sardines),
- others (sesame seeds, blackstrap molasses, corn tortillas, almonds, brown sugar).

It can be difficult to get enough calcium and vitamin D in the diet. For example, it takes about three servings of milk or dairy equivalents daily to get enough calcium

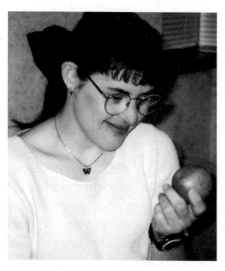

and vitamin D. If dietary intake is inadequate, teens and adults with DS should take a calcium and vitamin D supplement. Keep in mind that calcium seems to be best absorbed if taken at the same time as vitamin D and taken throughout the day, rather than all at once.

Hormones and Medications: After women reach menopause, there is an increased risk of osteoporosis due to decreased estrogen. In women who have reached menopause, estrogen replacement therapy is available to help maintain bone strength. However, studies have now found an increase in other health problems in women who take hormones. Therefore, we generally don't prescribe hormones for bone health in menopausal women with DS. Instead, we emphasize the exercise and dietary strategies described above. We also consider a referral to a dietitian or nutritionist if the woman is having trouble eating the right types of foods, or a referral to a physical therapist if she has trouble with movements or inadequate strength needed for bone health.

DIAGNOSIS OF OSTEOPOROSIS

A special type of x-ray known as a DEXA (dual-energy x-ray absorptiometry) scan is used to diagnose both osteoporosis and thinning of the bone that can lead to osteoporosis. This is a painless scan that requires the person to lie still for about five to ten minutes.

We recommend starting them once a woman has reached menopause. We also recommend them when we diagnose celiac disease and for those on high-risk medications. If the DEXA is normal, we consider repeating it in a few years.

The score on the scan is called a T-score. It is a comparison to the average score for a young, healthy person. The number is the number of standard deviations (a statistical measure) the person's score differs from the average of the young, healthy individuals. The results are classified as:
- ◆ normal, if the T-score is –1.0 and above,
- ◆ osteopenia, if between –1.0 and –2.4,
- ◆ osteoporosis, if less than or equal to –2.5.

Osteopenia means that there has been some thinning of the bones, but not to the extent seen in osteoporosis. The risk for fracture is not as great but it certainly is a warning stage to work on improving bone health.

TREATMENT OF OSTEOPOROSIS AND OSTEOPENIA

The goal of treatment is to increase bone density and to reduce fractures that are associated with decreased bone density.

Osteopenia: Treatment for osteopenia includes the measures outlined in the section on prevention. A repeat scan should be done in one or two years to assess whether the bones have improved or whether the disease has progressed.

Osteoporosis: Treatment for osteoporosis also includes all of the recommendations in the prevention section. In addition, the following medications should be considered:

- Biophosphates such as alendronate (Fosamax), risedronate (Actonel), and ibandronate (Boniva): These should be taken with a full glass of water first thing in the morning, 30 minutes before the first food or drink. Afterwards, the person should avoid lying down for 30 minutes. These medications have been shown to increase bone density and reduce fractures. However, they can cause inflammation and bleeding in the esophagus. They have also been implicated in *osteonecrosis* (damage to the bone) of the jaw. Various forms of these medications can be taken daily, weekly or monthly.
- Calcitonin: This is a medication given as a nasal spray that has been shown to increase bone density but not reduce fractures. One spray is given each day and nostrils are alternated (give in one nostril one day, the other the next day).
- Raloxifene (Evista): This medication effects estrogen receptors. It has been shown to increase bone density and to decrease vertebral fractures but not hip fractures. It can cause blood clots in the legs or lungs. (We have seen an increased susceptibility to blood clots in our patients with DS who are on birth control pills, so we don't usually use Evista because of the blood clot concerns).
- Teriparatide (Forteo): It promotes new bone formation and reduces vertebral fractures. It requires a daily injection and to date we have not used it with our patients with DS.

Osteoporosis can be a very serious medical problem that can lead to very disabling, and even life-threatening, fractures. Regular exercise and good nutrition are readily available preventative measures for people of all ages.

AUTOIMMUNE ARTHRITIS CONDITIONS

Autoimmune conditions are diseases in which the body's immune system attacks parts of the body, similar to the way the body fights an invading germ. These types of diseases are thought to be more common in people with DS. Some of these conditions can cause arthritis. Arthritis due to an autoimmune condition is different from osteoarthritis. These conditions include:

- **rheumatoid arthritis:** an inflammatory condition that causes:
  - morning stiffness of joints,
  - swelling of the joints (especially the hands and wrists) that is associated with pain,

> ➤ nodules (swellings) under the skin,
> ➤ damage to the joints,
> ➤ an elevation of the Rheumatoid factor (detected with a blood test), and sometimes
> ➤ symptoms not associated with the joints.

Lab Tests for Autoimmune Conditions

One indication that a person with DS may have an autoimmune disorder is an elevated level of globulins in his blood work. Globulins are proteins in the blood that help fight infections. They can be abnormally elevated in inflammatory conditions such as autoimmune diseases. However, elevated globulins may also indicate the presence of another disorder, or may be normal for that particular individual.

It is not uncommon to find an elevation of globulins on blood work drawn from a person with DS. An elevated globulin can be indicative of many health issues:

- ◆ autoimmune conditions such as rheumatoid arthritis, systemic lupus erythematosus, and others;
- ◆ liver disease;
- ◆ acute inflammation/infection;
- ◆ multiple myeloma (malignant tumor of the plasma cells—plasma cells are formed in the bone marrow, are released into the bloodstream, and produce globulins to help fight infections);
- ◆ celiac disease (as indicated in Chapter 11, we have found several people with an elevated globulin to have celiac disease).

Anabolic steroids, as well as estrogen and progesterone (for example, in birth control pills), can also cause an increase in the globulin level.

If globulin levels are high, follow-up testing will be done. This usually involves sending a blood sample and possibly a urine sample to assess the subtypes of globulins. These tests are called serum protein electrophoreses and urine protein electrophoresis. In addition, specific urine testing for multiple myeloma (urine for Bence-Jones protein) may also be done, or blood tests for celiac disease. Additional testing for other autoimmune conditions may also be indicated. The decision to do these or other tests may be based on the findings in the history, physical exam, or other lab tests.

Most often, we have found the result of the serum protein electrophoresis to be non-specific (that is, no clear disease is found). The decision to do additional testing in that situation is again based on findings in the history, physical exam, and other lab tests, as well as the physician's suspicion that there may be a underlying problem. Sometimes, however, we just conclude that the person with DS has no abnormal conditions that explain the elevated globulins.

- **systemic lupus erythematosus:** a condition that affects multiple organ systems and causes:
  - ➤ inflammation of the joints,
  - ➤ fever,
  - ➤ decreased appetite,
  - ➤ weight loss,
  - ➤ skin lesions,
  - ➤ muscle aches,
  - ➤ neurologic symptoms including confusion, and
  - ➤ many other possible symptoms.
- **psoriatic arthritis:** an arthritis condition that sometimes occurs in people who have psoriasis (see Chapter 6). Symptoms include:
  - ➤ psoriasis skin lesions,
  - ➤ arthritis with joint swelling and pain,
  - ➤ changes of the nails (pitting, discoloration, separation of the nail bed from the underlying tissue),
  - ➤ fever,
  - ➤ fatigue,
  - ➤ other symptoms.

Rheumatoid arthritis can occur in childhood as well as adulthood. Systemic lupus and psoriatic arthritis more commonly occur in adulthood.

These conditions are diagnosed through history and physical as well as blood work and, often, x-rays.

The treatment approaches for osteoarthritis discussed earlier in the chapter can be used to reduce the joint pain associated with these autoimmune conditions. There are also a number of medications available that can prevent these diseases from worsening by reducing the immune system action on the joint. These treatments include:

- ◆ methotrexate,
- ◆ steroids (e.g., prednisone),
- ◆ hyroxychloroquine,
- ◆ azathioprine,
- ◆ infliximab (Remicade),
- ◆ adalimumab (Humira),
- ◆ and others.

It is now recognized that early treatment with these medications can prevent damage to the joints. Consider a consultation with a rheumatologist early in the course of the disease for advice on, and treatment of, one of these autoimmune arthritis conditions.

Chapter 14

Cancer

· · · · · · · ·

When she was 47, Janice had an unexpected weight loss. Her bowel movements had become smaller in size and she often had diarrhea. She was evaluated by her local physician, who sent her for a CBC (blood count), chemistry panel, and thyroid blood tests. The only abnormality found was that her hemoglobin was low. Additional testing determined that her anemia was due to iron deficiency.

Janice's physician referred her to a gastroenterologist, who recommended a colonoscopy to assess for colon cancer. Janice and her parents came to the Adult Down Syndrome Center for our opinion prior to consenting to the colonoscopy. We discussed the lower incidence of colon cancer in people with Down syndrome. We also discussed the higher incidence of celiac disease. We then drew blood work for celiac disease. The results were borderline—not clearly consistent with celiac disease. We agreed with the plan to proceed with colonoscopy. Particularly since Janice would require general anesthesia for the procedure, we recommended that she also undergo an upper endoscopy (EGD) with a small bowel biopsy to test for celiac disease while under general anesthesia.

Fortunately, the colonoscopy was normal and no colon cancer was found. The upper endoscopy (EGD) also did not show any abnormalities, but the biopsy of the small intestine was abnormal and consistent with celiac disease. Janice started taking oral iron supplements and switched to a gluten-free diet. Her anemia and diarrhea resolved and her weight returned to normal.

Many people are aware that leukemia is more common in children with Down syndrome (DS). There are also a few other cancers that are more common in people with DS. However, studies have found that many other forms of cancer are less common in people with DS than in the general population. It has been postulated that an extra copy of the gene Ets2 on the 21st chromosome may repress cancer (Reeves Nature, 2008). Other genes are also being evaluated to determine whether they are involved in decreasing cancer incidence in people with DS.

It is important to be aware of the relative rarity of the different types of cancer when making decisions about healthcare for people with DS. In the example of Janice, our knowledge that colon cancer is less common in people with DS led us to look for another cause for her iron deficiency anemia. In contrast, in older people who do not have DS, colon cancer is near the top of the list of diseases to assess for if iron deficiency anemia is diagnosed. In that situation, proceeding with the colonoscopy alone as the initial step could be appropriate.

Another important point related to Janice's case story is that she did undergo the colonoscopy to assess for colon cancer. Although DS does appear to protect against developing cancer, it doesn't completely eliminate the risk. In addition, as the life spans of adults with DS continue to increase, it will be important to continue to monitor to see whether the incidence of cancers (which often increases with age) increases. For now, however, our approach is guided by the knowledge that most cancers are less common in people with DS, but that cancer is not nonexistent in people with DS.

LESS COMMON CANCERS

A number of cancers seem to be less common in DS. These cancers are associated with solid tumors—masses of abnormal tissue that do not contain cysts or liquid areas. The following are examples of types of cancers that appear to be less common:

◆ brain tumors,
◆ lung cancer,
◆ colon cancer,
◆ stomach cancer,
◆ prostate cancer,
◆ kidney cancer, and
◆ breast cancer.

Again, it is not out of the realm of possibility that an adult with DS would develop one of these types of cancer. Signs that someone might have one of these types of cancer (a breast lump, blood in the stool, difficulty urinating, etc.) should not be ignored. In addition, if there is a family history of a particular type of cancer, this should always be mentioned to the doctor so that he or she can make a note of it in the medical history and determine whether screening tests are warranted.

More Common Cancers

Leukemia

A few types of cancer are more common in people with DS than in the general population. For example, research has shown that leukemia is more common in children with DS. Several studies have indicated that the incidence is increased only in the first few years of life, but studies have indicated that the increased incidence lasts until the late teens. By adulthood, however, the incidence of leukemia is no longer higher than usual.

Leukemia is cancer that causes an increase in the formation and accumulation of abnormal immature blood cells. For example, a normal white blood cell count is in the 5,000 to 11,000 range. In leukemia, the count can be over 100,000. In a patient with leukemia, the white blood cells are immature, don't function as well as usual, and accumulate in the bone marrow and other locations. When this happens, the bone marrow is not able to produce other cells (red blood cells and platelets).

Symptoms of leukemia include:

- ◆ fever,
- ◆ infections (including serious, life-threatening infections),
- ◆ bleeding and bruising, often with no apparent cause,
- ◆ bone pain,
- ◆ fatigue,
- ◆ enlarged liver, spleen, and lymph nodes.

The primary treatment is chemotherapy. Chemotherapy may involve intravenous injections, intramuscular injections, and/or oral medications. There are likely to be several cycles of medications given over several months. Supportive therapy is also essential. Supportive therapy includes good nutrition, adequate hydration, prompt treatment of infections, and transfusions as needed (e.g., platelets and red blood cells). Sometimes, a bone marrow transplant may also be needed.

Although children with DS are more likely to get leukemia, they also respond better to treatment. The survival rate for acute myelogenous leukemia (AML) is about 85 percent for children with Down syndrome, which is greater than for children without Down syndrome. The survival rate for acute lymphocytic leukemia (ALL), however, is similar for the two groups.

Adults (without DS) who survived childhood leukemia have an increased risk for other medical conditions, especially musculoskeletal, cardiac, and neurologic conditions. This risk is particularly high for those who had radiation therapy, which is less often used now to treat leukemia. Less information is available about adults with DS who survived childhood leukemia. However, since they *may* also be at higher risk of these medical conditions, it may be prudent to monitor for these conditions, particularly if the adult received any radiation therapy. It is important to mention to any health care practitioner unfamiliar with the person's history that she is a leukemia survivor and discuss the treatments she received.

CANCER OF THE TESTICLE

Cancer of the testicle—the male organ that produces sperm and hormones such as testosterone—is more common in men with DS. Fortunately, cancer of the testicle can usually be found on a physical exam.

There are two reasons that cancer of the testicle is more common in men with DS:
1. Cancer of the testicle appears to be linked to having Down syndrome.
2. The incidence of cancer of the testicle is higher in men who have (or had) an undescended testicle, and undescended testicles are more common in males with DS.

Before a boy is born, his testicles are in his abdomen. Ordinarily, they migrate into his scrotum, their normal position, before birth. Sometimes, however, the testicles have not migrated into the scrotum by the time a boy is born. If they have not descended at birth, they often will do so by three months of age. However, in boys with DS born with undescended testicles, they more commonly don't descend at all.

Treatment for an undescended testicle is to surgically (under general anesthesia in the operating room) bring the testicle(s) into the scrotum. However, even if brought down into the scrotum surgically, there remains a higher incidence of cancer. If the surgery is done, however, the testicles can be palpated during the physical exam, making it easier to detect cancerous lumps.

If an adolescent or adult male has not had one or both testicles surgically brought down into the scrotum as a young child, the recommended treatment is usually to surgically remove the testicle. Alternatively, regular screening with a CT (computed tomography) scan or ultrasound may be considered. Although this does not prevent the development of cancer, it may enable it to be detected sooner.

It should be noted that the fertility of an undescended testicle is reduced even if surgically corrected. However, the longer the testicle remains undescended, the worse the fertility. This means that surgery to bring an adult's testicle into the scrotum may not improve his fertility, and the testicle will still be at greater risk for developing cancer.

Fortunately, cancer of the testicle is generally curable, particularly if found early. In addition, no invasive testing is needed for screening (if both testicles are descended). Reviewing the appropriate history from the patient and family and a good physical exam are the evaluations that are required to screen for testicular cancer.

Self-examination can also be useful in detecting testicular cancer. Teaching a man how to examine his testicles and the abnormalities to palpate (feel) for can be part of the annual physical exam. However, many men with DS have trouble understanding what changes they should be checking for. Some men with DS also find discussions about testicular cancer or testicular abnormalities disturbing. They can become overly focused on the exam and perseverate about their concern of finding an abnormality. These challenges make it especially important for men with DS to have a testicular exam performed by a medical practitioner each year.

The exam by a medical practitioner is the key component of the evaluation. The findings that require further assessment include:

- an enlarged testicle,
- a change in the texture (firmer, harder),
- a palpable mass or lump.

Testicular cancer is usually painless. However, sometimes the abnormality is inadvertently found after a man sustains an injury that causes a painful testicle. If an abnormality is found on the exam, an ultrasound of the testicles can be helpful in further assessment. This is a painless procedure. Referral to a urologist is recommended to confirm the abnormality and to discuss treatment. If cancer is suspected, CT scans and blood tests will be ordered to check for possible spread of the disease.

Treatment of testicular cancer (and a mass suspected to be cancer) involves surgically removing the testicle. An incision is made in the groin, the testicle is pulled out of the scrotum, and surgically removed. In other words, even if a mass is suspected of being cancerous, the testicle is removed completely and not biopsied. This is because there are concerns that taking a biopsy of the testicle (while the testicle is still in the body) may cause spread of the cancer.

After surgery, radiation and/or chemotherapy may be recommended. Regular follow-up care with a urologist and/or oncologist (a physician who specializes in treating cancer) is recommended to monitor for the spread of the disease that could not be previously detected. If both testicles are removed, testosterone supplements may be needed.

Since removing a testicle impairs fertility, collection of sperm prior to surgery may be considered if there is a chance the patient might like to try to father a child in the future. See Chapter 16 for information about male fertility.

LYMPHOMA

Some data suggest that lymphoma may be more common in people with DS. Lymphoma is a cancer of the lymph system, which ordinarily has several functions, including helping the body fight infections. Lymph nodes are present in many areas in the body, including the neck, in the axilla (armpits), in the abdomen, and in the groin. The lymph nodes most commonly noted (in people without lymphoma) are the ones in the neck, which often become inflamed and enlarged with an upper respiratory infection or sore throat.

People who develop lymphoma usually present with one or more enlarged lymph nodes. These enlarged lymph nodes may be first noted when the person has an illness or infection, but they persist. Sometimes the enlarged lymph nodes may be found in the absence of an infection. Other symptoms include:

- chest pain,
- unexplained weight loss,

◆ recurring fevers,
◆ night sweats,
◆ fatigue,
◆ rashes (which can be anywhere on the body)
◆ lower back pain.

Treatment of lymphoma consists of one or more of the following:
◆ chemotherapy,
◆ radiation,
◆ biologic treatments (such as injections of cytokines or antibodies) to stimulate the body's immune system to fight the tumor.

There are many subtypes of lymphoma. The cure rate of lymphoma depends on the type, the person's age, the stage of the lymphoma (how far the cancer has progressed), and the individual's overall health. Although there is not much information available as to the prognosis for adults with DS, the survival rate in some situations for people without DS is as high as 95 percent. The earlier treatment is begun, the better the prognosis. So, it's very important to seek medical attention as soon as enlarged lymph nodes are found.

MALIGNANT MELANOMA

There is some speculation that malignant melanoma may also be more common in people with DS. It is a cancer of the cells of the melanocytes. Melanocytes are the pigment-producing cells of the skin (and some other parts of the body). Sun exposure, especially if it leads to bad sunburns early in life, increases the risk of melanoma. Genetic factors may also increase the risk. In general, risk is higher for people with fair skin.

Prevention includes wearing clothing that protects against the sun, wearing sunscreen of at least SPF 15 (and perhaps even higher), and limiting sun exposure, particularly in the mid-day.

Malignant melanoma may start from a mole (nevus)—a raised darker-pigmented area of the skin. It may also appear on previously normal skin.

As part of every physical exam, the skin should be examined for new lesions or changes in a mole. People who have moles should also be taught to keep an eye on them for changes in appearance. Changes in a mole that need further investigation include:
◆ bleeding,
◆ irregular shape,
◆ irregular pigmentation (several colors or shades of color in a mole that was previously one color),
◆ increasing size or depth,
◆ asymmetry.

Treatment for malignant melanoma consists of surgically removing the lesion. Based on the microscopic assessment of the tissue, additional testing such as MRI, CT, or PET scans may be necessary to determine whether the disease has spread to other parts of the body, including internal organs or lymph nodes. If the melanoma has spread, chemotherapy, radiation, and/or biologic treatments (see section above) to stimulate the body's immune system to fight the cancer may be recommended.

The cure rate for melanoma is good—as high as 90 percent—if it is treated before the melanoma has spread. The survival rate is much lower if the melanoma has already spread when the diagnosis is made. People who have had one melanoma should definitely take extra precautions against sun exposure and be monitored closely for the development of new cancerous lesions.

CANCER SCREENING

Overall, the risk of cancer is reduced for people with DS, although some cancers are more common. The benefits of screening must be balanced with the risks of the screening test, the risks of follow-up testing required for an abnormal screening test,

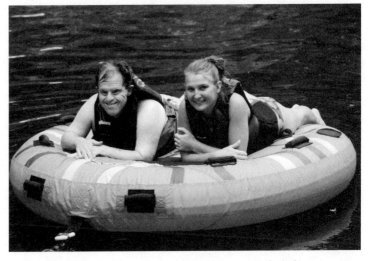

and the risk of anesthesia that may be required for an adult with DS to complete testing. In addition, the risks that family history or other health factors (such as cigarette smoking) contribute to the incidence of the disease must be considered. With limited data available regarding the overall benefit and risk of screening people with DS for cancer, each individual and her own health, risk factors, and ability to manage testing must be carefully considered. Screening tests, including cancer screening, are discussed in more detail in Chapter 3.

Chapter 15

Thyroid Disorders
and Diabetes

Jenny, age 27, came to the Adult Down Syndrome Center because she and her mom were concerned about her mood. She was described as having become "moody" over the preceding three months. She was anxious and was having a hard time sitting at her desk at work, where her job was to greet customers and answer the phone. She was also having trouble falling asleep and had lost eight pounds. Jenny's brother, who does not have Down syndrome, had a history of depression that had presented in a similar fashion. Not surprisingly, Jenny and her mom were worried that Jenny could also be developing depression.

Jenny's physical exam did not uncover any abnormalities except a mild increase in her reflexes. Blood tests, however, revealed that her thyroid stimulating hormone (TSH) was low and her T4 was high, consistent with hyperthyroidism (overactive thyroid). A thyroid scan was also consistent with hyperthyroidism, but showed no other abnormalities.

After treatment options were discussed, Jenny started taking two medications for hyperthyroidism, methimazole (Tapazole) and propranolol (Inderal), which reduced her symptoms. When she was reevaluated in two months, she had regained three pounds and her symptoms had resolved. Her blood work demonstrated normal thyroid function. The propranolol was discontinued and she continued to do well. Three months later, she was still doing well and her thyroid function remained normal.

However, when Jenny returned for a check-up three months later, she had gained ten pounds, was feeling "sluggish," and had developed constipation. Her exam revealed increased dry skin and slow reflexes. Blood work showed an elevated TSH and low T4 consistent with hypothyroidism (underactive thyroid). Her methimazole was discontinued at this point, but her symptoms persisted. Six weeks later, Jenny's labs were repeated and they remained consistent with hypothyroidism. She was then started on a medication for hypothyroidism, levothyroxine (Synthroid). Afterwards, her symptoms improved and her labs normalized. Jenny continues taking this medication and she has remained symptom free. Her lab values have also remained normal.

The endocrine system is one of those body systems that is usually out of sight, out of mind. It consists of glands that produce hormones—chemical messengers that transport a signal from one cell to the other and affect the function of the receiving cell. When something goes wrong with a gland, the level of hormones made by that gland increases or decreases above normal levels. This leads to endocrine disorders that can oftentimes be very serious.

Two endocrine disorders are more common in people with Down syndrome—thyroid dysfunction and diabetes mellitus. They are the subject of this chapter.

THYROID DISORDERS

Thyroid hormones affect nearly every cell in the body. They increase the basic metabolic rate (the rate calories are burned at rest), affect the synthesis of proteins, and help regulate bone growth, the maturation of nerve cells, and other functions. Thyroid hormones are produced in the thyroid gland in the neck.

The human body produces two types of thyroid hormones—T3 and T4 (the first has three iodine groups attached, and the second has four). The thyroid gland is stimulated to make these hormones by thyroid stimulating hormone (TSH), which is made in the pituitary gland in the brain. The hypothalamus of the brain signals the pituitary gland to release TSH by releasing TSH-releasing hormone (TRH). Ordinarily, when there is enough thyroid hormone present in the body, the thyroid hormones loop back to the hypothalamus to decrease TRH production, which reduces TSH production by the pituitary. This in turn reduces T3 and T4 production by the thyroid gland. Sometimes, however, the body makes too much or too little of the thyroid hormones (T3 and T4) or TSH.

The following are possible patterns of TSH and thyroid hormones (TRH is less commonly measured):
- normal TSH, normal thyroid hormones: normal thyroid function;
- elevated TSH, lower thyroid hormones: hypothyroidism (due to thyroid's dysfunction);

- low TSH, low thyroid hormones: hypothyroidism due to decreased pituitary production of TSH;
- high TSH, normal thyroid hormones: borderline (or subclinical or compensated) hypothyroidism;
- low TSH, elevated thyroid hormones: hyperthyroidism.

All of the thyroid problems listed above are more common in people with DS than in those without DS. Early signs of these problems can be difficult to detect, as some of the symptoms such as dry skin often occur in people with DS who do not have thyroid problems. For this reason, thyroid tests are recommended annually. In our patients who do not have a thyroid disorder, we recommend doing an annual blood test known as a TSH with reflex. The reflex part indicates that the lab automatically determines the T4 level if the TSH is abnormal. (If the TSH is normal, the T4 is not measured.)

Hypothyroidism

Hypothyroidism (underactive thyroid) is common in people with DS. About 40 percent of our patients at the Adult Down Syndrome Center have hypothyroidism. It can start at any time in life. Some infants are born with hypothyroidism, but it can also occur throughout childhood and adulthood.

Causes of Hypothyroidism

Worldwide, the most common cause of hypothyroidism is iodine deficiency in the diet . (The thyroid needs iodine to function, so if there is inadequate iodine in the diet, the thyroid doesn't work right.) In the United States, however, iodine deficiency is uncommon and the cause is more often the result of autoimmune destruction of the thyroid gland. (For unknown reasons, the body's defense system "sees" the thyroid gland as an enemy to be fought.) This condition is known as *Hashimoto's Thyroiditis.*

Hashimoto's thyroiditis appears to be the most common cause of hypothyroidism in people with DS. Less common causes include dysfunction related to x-ray/radiation injury, surgical injury, medication side effect, and pituitary or hypothalamic disorders.

Common symptoms of hypothyroidism include:
- weakness,
- dry skin,
- lethargy,
- slowed speech,
- puffy eyelids,
- cold intolerance,
- decreased sweating,

- cold skin,
- thickened tongue,
- facial puffiness,
- weight gain,
- coarse hair,
- pale skin,
- forgetfulness,
- constipation,
- impaired cognition (thinking),
- menstrual irregularities.

Because many of these complaints can be associated with other health problems and many of them are common in people with DS who don't have hypothyroidism, annual thyroid testing is recommended. This can be done through thyroid blood tests of TSH and possibly T3 and T4. Testing should also be done any time there is a sudden onset of these symptoms and they are serious enough to interfere with the person's daily life.

TREATMENT OF HYPOTHYROIDISM

Treatment of hypothyroidism involves using synthetically prepared medications (Synthroid, Levoxyl, or available generics) to replace the body's missing thyroid hormone. The starting dose can be calculated based on the patient's weight or based on nationally recognized "middle-of-the-road" doses such as 75 or 88 micrograms (for adults). Thyroid hormone can increase blood pressure and resting heart rate; therefore, patients who are elderly or who have underlying heart disease should start at lower doses.

Thyroid hormone level should be checked six to eight weeks after starting the medication or changing the dose to document that normal hormone levels are achieved. If normal levels have not yet been reached, the dose should be adjusted and the blood test should be repeated again in six to eight weeks.

After the appropriate dose of medication has been achieved, the patient will need to take the medication for the rest of his life. A thyroid hormone level (TSH) should be checked at least annually to follow the patient's hormone requirements.

Usually the person's primary physician can appropriately manage hypothyroidism. In more complicated or difficult-to-manage cases, a referral to an endocrinologist may be necessary.

Once the medication brings hormone levels back to normal, the symptoms of hypothyroidism usually improve and the person should feel like his normal self. Remember, however, that many of the symptoms of hypothyroidism are also characteristics of people with DS. These concerns may improve but usually don't disappear. For example, dry skin is a symptom of hypothyroidism but also a common characteristic of DS. Treating hypothyroidism may improve the dry skin but probably won't resolve it.

CONDITIONS THAT CHANGE THYROID HORMONE REQUIREMENTS

ADVANCED AGE AND MALNOURISHMENT

As people with hypothyroidism get older, it is often necessary to decrease the dose of medication. This is because the thyroid hormone becomes less tightly bound to proteins in the bloodstream (many hormones in the body "hitch a ride" on proteins in the blood in order to travel throughout the body). Therefore, more hormone is available to be plucked out of the bloodstream and used by the body. The age this occurs varies, so regular monitoring of thyroid blood tests is important.

Patients who are malnourished also may need their thyroid medication decreased, because as the body's nutrition is compromised, it is less able to make the proteins the thyroid hormone binds to in the bloodstream. For adults with DS, conditions that may lead to nutritional deficiencies and therefore may require changes in thyroid medication include celiac disease, severe gastroesophageal reflux disease (GERD), and decreased appetite due to Alzheimer disease.

MEDICATION SIDE-EFFECTS

Some medications decrease the availability of thyroid hormone for use by the body, while others cause the hormone to be used more quickly. The table below lists medications that could affect hormone levels.

Medications that may **DECREASE** the hormone level (larger dose of thyroid medication may be needed)	Medications that may **INCREASE** the hormone level (smaller dose of thyroid medication may be needed)
lithium	furosemide (Lasix)
iodine-containing medications	mefenamic acid (Ponstel)
amiodarone (Cordarone)	aspirin
sucralfate (Carafate)	
iron supplements	
cholestyramine (Questran)	
colestipol (Colestid)	
antacids with aluminum	
calcium supplements	
rifampin (Rifaidin)	
phenobarbitol	
carbamazepine (Tegratol)	
warfarin (Coumadin)	
oral anti-diabetic medications	

BORDERLINE HYPOTHYROIDISM

Borderline hypothyroidism (also called subclinical hypothyroidism or compensated hypothyroidism) is often seen in individuals with DS. In this condition, the level of TSH is high, but the thyroid hormones are not decreased. In hypothyroidism, usually the T3 and/or T4 are low. The low level of the hormones loop back to the brain to signal it to raise the level of TSH, which functions to stimulate the thyroid to make more thyroid hormone (T3/T4). However, the significance of the situation in borderline hypothyroidism with the elevated TSH but normal T3 and T4 is less clear.

Endocrinologists disagree about treatment for borderline hypothyroidism. Some think it should be treated with thyroid hormone. Others think it should just be monitored. One reason for the uncertainty is that it is not uncommon for people with DS to have a slightly abnormal TSH level (with normal thyroid function–T3/T4) and then later, without treatment, the TSH can become normal.

This is the approach we follow at the Adult Down Syndrome Clinic when a patient is found to have an elevated TSH and normal hormones:

- ◆ If the person has symptoms consistent with hypothyroidism, treat with thyroid hormone.
- ◆ If the TSH is more than a little elevated, treat with thyroid hormone, even if the person does not have symptoms of hypothyroidism. (For example, if normal is 1—5, consider treating if TSH is greater than 10.)
- ◆ Consider drawing blood to test for thyroid antibodies (anti-thyroglobulin antibody and anti-microsomal antibodies). An elevation of these antibodies is consistent with an autoimmune cause of the thyroid dysfunction. (These antibodies attack the thyroid causing a decrease in thyroid function.) One study demonstrated that if people with DS who have an elevated TSH and normal thyroid hormones also have elevated antibodies, they are likely to develop hypothyroidism (elevated TSH and low thyroid hormones). The study concluded that it was, therefore, reasonable to treat for hypothyroidism if the antibodies were elevated.
- ◆ Particularly if none of the above are present (the person does not have symptoms, the TSH is only minimally elevated, and the antibodies are normal), regular monitoring is a reasonable approach. More frequent monitoring (every three to six months) may initially be considered, but if the thyroid normalizes or remains stable with borderline hypothyroidism, annual monitoring may be appropriate. If the symptoms of hypothyroidism do occur, however, a repeat blood test should be considered at that time.

HYPERTHYROIDISM

Hyperthyroidism (overactive thyroid) is a little more common in people with DS than in people without DS, but nowhere near as common as hypothyroidism. Less than 1 percent of the 4500 adolescents and adults seen at the Adult Down Syndrome Center have been diagnosed with hyperthyroidism.

In the early stages of Hashimoto's thyroiditis, the thyroid may be initially overactive. Often it later "burns out" and becomes underactive (hypothyroidism). Grave's disease, another autoimmune disorder, can also cause hyperthyroidism.

Symptoms of hyperthyroidism include:

- nervousness,
- increased sweating,
- heat intolerance,
- palpitations (a sense of an abnormal or fast heart rate—usually noted as above 100 beats per minute or higher than usual for that person),
- fatigue and weakness,
- weight loss,
- increased appetite,
- tremor,
- emotional lability (frequent mood swings),
- sleep disturbance (often sleeping less or more restlessly).

Diagnosis of hyperthyroidism is made on the basis of blood tests (a low TSH level and high T3 and/or T4). Additional diagnostic testing may include an I-123 thyroid scan. This test involves injecting a small amount of radioactive iodine into the bloodstream and then doing a nuclear medicine scan. This is a painless test, except for the IV used to inject the iodine. This scan can help look for abnormal nodules and assess thyroid function. If any suspicious nodules are found on the thyroid during the physical exam or on the scan, an ultrasound and a fine needle aspiration may be recommended in order to assess for cancer in the nodule. If necessary, the skin can be "numbed" with local anesthetic. In some cases, the person may need to be sedated to allow this test to be done.

Treatment for hyperthyroidism may include medications to treat symptoms and/ or medication or other modalities to reduce thyroid hormone.

Medications known as beta blockers are used to treat symptoms. Propranol (Inderal) is most commonly recommended. It is usually used temporarily while other treatment is being implemented to reduce thyroid hormone.

Medications to reduce thyroid hormone include:

- methimazole (Tapazole), and
- propylthiouracil (also referred to as PTU).

Patients taking these medications should have complete blood count (CBC) and liver blood tests done to monitor for side effects. Possible side effects include a decrease in red and white blood cells and platelets and toxicity (damage) to the liver.

If medications alone cannot control the thyroid hormone, other treatments include:
- ◆ ablating (destroying) the thyroid gland with an injection of radioactive (I–131) iodine;
- ◆ surgically removing the thyroid. This would be the choice if the thyroid was causing serious symptoms, such as compressing the airway due to enlargement of the thyroid.

If the thyroid is removed or destroyed, the person will have to take medication for hypothyroidism (levothyroxine, levoxyl, Synthroid).

In many of our patients at the Center who have been diagnosed with hyperthyroidism, the thyroid eventually "burns out," as in the case of Jenny at the beginning of the chapter. Therefore, for many, the treatment has been temporary, although it may need to continue for months to even years. Eventually most have developed hypothyroidism, as in Jenny's case, but some of them regained normal thyroid function.

DIABETES MELLITUS (DM)

Diabetes mellitus is another disorder caused by difficulties with the endocrine system. In this case, it is the hormone insulin that is at the root of the disorder. Insulin is produced by the pancreas and ordinarily helps sugar enter into cells (so cells can use the sugar to produce energy). If the body doesn't make enough insulin or if the cells are resistant to insulin, sugar builds up in the blood and the cells have a reduced amount of sugar in them to produce energy.

There are two types of diabetes mellitus. Type I is more common in DS; Type II is frequently diagnosed, but not more common.

1. *Type I DM, previously called juvenile diabetes or insulin dependent diabetes,* most often starts in childhood and is due to insufficient production of insulin by the pancreas. Susceptibility to developing Type I DM seem to have a genetic component (having a family member with Type 1 DM does increase the chance of developing the disease).

2. *Type II DM, previously called adult onset DM or non-insulin dependent DM,* is caused by increased resistance to insulin. The body needs increasingly larger amounts of insulin to function because the cells don't respond normally to insulin. Type II DM is often associated with obesity. In people without DS, it is now even being found in children. Our youngest patient with Type II DM developed it at age 15 years.

At present there are no preventative measures available for Type I DM. Type II DM can often be prevented if the person loses weight (if overweight) or maintains an ideal body weight and exercises regularly.

Symptoms of both types of DM include:
- increased urination,
- increased thirst,
- weight loss,
- fatigue,
- muscle cramps,
- mood changes,
- vision changes (such as blurred vision),
- headaches,
- abdominal pain,
- nausea, diarrhea, or constipation.

TREATMENT FOR DIABETES

The basic goals of treatment of DM include: 1) helping the body get sugar (glucose) into the cells so they can function, and 2) reducing the sugar in the blood to reduce the damaging effects of high blood sugar. The medications used to accomplish these goals are different from types I and II and are discussed below.

Paying careful attention to nutrition and exercise is important for adults with both types I & II DM. Recommended guidelines include:
- reaching or maintaining ideal body weight and exercising regularly;
- eating a diet low in saturated fats;
- limiting simple sugars (such as those found in candy, cake, cookies, and donuts); and
- for patients with type I DM, counting carbohydrates—limiting carbohydrates and knowing the amount to be eaten so the proper dose of insulin can be given (see below).

TREATMENT FOR TYPE I

In Type I DM, the insulin level is low, so the treatment is to provide extra insulin. This has traditionally been accomplished by injecting insulin into the body (under the skin where it is absorbed into the bloodstream). The insulin that is used is human insulin that is made by putting the human gene (that codes for the making of insulin) into bacteria. The bacteria then make human insulin, which is collected and prepared for use in humans. There are several types of insulin that have differing onsets (or quickness) of action and that last for varying lengths of time. These are usually injected before a meal. This replicates the normal body response of increasing insulin in response to consuming food or drink. When using this method of giving insulin, the individual's blood sugar must be measured multiple times a day to ensure that the correct dosage of insulin is being given. Often the level is checked before each meal and in the evening before bedtime.

A more recent approach to treating Type I DM has been to use glargine insulin (Lantus) or detemir insulin (Levemir), which provide a steady basal level of insulin throughout the day (after a daily or twice daily dose). This is given along with a rapid acting insulin just before or with a meal. Insulin pumps are also available that provide a continuous, basal level of insulin, as well as bolus (an increased amount) doses that are given before meals and snacks. These doses are injected under the skin. When using these approaches, the individual still needs to measure his blood sugar levels. At this time, pumps are not available for patient care that both automatically measure and deliver insulin in response to the measured sugar.

TREATMENT FOR TYPE II

In Type II DM, treatment is designed to help the cells get the sugar they need to function and to reduce the amount of sugar in the blood. Medications with a variety of actions on the body may be prescribed in order to meet these goals. These medications can:
- decrease the amount of glucose made by the liver;
- reduce absorption of glucose from the food in the intestines;
- increase the sensitivity of the cells to insulin (so the insulin present is more effective);
- stimulate the islet beta cells in the pancreas (where insulin is made) to make more insulin;
- provide additional insulin (via insulin injections).

Medications used to treat Type II DM include:
- Metformin (Glucophage, Glumetza, Riomet) is an oral medication that decreases glucose production in the liver, decreases glucose absorption in the intestine, and increases sensitivity to insulin. It is often considered the preferred first medication because some people lose weight with metformin and it increases sensitivity to insulin. One potential side effect that is uncommon but can be very serious is lactic acidosis, the build-up of lactic acid. This is more common when the individual has kidney disease, is dehydrated, gets a serious infection (sepsis), or has insufficient liver function. It is recommended to temporarily stop metformin prior to an x-ray study that includes IV contrast, before surgery, and if the person develops a serious infection or dehydration. Avoid using metformin if the person has kidney or liver disease. Diarrhea is a more common side effect.
- Sulfonylurea medications are oral medications that stimulate the pancreas to make more insulin. Examples include:
  - glimepiride (Amaryl),
  - glipizide (Glucotrol), and
  - glyburide (DiaBeta, micronase).
- Thiazolidinediones are oral medications that increase insulin sensitivity. Thiazolidinediones can affect the liver, so for the first year of use, having blood tests to monitor liver function every two months is recommended. Examples include:

> ➤ pioglitazone (Actos), and
> ➤ rosiglitazone (Avandia).
- ◆ (Alpha)-glycosidase inhibitors are oral medications that delay glucose absorption by inhibiting alpha-amylase, an enzyme in the pancreas, and alpha glucoside hydrolase, an enzyme in the intestines. These are often considered the last oral medication of choice because of gastro-intestinal side effects. Examples include:
>   ➤ acarbose (Precose), and
>   ➤ migitol (Glyset).
- ◆ Insulin may need to be given via injection, as described above for Type I DM.
- ◆ Pramlintide (Symlin) decreases blood sugar after a meal, suppresses the secretion of glucagon (a hormone that raises blood sugar), slows emptying of the stomach after eating, and promotes satiety (the sensation of being full after eating). All of these effects reduce the amount of insulin needed. It is given by injection like insulin, but cannot be taken by someone who is taking insulin.

Metformin, pioglitizone, and rosiglitazone can be especially good choices for people with DS who have type II DM. This is because these medications do not cause low blood sugar (hypoglycemia), discussed below. Although acarbose and miglitol don't cause hypoglycemia either, they are often not well tolerated due to gastrointestinal side effects. Insulin and pramlintide are less attractive choices because they need to be injected.

HYPOGLYCEMIA

One significant complication of treatment of DM is hypoglycemia (low blood sugar). Low blood sugar may be related to improper dosing of medication, a sudden increase in the amount of exercise, a sudden decrease in the amount of food consumed without a decrease in the medication, and illness.

Symptoms of hypoglycemia include:
- ◆ hunger,
- ◆ trembling,
- ◆ pallor (pale color),
- ◆ sweating,
- ◆ shaking,
- ◆ pounding heart,
- ◆ anxiety,
- ◆ dizziness, lightheadedness,
- ◆ poor concentration,
- ◆ weakness,
- ◆ confusion,
- ◆ slurred speech,

  ◆ blurred or double vision,
  ◆ unsteadiness,
  ◆ poor coordination,
  ◆ fearfulness,
  ◆ fatigue,
  ◆ irritability, and
  ◆ aggressiveness.

Hypoglycemia is of particular concern in people with DS because many have difficulty self-reporting these symptoms. If these symptoms are not reported or noted, the situation may progress to include these more serious symptoms/signs:
  ◆ numbness (especially of the hands and feet),
  ◆ stupor and confusion,
  ◆ seizures, or
  ◆ coma.

The rate that the low blood sugar can develop into a seriously low level depends on the individual person's diabetes (his body chemistry), the medication used (e.g., insulin vs. an oral medication), and other factors. In people who are taking oral medications, seriously low blood sugar typically may develop over hours to several days. In people on insulin, however, this can occur in minutes to hours.

Treatment of hypoglycemia involves getting glucose (sugar) into the individual quickly. This can be given through:
  ◆ sugar-containing food or beverages that can be quickly absorbed (e.g., juice, hard candy, or regular soda),
  ◆ glucose tablets,
  ◆ glucagon—given as an injection (e.g., into the arm) or via an IV to raise blood sugar,
  ◆ IV dextrose—dextrose (sugar) given via IV by medical personnel.

If the person is too confused to swallow well or has lost consciousness, glucose should not be given by mouth. Instead, he will need glucagon or IV dextrose.

MONITORING DIABETES

People with DM need to be regularly stuck with needles in order to monitor their blood sugar and ensure that their diabetes is being optimally managed. For people with DS, as for everyone, frequent needle "sticks" can be challenging. The treatment of DM includes three such potential challenges:
  ◆ People with DM need to have regular blood draws through the health care practitioner's office to measure a variety of blood levels;
  ◆ Blood glucose monitoring—drawing a small amount of blood (usually) from the finger—is unavoidable. This may be done daily, several

times a day, or less frequently depending on the type of DM and the level of control. These tests are done at home, at restaurants, before exercise, and at other times.

◆ Everyone with type I DM and some people with type II DM need injections of insulin.

Some people with DS can participate in much of the management. Steps that need to be learned and mastered are listed below.

◆ To do the blood glucose monitoring, the person needs to stick his finger to draw blood (or allow someone else to stick him) and then place the blood onto a test strip. (Some machines allow the blood to be entered directly into the machine.) The test strip is then placed into a glucose-monitoring device (a small hand-held machine) that measures glucose level. The number is then usually written in the person's record, although some machines store the list of glucose levels. A normal blood glucose is in the range of about 75-105. "Tight" control of DM strives to keep the blood sugar in the range of 80-150. However, as discussed above, this increases the chance of developing hypoglycemia (low blood sugar), which can be very dangerous. An optimal level of control varies for each individual and may need to be less "tight" for a person with DS to avoid the potentially serious complication of hypoglycemia. It should be noted that recent studies have questioned whether doing regular home glucose monitoring in people with Type II DM actual helps prevent complications of the disease. Even if regular monitoring is not done, it will be necessary to check the sugar if hypoglycemia or hyperglycemia (elevated blood sugar) is suspected.

◆ For people with Type I DM (and some with Type II), the value of glucose may be used to determine how much insulin is given. This may require checking the glucose several times a day (for example, before meals and before bed) and adjusting the dose of insulin based on the level of the sugar and the anticipated amount of carbohydrates to be eaten.

◆ For people with Type I DM (and some with Type II), the insulin has to be measured. This can be done with a small syringe and needle to draw the insulin out of a bottle. Alternatively, some insulin is now available to be given via an insulin pen. A dial is turned to set the pen to deliver a set amount of insulin. The needle is then inserted under the skin (similar to injecting from the insulin syringe) and the insulin is injected. Additionally, insulin pumps are available. The pump is worn on a belt or in a pack around the waist or on the arm. The pump is (usually) attached to a tube that goes to a needle that is placed under the skin (and is replaced periodically). Insulin is continuously injected under the skin (usually in the waist). Before a meal, a bolus of insulin is usually injected. The amount needed for the meal is calculated and the information is entered into the pump. Over a relatively short period of time the bolus is injected under the skin. A bolus may also be given if the person's sugar level is running high in the blood.

Clearly, there may be multiple steps to monitoring and treating DM. Most adults with DS need some assistance with some or all of these steps. However, over time, some people with DS can learn to perform some or all of the steps. It usually works best if they work with a professional diabetes educator who uses a hands-on approach to teaching. Each step should be shown to the individual (usually repeatedly) and the person should practice in the presence of the educator. Family or care-providers should also learn the steps so they can support and reinforce what is learned and perform the steps when the person with DS may not be able (for example, if he is ill). Many people with DS and DM can benefit from using a picture guide of the steps involved in managing diabetes. Watching a video demonstrating the steps is also helpful.

For adults in residential or day programs, the rules outlined by state and federal policy will dictate the level of training required for the staff people who will assist with DM management. In some situations, a nurse may need to be present. This can limit the availability of choices for adults who have both DS and DM.

Monitoring in the Physician's Office: Periodically, individuals with DM need to have a Hemoglobin A1C (Hgb A1C) blood test. This test provides a reading that corresponds to the person's average blood glucose over the preceding 6 to 12 weeks. A person with good diabetic control will have less than 7 percent average blood glucose. If the Hgb A1C is higher, the individual's treatment regimen needs to be adjusted. Recommendations are that people with Type I DM have the Hgb A1C test done every three months, and those with Type II, every three to six months.

Diabetes and Nutrition

Good nutrition can be a challenge for people with DS even if they don't have diabetes. It can be even more challenging for people who must contend with the extra guidelines and monitoring required to manage diabetes. We recommend that adults with DS and DM consult with a nutritionist, dietitian, and/or diabetic educator. Periodic, regular visits may be required. Training needs to extend outside the classroom into the grocery store, the kitchen at home, restaurants, etc. to help the individual learn to use what he learns.

Many people with DS require assistance to take what they learn in one setting and apply it to another. Often visual supports can help them with this generalization. For example, it may be helpful to compile a book that contains labels or pictures of foods they can eat or foods they should avoid. Although a diagnosis of DM can reduce an individual's independence initially, with instruction and a reminder system, many people with DS can learn to make healthy choices for themselves.

POSSIBLE COMPLICATIONS OF DIABETES

A number of disorders can develop as a complication of diabetes. Anyone with diabetes should be regularly evaluated for signs of:

- eye disease, including diseases of the retina and cataracts (an annual eye exam should be performed by an ophthalmologist or optometrist);
- disease of the peripheral nerves (particularly the feet), which can decrease the ability to sense light touch or pain, to balance, and to perceive vibration;
- kidney disease;
- atherosclerotic disease (vascular disease, plaques in the arteries).

Due to vascular disease and disease of peripheral nerves, people with DM are more prone to developing non-healing skin ulcers, especially on the feet. The person's feet should be inspected daily to check for skin changes, signs of infection, or small ulcers. Regular evaluations in the medical office are also recommended. Other useful preventive strategies include taking good care of dry skin (see Chapter 6), wearing well-fitting shoes with adequate padding, and using orthotics. It is imperative to prevent skin problems or to find them early to prevent worsening that can lead to extensive ulcers, infections, amputations, and even death.

If non-healing skin ulcers do develop, aggressive management is strongly recommended. Treatment includes optimizing treatment of diabetes, addressing other nutritional issues, and local care of the wound. Referral to a wound care clinic, podiatrist, vascular surgeon, nutritionist, or other specialists may be necessary.

Tests that can be done in the medical office to check for complications of diabetes include:

- annual urine test (urine for microalbumin and/or assessment for protein in the urine for Type 2 DM) to monitor for kidney problems;
- lipid panel to assess for cholesterol every 6 to 12 months (the goal is for low-density lipoprotein—LDL—the "bad" cholesterol to be less than 100. Remember, as discussed in Chapter 9, total cholesterol is often high in people with DS but does not necessarily cause atherosclerotic disease. However, the risk of atherosclerotic disease is of greater concern in people with DM, so more attention needs to be paid to cholesterol and treating elevated cholesterol);
- screening for signs of depression—which is more common in people with DM and can result in individuals not taking as good care of their DM as they would otherwise;
- blood testing for kidney function (blood urea nitrogen and creatinine).

The risk of complications from diabetes in people with DS has not been as thoroughly studied as in those without DS. Generally speaking, however, although modifications may need to be made as noted above, the treatment and monitoring of the disease should be the same as in people without DS.

CONCLUSION

People with DS have a higher incidence of thyroid problems and Type I diabetes. Because of these potentially serious endocrine problems, adults with DS should be regularly screened through blood tests, and parents and other caregivers should be aware of the warning signs for thyroid problems and diabetes. If these problems develop, treatment can often be managed by the individual's primary health care provider. However, the person may need a consult with an endocrinologist for one evaluation or on an ongoing basis, depending on difficulties in diagnosing and treating the problem.

Chapter 16

Gynecology

· · · · · · · · · ·

Gwen was a 26-year-old woman with Down syndrome who was brought to the Center to be evaluated for behavioral concerns. Specifically, she was periodically becoming agitated and irritable. We determined that these behaviors only occurred when she was having her period (menses) each month. Gwen had limited verbal skills, so she could only provide limited information. However, it appeared likely that she was experiencing discomfort during her menses. After evaluating when the behavior change occurred in relation to her period, we recommended she take ibuprofen for 7 days each month, starting 21 days after her previous period began. Over the next few months, her agitation and irritability improved.

Gynecological problems seem to occur as frequently in women with Down syndrome (DS) as in women without DS. The difference is that when women with DS do have problems, they often have trouble expressing them to a medical professional. This means regular gynecological checkups are important, whether with a gynecologist or the primary health care provider.

THE GYNECOLOGICAL EXAM
· · · · · · · · · · · · · · · ·

At the Adult Down Syndrome Center, our guideline is to start gynecological exams for all women with DS aged 21 and over. We do these exams during their annual physical unless a patient prefers to see her gynecologist for the exam.

The first steps in the medical office in assessing for gynecologic issues are to take a history and do a physical exam. Pieces of history to discuss were outlined in Chapter 3 and also include issues that are discussed in this chapter. The physical exam can sometimes be much more challenging. As discussed in Chapter 3, we use little sedation and recommend caution.

To make the exam as comfortable as possible for the woman and to increase our success rate in completing the exam, we introduce elements of the exam gradually. We generally don't do a Pap smear or pelvic exam on the first office visit. We want the woman to develop some degree of comfort with coming to the Center before doing this part of the exam.

- ◆ When necessary, we "work our way up" to the complete exam. For example, we might have the woman wear a gown but not remove her undergarments at one exam, examine only the external genitalia at the next exam, and at subsequent exams do the internal exam and Pap smear. Also, we do not always do Pap smears, as discussed later in this chapter.

- ◆ We don't usually use the stirrups. We have the woman lie on the exam table with her knees raised and her feet together, and then spread her knees apart. Many women with and without DS find this position less uncomfortable and less anxiety-provoking.

- ◆ When possible, we use a speculum to view the vagina and cervix and perform the Pap smear. Some women don't tolerate the speculum. In those instances, we will either:
  - ➤ do a one-finger exam in an effort to touch the cervix and then pass the brush along the finger to collect the cells from the cervix; or
  - ➤ do a blind Pap smear by passing the brush into the vagina towards the cervix without either visualizing or palpating the cervix. Interestingly, a high percentage of the time we get a good collection of cells needed for an adequate Pap smear (that includes endocervical cells from the cervix).

- ◆ For the bimanual (internal) exam done with the examiner's hands, ideally one hand is placed on the abdomen and two fingers of the other hand are placed into the vagina to palpate (feel) the pelvic organs. For women who have an intact hymen and/or a small introitus (opening to the vagina), it is often necessary to do the exam with one finger. This may limit the exam but make it possible to get some information that would not be possible if the patient was not able to cooperate with a two-finger exam.

Pictures or models can be used to prepare the woman for the exam. In addition, we require that the patient's mother, sister, other female relative, female caregiver, or female nursing staff be present for support.

Helpful Resources

There are several resources that can be helpful in educating young women with DS about caring for their periods. We suggest considering:
- *Teaching Children with Down Syndrome about Their Bodies, Boundaries, and Sexuality: A Guide for Parents and Professionals,* by Terri Couwenhoven, published by Woodbine House (www.woodbinehouse.com)
- *A Girl's Guide to Growing Up,* by Liz Smith (booklet and video), available in English and Spanish from MarshMedia (www.marshmedia.com); a male version is also available

MENSTRUATION

The onset of menses (periods) can occur at a younger age in girls with DS, sometimes as early as 8 years of age. Often, however, periods begin around the same age as in girls without DS, or between about ages 10½ and 14½ . In our experience at the Adult Down Syndrome Center, nearly all women with DS aged 16 to 17 and older have at least irregular periods.

The hygiene care of periods can be challenging for some girls and women with DS. Information on educating girls and young woman about the care of their periods is available from several sources (see box).

Irregular periods are quite common in girls with and without DS for the first few years. This can certainly make hygiene more difficult due to the lack of predictability. Some girls and women use birth control pills (oral contraceptive pills—OCPs) to improve regularity or reduce blood flow to make their period more manageable. Use of OCP's is discussed below.

PAINFUL PERIODS

Dysmenorrhea (painful periods) is common in women with DS, just as it is in women in general. The pain can usually be effectively controlled with ibuprofen (Advil, Nuprin, or Motrin), acetaminophen (Tylenol), or similar medications. If ibuprofen is started several days before the woman's period is expected to start, it can reduce the heaviness of the period, as well as discomfort.

Sometimes a woman with DS may have difficulty communicating her pain and the only outward sign of dysmenorrhea will be a behavior change around the time of her period (as with Gwen at the beginning of this chapter). Use of medication to decrease cramping can be extremely helpful in reducing the behavior changes. Oral contraceptive pills (OCPs) can also significantly improve dysmenorrhea. OCPs are discussed further below.

Additional treatments for dysmenorrhea include:
- regular exercise (to raise endorphins);
- supplementation with 100 mg of vitamin B1 (thiamine) daily;
- supplementation with fish oil (specifically, one gram per day of omega-3 fatty acids);
- a low fat, vegetarian diet.

If symptoms don't respond to treatment or are more severe, it is important to look for other possible causes of dysmenorrhea. Conditions such as endometriosis (uterine tissue found outside the uterus) and fibroids (benign tumors of the uterus) can cause discomfort. To check for these conditions, a gynecologist might conduct tests such as an ultrasound, or laparoscopy (passing a scope through the abdominal wall into the abdominal and pelvic cavity).

PMS

In our clinical experience at the Adult Down Syndrome Center, premenstrual syndrome (PMS) seems to be about as common among women with DS as in those without DS (approximately 5 percent).

PMS symptoms include:
- mood changes (mood swings, depressed mood, anxiety, and others),
- bloating,
- food cravings,
- edema (swelling in legs and/or hands)
- headaches, and
- breast swelling and tenderness.

The symptoms start about a week before the period begins and are not present the rest of the month. PMS is diagnosed when these symptoms are severe enough to interfere with everyday life. Again, we have found that some women with DS are not able to articulate their discomfort. However, parents and other caregivers are often able to observe signs such as irritability, intolerance of annoyances that are usually tolerated, and less interest in participating in activities. The timing of the behavioral change is the big difference between PMS and dysmenorrhea for women who can't explain their symptoms.

A more severe form of PMS is premenstrual dysphoric syndrome. This condition causes severe, recurrent depressive and anxiety symptoms, occurring about a week before the period begins. Physical symptoms of PMS may also be present. It seems to occur in a small percentage of our female patients (less than 1 percent).

Treatment for PMS includes:
- increased daily exercise;
- eating regular, balanced meals (frequent smaller meals high in complex carbohydrates and low in fat and caffeine);

- getting regular sleep;
- supplementation with
    - vitamin B6 (100 mg daily),
    - calcium (600 mg twice a day),
    - omega-3 fatty acids (one gram daily as a supplement or from the diet—but it can be difficult to get enough from the diet),
    - vitamin E (400 International Units daily),
    - magnesium (200-400 mg daily),
    - manganese (1.8 mg daily);
- oral contraceptive pills containing drospirenone (such as Yaz or Angeliq);
- selective serotonin reuptake inhibitor (SSRI) antidepressants such as fluoxetine (Prozac) or sertraline (Zoloft) (these can be taken during appropriate time in the cycle or daily; it is generally easier for our patients to take daily rather than try to figure out when to take the pills each month);
- ibuprofen and other antiinflammatory medication for cramping;
- spironolactone (Aldactone) for swelling;
- bromocriptine (Parlodel) for breast tenderness;
- buspirone (Buspar) for anxiety (taken in the same way as the SSRIs above).

LACK OF MENSTRUATION IN PREMENOPAUSAL WOMEN

Once a woman has begun having periods fairly regularly, she should always consult with her healthcare provider if her periods stop. The absence of menses (amenorrhea) in a woman who has not gone through menopause can be caused by several conditions. Hypothyroidism, weight change, and medication side effects are the common reasons seen at the Adult Down Syndrome Center. Pregnancy is, of course, another cause, but one we have encountered infrequently. It is important to assess for and treat causes of amenorrhea to prevent long-term complications.

Women who are not pregnant and still producing estrogen but not having periods are at risk for changes in the endometrium (tissue of the inside of the uterus). These changes can progress to cancer of the uterus. Therefore, when we are evaluating a woman whose periods have stopped, we generally recommend a pelvic ultrasound to assess the uterus. Ideally the ultrasound should be done both transabdominally (a scan done through the abdominal wall) and transvaginally (done through the wall of the vagina by passing a small ultrasound transducer into the vagina). Some women with DS, however, find it difficult or impossible to cooperate with the transvaginal ultrasound, so only the transabdominal can be performed.

If the endometrium is thickened, this can be a sign of uterine cancer and should be further evaluated. Tissue from the endometrium must be collected either via endometrial aspiration or dilatation and curettage (D and C) to assess the cells of the uterine lining. Both procedures can be painful. If the endometrial aspiration cannot be done in the office, a D and C can be performed in the operating room under anesthesia. As discussed in Chapter 14, most cancers are less common in adults with DS, and we have found the rate of uterine cancer to be low in women with DS.

As discussed in Chapter 15, hypothyroidism is relatively common in adults with Down syndrome. One symptom of hypothyroidism in women is menstrual irregularities, including periods that are lighter or heavier than usual or missed entirely. Treating the hypothyroidism usually resolves the menstrual irregularities.

Women who have lost or gained a significant amount of weight can also stop having periods. If the weight change is inappropriate, the first step in treatment is to work with the woman to lose or gain weight.

Additionally, oral progesterone (Provera) can be used to regulate periods when a woman is experiencing amenorrhea. We generally prescribe 10 mg tablets once a day for the first 10 days of the month. Most women will have a period near the end of the 10 days or just after. We usually recommend using the Provera every other month or every third month. If the woman starts having periods with the Provera, sometimes it will "jump start" her cycle. Therefore, if she continues to have her period during the months she is not taking Provera, the Provera can often be discontinued.

In our experience the medications that most often cause amenorrhea (absence of menses) in women with DS are the antipsychotics. Medications such as risperidone (Risperdal), olanzapine (Zyprexa), quetiapine (Seroquel), and others can cause menstrual irregularities. This may be related to weight gain, an increase in the hormone prolactin, or other causes. We generally recommend checking a prolactin level before prescribing these medications for our female patients. If the prolactin is normal before starting the medication and elevated if/when her periods stop, the elevation of prolactin is more likely to have been caused by the medication. Our approach to assessing and treating amenorrhea in women who are taking these medications is the same as described in the paragraph above. We may also change the medication that is causing the amenorrhea to see if periods will resume.

MENOPAUSE

Menopause (the cessation of menstrual periods) can occur at a younger age than usual for women with DS. In American women without Down syndrome, the average age of menopause is about 51. The average age of menopause in the women seen at the Adult Down Syndrome Center is 42 years of age. We have, however, diagnosed menopause in some women who were in their early to mid 30s.

Menopause is defined to have occurred when a woman has missed twelve consecutive menstrual cycles. Ovarian production of estrogen declines with age until a woman makes insufficient estrogen to stimulate the development of the endometrium and her periods stop.

Technically, the years leading up to menopause are known as perimenopause. Women in the general population report a wide range of symptoms during this time, including:

- ◆ hot flashes,
- ◆ sleep disturbances,
- ◆ heart palpitations,
- ◆ vaginal dryness,
- ◆ breast tenderness,
- ◆ and others.

Women who visit our clinic do not commonly complain of these symptoms. It should be noted, though, that it is difficult to get a clear complaint of a hot flash. It seems to be a difficult concept for most women with DS to comprehend. However, occasionally someone else will note that a woman with DS has sweating or flushing episodes. In addition, one of our women patients with DS would regularly fan herself in an apparent effort to "cool off" from a hot flash.

Mood changes, sleep disturbance, and urinary incontinence can also occur during the years leading up to menopause. Some women have irregular periods for several months to a few years before their periods completely stop. Periods may occur more or less frequently than usual or be significantly heavier or lighter than usual. Osteoporosis (thinning of the bones) also increases with menopause (see Chapter 13).

The treatment of perimenopausal symptoms has significantly changed in the last several years since a study indicated that using hormone replacement therapy (HRT) (estrogen and progesterone) increases the risk of breast cancer, coronary heart disease, stroke, and pulmonary embolism after five years of use. Therefore, the use of HRT is less common than in the past. Smaller doses for shorter periods of time are still used for symptomatic menopause, especially when 1) symptoms such as hot flashes and mood changes are more severe, and 2) the hormones can be used for less than five years. However, other treatments are now used to prevent osteoporosis in women who aren't having symptoms. These preventative treatments are discussed in Chapters 2 and 13.

Sometimes treatments are prescribed for one or more specific menopausal symptoms. For example:

- ◆ Soy (flavinoids) may be used to treat hot flashes and vaginal dryness. (It is difficult to get enough soy in the diet, so this can be taken as a supplement.)
- ◆ Medications can be used for sleep disturbance (see Chapter 18).
- ◆ Antidepressant medications such as paroxetine (Paxil) and venlafaxine (Effexor) may be prescribed to reduce flushing and hot flashes (although this is not an FDA-approved indication). Antidepressants can also be used for depression associated with menopause.

If there is any doubt that a woman has reached menopause, a blood test for follicle stimulating hormone (FSH) can be done. When the FSH rises above a certain level, it signifies that the woman has reached menopause. This test may be done if the physician needs to determine whether to look for other possible causes for the cessation of periods.

FERTILITY

Women with DS are thought to have a fertility rate that is a little lower than normal. This reduced rate is probably due to a higher miscarriage (spontaneous abortion) rate.

Theoretically, 50 percent of the children conceived by women with trisomy-21 will have DS (assuming the father does not have DS). This is because a woman's egg cells ordinarily contain half the chromosomal material found in her other cells—that is, they contain one copy of each chromosome, rather than the two copies found elsewhere in her body. Because women with trisomy-21 have three copies of the 21st chromosome in their cells, rather than two, approximately half of their eggs will have two copies of the chromosome and half will have one. If they conceive a baby with a father who has the normal complement of chromosomes in his sperm (i.e., one copy of the 21st chromosome), that means they might have a baby with either two or three 21st chromosomes, depending on whether an egg with one or two 21st chromosomes is fertilized.

The fertility rate and percentage of children with DS born to a woman with DS due to mosaicism would theoretically depend on which cells in her body have trisomy-21. That is, it would depend on the percentage of her egg cells that have an extra chromosome.

Men with DS are thought to have a significantly reduced fertility rate. This may be due to abnormal sperm. However, lack of information about sex, as well as decreased opportunities to have sex, may also contribute to a decreased fertility rate. For a long time, men with DS were thought to be infertile, but there are now several reported instances of men with DS impregnating women and fathering a child. If it is important to determine a man's fertility, a semen analysis can be done on his ejaculate to assess sperm count and viability of the sperm.

RELATIONSHIPS AND HEALTHY SEXUALITY

Education about sexuality, sexual activity, relationships, and birth control is the first and most important cornerstone to healthy sexuality. It is not a subject that can be dealt with well in a short office visit or in this book. A more thorough approach that takes into account the person's ability to understand, as well as his or her present level of knowledge, is recommended. We recommend that you consult resources such as Terri Couwenhoven's book, *Teaching Children with Down Syndrome about Their*

Bodies, Boundaries, and Sexuality: A Guide for Parents and Professionals.

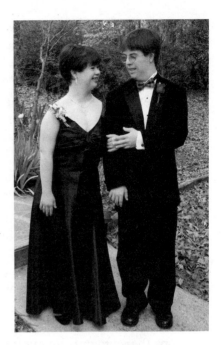

You may also want to consult with professionals in your community who are experienced in instructing teens and adults with developmental disabilities about sexuality and relationships. To locate someone who can provide this instruction, contact the following types of agencies or individuals:

- ◆ Local disability organizations such as the ARC, Down syndrome support group, or UCP may have lists of classes, experts, or other resources.
- ◆ Planned Parenthood clinics or other family planning agencies have specialists on staff who provide information about pregnancy, sexually transmitted diseases, consent, etc., and may have experience explaining these topics to people with disabilities.
- ◆ AASECT professionals are certified by the American Association of Sex Educators, Counselors, and Therapists and are trained in teaching about all aspects of sexuality. Not all are experienced in working with people with disabilities, however. A list of AASECT certified professionals is available at www.aasect.org.
- ◆ Family physicians may feel comfortable with providing individualized education sessions on sexuality to their patients, or may be able to refer you to classes, counseling services, or other resources in your community.

BIRTH CONTROL
◆ ◆ ◆ ◆ ◆ ◆ ◆ ◆ ◆ ◆ ◆ ◆ ◆ ◆ ◆ ◆

Most of our patients are not sexually active (having sexual intercourse). However, as opportunities for sexual activity and marriage increase for adults with DS, we anticipate that more of our patients will become sexually active.

If the adult with DS is sexually active or likely to become sexually active, here are some methods of birth control to consider:

- ◆ **Natural Family Planning (NFP)** methods rely on regular observations of a variety of changes in the woman's body (e.g., temperature, vaginal mucous, and others) to determine which days the woman is more likely to be fertile. Sexual activity is avoided at these times to prevent pregnancy. We are not aware of anyone with

DS using this method and would expect that most people with DS would not be able to monitor the changes and determine the times of increased fertility without significant assistance.

◆ **Barrier methods** are so called because they are designed to prevent sperm from reaching the egg. Common methods include using condoms or diaphragms. These can be effective in preventing pregnancy but can be challenging to use for many people with DS.

◆ **Intra-uterine devices (IUD's)** consist of a small T-shaped device that is inserted into the uterus by a medical practitioner. An IUD could theoretically be effective for an adult with DS, although we have no experience with them in women with DS. Side effects may include increased discomfort during menstruation, heavier bleeding, and increased risk of pelvic inflammatory disease (pelvic infection due to sexually transmitted disease).

◆ **Depo-Provera** is an injection of progesterone that is given every three months and stops the woman from ovulating. This is generally well tolerated by women with DS, but it does require an intramuscular injection every three months. Most women on Depo-Provera stop having periods, although they may have irregular periods in the first year. Bone density loss is a possible side effect, particularly when Depo-Provera is used for a longer duration. This may be of greater concern in women with DS because they are more likely to develop osteoporosis anyway. In addition, blood clots (thromboembolism) can be a side effect. Other possible side effects are deep venous thrombosis (blood clots, particularly of the veins of the legs) and pulmonary embolism (blood clots that go into the vascular system of the lungs), which are serious and potentially life-threatening. The risk is increased for women who smoke.

◆ **Oral contraceptive pills (OCPs),** otherwise known as birth control pills (BCPs), are taken daily and prevent the woman from ovulating. Our patients at the Adult Down Syndrome Center generally tolerate them well. Nausea, breast tenderness, and irregular bleeding are common side effects that usually resolve in the first several months of use. The side effects of blood clots (mentioned above) are also a serious concern for OCPs. Theoretically, pills containing a lower amount of estrogen may have a lower risk of blood clots. Gall bladder disease (which is more common in people with DS) is also a potential side effect. BCPs can also raise blood pressure. Because of these possible health risks, we are cautious in prescribing BCPs for our patients. We screen them to make sure they are not at high risk for blood clots, as described in the box below. We also regularly evaluate our patients who are on BCPs by checking blood pressure and evaluating how well the BCPs are being tolerated. We consider stopping BCPs after age 35 because of the potential for increased risk of clotting with age documented in women without DS (although this has not documented in women with DS).

Blood Clots and Down Syndrome

We have seen a few women with DS develop blood clots when taking oral contraceptive pills. This includes a woman with DS who had a pulmonary embolism (PE)—a blood clot that traveled to the vascular system of the lungs. A PE has the potential to be life-threatening. After this occurred, we reevaluated the use of OCPs in our patients. Now, prior to prescribing them for our patients, we evaluate them with blood tests to assess for hypercoagulability (a tendency toward developing blood clots).

We have found several women with DS who had one form or another of a hypercoagulability condition. If a patient has any of a number of hypercoagulable conditions, we don't prescribe OCPs or Depo-Provera. We may also refer the patient to a hematologist for possible further work-up or long-term use of an anticoagulant medication, such as warfarin (Coumadin).

Certainly pregnancy is not the only potential concern related to sexual activity, given the possibility of developing AIDS (Acquired Immune Deficiency Syndrome) or other sexually transmitted diseases as possible complications of sexual activity. Education is again the most important piece of preventing sexually transmitted diseases. Condoms when used appropriately can also prevent sexually transmitted diseases. Unfortunately, many people with DS would find the use of condoms challenging. If an adult with DS is in a long-term relationship that might develop into a sexually active one, it may therefore be wise to ensure that both partners be tested for AIDS and other sexually transmitted diseases to make sure it's safe.

PREGNANCY

Little information is known about pregnancy in women with DS. We have not personally cared for any women with DS during their pregnancies, although to date, we have had two patients who became pregnant and delivered healthy infants who didn't have Down syndrome. (Both patients delivered their babies before we met them.)

According to the limited research done, women with DS are more likely to have babies with DS themselves (see the section on Fertility, above), and babies with DS have a higher incidence of being born prematurely and with medical complications such as heart defects. Emotional supports as well as careful monitoring are very important elements of prenatal care. It may be advisable to seek care from an obstetrician who specializes in high risk pregnancies to ensure that the woman receives appropriate prenatal care.

PAP SMEARS

Cervical cancer is now known to be related to infection with the human papilloma virus (HPV). This is a virus that is sexually transmitted. Pap smears are done to look for changes in the tissue of the cervix that are indicative of infection with HPV, precancerous changes, or cancer of the cervix.

If a woman is not sexually active, the risk of cancer of the cervix should be negligible. As indicated in Chapter 3, we recommend a Pap smear every three years for our female patients who are not sexually active and who are not having symptoms. If the woman is sexually active, we consider an annual Pap smear. The use of the HPV vaccine to prevent cervical cancer is discussed in Chapter 3.

Some women with DS have a difficult time complying with a Pap smear. Although it would be possible to sedate these patients and perform a pap smear, as discussed in Chapter 3, we limit the use of sedation. For our female patients who are not sexually active and who aren't having symptoms, the risk of sedation seems to exceed the benefit of doing a Pap smear (since cancer of the cervix is theoretically not possible if a woman is not sexually active).

In fact, researcher have demonstrated a very low incidence of abnormal Pap smears in women with intellectual disabilities who are not sexually active and not having symptoms (Quint and Elkins, 1997). Therefore, if a woman who is not sexually active cannot comply with a Pap smear or pelvic exam without sedation, we simply don't do the Pap smear or exam. However, if the woman is sexually active or having symptoms such as abnormal bleeding, we consider sedation and even anesthesia to complete the exam. If possible, we coordinate the Pap smear and pelvic exam with some other procedure that requires anesthesia.

Some physicians recommend doing screening pelvic ultrasounds for women who are not able to cooperate with a pelvic exam. The ultrasound does not provide the same information as a Pap smear, however, and therefore does not take the place of a Pap smear. Furthermore, there have been no studies that concluded that an ultrasound should replace a pelvic exam for women who cannot tolerate a pelvic exam. Consequently, we don't recommend using ultrasounds as a routine screening tool. However, if the woman is having symptoms such as pain or abnormal bleeding, we recommend an ultrasound if it is an appropriate tool to assess the cause of the symptoms.

YEAST INFECTIONS

Vaginal yeast infections don't seem to be more common in women with DS. However, they may take longer to diagnose and treat if the woman does not recognize what is wrong and seek medical treatment.

Symptoms of vaginal yeast infections include:
- ◆ Irritation and redness of the vulvae,
- ◆ vaginal discharge,
- ◆ unpleasant odor,
- ◆ itching,
- ◆ discomfort with urination,
- ◆ bleeding.

Poor hygiene may contribute to the development of infections. Instruction on personal hygiene is important and may need to be demonstrated if the woman has recurrent yeast infections. The keys are to teach the woman to gently wash the vulva using mild soap and water and to limit soaking in soapy bath water.

In our practice, the most common cause of yeast vaginal infections seems to be the use of oral antibiotics. Antibiotics not only kill the intended bacteria but also kill "good bacteria" in the intestines, vagina, mouth, and other places. It may be helpful to take acidophilus ("good bacteria") tablets or eat yogurt while on antibiotics to replenish helpful bacteria. It may also help to start treatment for yeast infections as soon as symptoms arise when taking antibiotics or to start antifungal treatment at the time of starting the antibiotic.

Antifungal treatments include:
- ◆ topical creams: nystatin (Mycostatin), clotrimazole (Gyne-Lotrimin, Mycelex), terconazole (Terazol);
- ◆ vaginal suppositories: miconazole (Monistat), terconazole (Terazol);
- ◆ oral medication: fluconazole (Diflucan).

The oral medication fluconazole tends to be the easiest for women with DS to use. It is one pill that is taken one time.

Yeast infections are diagnosed on the basis of:
- ◆ the history and physical exam, and
- ◆ collecting a sample of the vaginal discharge and examining it under the microscope.

Some women with DS have difficulty cooperating with the physical exam and collection of the vaginal discharge sample. If the description of the discharge sounds like yeast (white, curd-like), there is itching, and the person has recently been on antibiotics, there is a good chance it is a yeast infection. In that situation, we may treat the woman on the basis of the history and only push forward to do the exam if her condition fails to improve after a course of fluconazole treatment.

We don't typically see recurrent yeast infections in women with DS (except those caused by repeatedly taking antibiotics). When they do recur, however, it is important to test the woman for diabetes mellitus, since diabetes is associated with recurrent yeast infections.

Chapter 17

Seizures, Headaches, and Other Neurological Problems

Eduardo, age 35, was brought to the Center for an evaluation for headaches. The headaches had been occurring daily for about two months. They were primarily in the occiput (back) of his head. The pain responded to ibuprofen but would return a few hours later. He denied having any neck pain, vision changes, weakness, gait changes, or incontinence of urine or stool.

During the physical exam, we found that Eduardo's arms and legs had increased deep tendon reflexes. There was no weakness. The lateral cervical (neck) spine x-ray showed subluxation (abnormal movement) of the first cervical vertebrae on the second (atlantoaxial instability). An MRI showed pressure of the vertebrae on the spinal cord at the C1-2 level (level of the first and second vertebrae in the neck). Eduardo was referred to an orthopedic surgeon and neurosurgeon, who operated on Eduardo and stabilized his neck bones. After a period of recovery, Eduardo did well and no longer experienced headaches.

Neurology involves the study of the brain, nerves, and spinal cord. Because Down syndrome (DS) causes structural abnormalities in these parts of the body, it is not surprising that people with DS have a higher incidence of some neurological problems such as seizures. Perhaps more surprising is that the incidence of neurological problems is not higher. In addition, when neurological problems do occur, they may be due to causes that are less common in the general population.

This chapter focuses on one neurological problem—seizures—that is more common in people with Down syndrome, as well as on two neurological problems that are relatively rare in adults with Down syndrome, but can be serious when they occur—headaches and strokes.

HEADACHES

People with DS do not often complain of headaches, in our experience. In the 18 years that the Adult Down Syndrome Center has been in operation, it has not been common for our patients to complain of headaches. It is possible that the incidence is underreported because some people with DS can't articulate the problem or because people with DS have a higher tolerance for pain.

In the relatively few individuals who complain of headache at the Center, the underlying cause is usually not one of the more common causes such as migraine headaches or muscle contraction headaches. In a random review of 400 of our patients who were evaluated over a one-year period, only 6 reported a complaint of headaches. Two of the individuals had headaches due to head trauma they had sustained in a motor vehicle accident. Two had headaches due to atlantoaxial instability (cervical subluxation). One had headaches due to a hemorrhagic stroke (stroke due to bleeding into the brain), and another due to an acute epidural hemorrhage (bleeding between the outer covering of the brain and the skull, usually caused by trauma).

Other patients at the Center have reported headaches due to sinus infections, allergies, or strep throat. These headaches are not usually persistent or recurrent. Very few patients have been diagnosed with migraine headaches or muscle contraction headaches. Therefore, a complaint of headache by a person with DS deserves careful evaluation.

An evaluation should include checking for the problems noted above, including:
- ◆ head trauma,
- ◆ atlanto-axial instability (see Chapter 13),
- ◆ stroke (see below),
- ◆ epidural hemorrhage (uncommon in DS),
- ◆ sinus infection,
- ◆ allergies, and
- ◆ strep throat.

Another possible cause of headaches is eye strain, which may be due to impaired vision. Although eye strain as a cause of headaches tends to be overestimated in people without DS, it should at least be considered as a possible cause. As discussed in Chapter 8, teens and adults with DS should have regular eye exams. Headaches may also be a side effect of many medications. In addition, headaches may occur if the person misses a dose of a medication taken on a regular basis.

To look for underlying causes of headaches, the physician should take a history and perform a physical exam that includes looking for sinus or allergy complaints and assessing for neurological changes that could be caused by stroke, hemorrhage, or cervical subluxation. He or she might also consider imaging of the neck (lateral cervical spine x-rays, CT, or MRI) and/or the brain (CT or MRI).

Headaches Due to Allergies or Sinus Congestion

People with DS frequently have problems with nasal congestion, sneezing, and runny nose. However, people with DS appear to be less likely than those without DS to have these symptoms as a result of allergies. More often, these symptoms are related to infections or irritants such as smoke (see Chapter 7). Whatever the cause of sinus congestion, one of the symptoms can be headaches. However, once again a complaint of headache does not appear to be as common in people with Down syndrome.

If a headache is due to sinus problems or allergies, part of the treatment will be to reduce sinus congestion (see Chapter 7). Allergy treatments include:

- ◆ antihistamine medications such as diphenhydramine (Benadryl) or loratadine (Claritin),
- ◆ nasal steroid sprays such as fluticasone (Flonase),
- ◆ montelukast sodium (Singulair), which blocks leukotriene—a substance the body releases in response to exposure to an allergen.

If these treatment are not effective, the person may need a consult with an allergist to consider allergy testing. Allergy testing may include blood testing and/or skin testing. Skin tests are done with small pricks of the skin to introduce a variety of allergens (substances a person may be allergic to) into the body. If it is discovered what the person is allergic to and other treatments are not effective, desensitization shots may be considered. This treatment consists of regularly scheduled injections of a small but increasing amount of the allergen to decrease the body's sensitivity to it. Treatment of the allergies should help reduce or eliminate the headaches.

Seizures

A seizure is a sudden change in the electrical activity in the cortex of the brain. When a person has two or more unprovoked seizures, the diagnosis of epilepsy or a seizure disorder is made. The term seizure disorder is more commonly used now.

Unlike headaches, which are less common in people with DS, seizures are more common. Seizures can develop at any age, but they are more likely to begin either in childhood (usually in the first two years of life) or later in adulthood (often after age 35). The seizures that develop in late adulthood are often, although not always, associated with Alzheimer disease (see Chapter 19). A family history of seizures may increase the risk of having seizures in people with DS just as it does in people without DS.

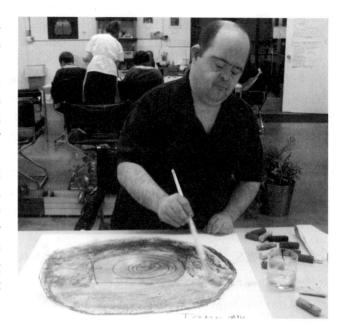

Types of Seizures

There are many types of seizures, and people with DS can have any of the types:

◆ **Generalized seizures** (affecting both sides of the brain):

  ➤ *Absence:* seizures that cause a brief (seconds to minutes) loss of consciousness or changes in posture. The person usually does not fall down, but may appear to stare blankly and be unresponsive for a few seconds. If postural changes are part of the symptoms, the person may fall.

  ➤ *Myoclonic:* seizures that result in repetitive muscle contractions; the person's arms and/or legs may jerk, but he does not usually fall down or lose consciousness. Some people will fall if the contractions are severe enough to knock them off-balance.

  ➤ *Tonic-clonic:* seizures that cause rhythmic contractions of muscles of all four extremities; the person usually loses consciousness and falls to the ground. During a general tonic-clonic seizure, the person often loses bowel or urinary control.

◆ **Partial seizures** (affecting particular areas of the brain)

  ➤ *Simple:* focal seizures (that affect one area of the brain) that are not associated with change in awareness or consciousness; examples include twitching of fingers, smelling an unpleasant smell that isn't there, or experiencing mood changes.

> ➤ Complex: focal seizures that result in an alteration of aware-
> ness or consciousness; examples include automatic repeti-
> tive behavior such as walking or uncontrollable laughter.

There are also febrile seizures, which are triggered by a fever and occur only in childhood. They will not be addressed in this book.

Before a seizure, a person may experience an aura—an altered state of conscious-ness or unusual sensation that provides a warning that a seizure is coming. For exam-ple, he may see flashing lights or imagine he smells a particular scent.

Some seizures (partial complex seizures) look "behavioral." For example, the person may make repetitive movements that appear to be under his voluntary control, but are not. For example, the person may walk about, but seem unresponsive while walking. Lip smacking is another example of a movement that may appear to be under the person's control when in reality it is not.

Other people may have sudden changes in mood, aggressive behavior, or other behavioral changes as the result of a seizure. Seizures should therefore always be con-sidered as a possible cause of sudden behavioral changes in an adult with DS, espe-cially if the person won't respond.

After a seizure is over, the person often has a post-ictal state—a period of fatigue and/or confusion.

Causes of Seizures

When people with normal brains have seizures, about a third of the time the cause for seizures is not clearly known (idiopathic seizures). In people who have ab-normalities of the brain (including those associated with DS), however, those brain abnormalities can be a cause of seizures. The specific brain abnormalities in people with DS that are thought to be associated with seizures include:

- ◆ structural abnormalities, which can cause electrical overstimulation;
- ◆ increased excitation of brain cells;
- ◆ decreased inhibition of electrical pathways (ordinarily, the brain has a system of checks and balances with pathways that excite and path-ways that inhibit or repress electrical activity);
- ◆ changes in the amount of neurotransmitters (the chemicals in the brain such as dopamine and serotonin that pass the electrical signal from brain cell to brain cell).

Other factors that may cause or contribute to seizures include:

- ◆ infections, especially of the central nervous system (e.g., meningitis, brain abscess);
- ◆ trauma to the head;
- ◆ metabolic disorders such as hyponatremia (low sodium);

◆ certain medications such as theophylline (used for asthma), isoniazid (used for tuberculosis), antidepressants, amphetamines (used for attention-deficit/hyperactivity disorder), anti-cholinesterase medications (such as donezepril/Aricept used for Alzheimer disease), and lithium;
◆ history of brain injury such as stroke.

The above factors can be a primary cause of seizures or can "lower the seizure threshold," causing someone who has a seizure disorder to have a seizure.

Other potential causes of seizures in the general population that have not been identified as the cause of seizures in our patients at the Adult Down Syndrome Center include:

◆ alcohol or drug withdrawal, and
◆ drug abuse.

RISKS OF SEIZURES

A significant concern for someone having a seizure is the potential for injury or even death. During certain types of seizures, individuals may fall or have body movements that can lead to injury if they strike the ground or other hard objects. In addition, the alteration in consciousness during a seizure can be dangerous in many situations. For example, serious injury can occur if someone has a seizure while driving, swimming, or walking on stairs.

Repeated or prolonged seizures can contribute to permanent neurologic (brain) injury. Brain cells can be damaged.

Some people with seizure disorders may sometimes experience back-to-back or continuous seizures. That is, before they have regained normal consciousness after one seizure, they have one or more additional seizures. This situation is defined as *status epilepticus.* This is considered a neurologic emergency and if not quickly controlled, can cause severe injury to the brain or even death. ***Call 911 or take the person to the emergency room if he is having continuous seizures.***

DIAGNOSIS OF SEIZURES

Adults with and without DS who develop seizures may not even be aware that they are having them. One reason is because seizures most often cause changes in consciousness. Another is that many seizures occur during sleep. Consequently, a good eyewitness account can be the most important clue to the diagnosis. Signs that an individual may be experiencing seizures include:

◆ episodes of "blacking out" (losing consciousness, as in fainting or forgetting what happened),
◆ episodes of difficulty talking or confusion,
◆ eyes rolling up,
◆ shaking movements,

- ◆ staring spells,
- ◆ jerking movements of an extremity,
- ◆ eye fluttering,
- ◆ making sounds that don't make sense in the context of the situation,
- ◆ unexplained injuries such as a tongue bite, a fracture, or bruising that are noted upon awakening (these can be signs that seizures are occurring during sleep).

If seizures are suspected, the person should see his primary provider and/or a neurologist for an evaluation. If the diagnosis is unclear or the treatment ineffective, consultation with a neurologist is definitely recommended.

EEG: An electroencephalogram (EEG) can provide additional confirming information. An EEG is done by attaching electrodes (wires) to the head with tape and a glue substance. The electrical waves of the brain are then measured. If the person has a seizure during the EEG, the EEG should be abnormal. Even if the person doesn't have a seizure during the EEG, abnormalities may be noted during testing. Sometimes, however, 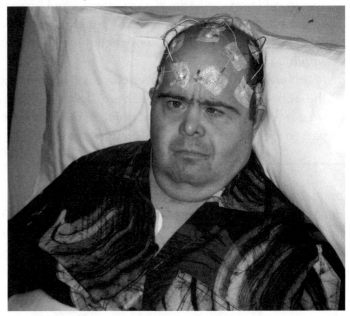 a person with a seizure disorder will have a normal EEG (if he does not experience a seizure during the EEG). While an EEG doesn't hurt, some people with DS have difficulty cooperating with this exam. Unfortunately, sedation can alter the results.

Doing an EEG while the individual is both awake and asleep can sometimes reveal abnormalities that do not show up if the EEG is only done while awake. However, as noted above, even when a person has a seizure disorder, the EEG may still not show the changes associated with seizures. Therefore, if the diagnosis is not clear, a prolonged EEG (for example for 24 hours) can be done. This may need to be done in the hospital. In addition, a prolonged EEG with video recording of the individual can provide additional information. If the person cannot cooperate with an EEG, just a video recording may be done to capture for the doctor what the concerning symptoms are.

CT Scan and MRI: If seizures are suspected, further testing should ideally be done to look for potential causes such as tumors, brain injury or trauma, or infection. Some of these things can be treated so seizures can be eliminated or reduced. A CT (computerized tomography) scan or MRI (magnetic resonance imaging) scan of the

What to Do If Someone Is Having a Seizure

The main goal is to prevent the person from injuring himself. How to best accomplish this will vary with the type of seizure. However, safety is of most concern with seizures that cause the person to fall or that cause shaking (tonic-clonic) movements. One way to prevent injury is to straddle the person having the seizure on the ground and put one leg on each side of him. This helps prevent the individual from bumping into furniture or other hard objects. Putting something soft under the person's head (like a soft pillow) if he is lying on concrete or a hard surface may also prevent injury.

In addition, sometimes diazepam rectal suppositories (Diastat) are prescribed. These can be given at the time of a seizure to stop a prolonged seizure. For most seizures, it is not necessary. The seizure will end spontaneously within a few minutes.

Note that you should never place a stick (such as a tongue depressor) into the person's mouth during a seizure. This was recommended in the past, but we now know that placing something in the mouth can cause injury to both the person having the seizure and to the person holding the tongue depressor.

brain is recommended. Both of these tests are painless but do require lying still on a table. An MRI can give more information than a CT scan but some people—both with and without DS—may find it more challenging to cooperate with because the scanner is more claustrophobic, makes more noise, and takes longer.

TREATMENT

There are a number of medications available to prevent seizures. The choice depends on the type of seizures, the person's tolerance to the side effects, and how well the seizures respond to the medication. For some individuals, more than one medication is necessary. Sometimes it is not possible to completely prevent seizures from occurring. However, medications can generally at least lessen the frequency or severity of seizures.

Medications include:

- ◆ carbamezepine (Tegretol, Carbatrol),
- ◆ clonazepam (Klonopin),
- ◆ valproic acid or valproate (Depakote, Depakene),
- ◆ phenytoin (Dilantin),
- ◆ ethosuximide,
- ◆ gabapentin (Neurontin),
- ◆ levetiracetam (Keppra),
- ◆ lamotrigine (Lamictal),
- ◆ topiramate (Topamax).

For some of the medications, blood tests can be done to measure the level of the medication in the blood to guide dosing the medication. Generally, the goal is to give the person the lowest dose possible that results in good seizure control with the fewest side effects. This may require some experimentation. Many of the side effects are subjective (e.g., effects on mood or energy) so adults with DS may not be able to report them. This means that family members or others may need to observe the person to get a sense of how he feels on the medication.

Some of the medications require that blood tests be done to check for side effects. These tests include:

- CBC (complete blood count) to monitor for a reduction in the white blood cell count, red blood cell count, and/or platelet count;
- liver tests (hepatic panel) to monitor for liver damage;
- electrolytes tests (blood test) to monitor for decreased sodium level;
- other tests to monitor for other changes.

We have found that most adults with DS tolerate anticonvulsant medications well. Sometimes, however, the medications make them quite sedated. Especially in older individuals, the medications may cause some confusion. This seems to be particularly a concern with phenytoin (Dilantin). If the person's current treatment is challenging, a good neurologist should be able to work with him until he or she finds the medication or combination of medications that will control the seizures best with the fewest troublesome side effects.

For severe, intractable seizures, surgery is another potential treatment option. The brain is "mapped" so the area causing the seizures can be found and removed. This is a treatment that is infrequently required and can result in cognitive or physical limitations or other changes to the person's abilities, depending on what area of the brain is removed. There is limited information available about the use of this surgery in people with DS. You might want to get a second or third opinion if this treatment is recommended.

PRECAUTIONS FOR PEOPLE WITH SEIZURES

For all people who have seizures, it makes sense to take precautions that can prevent injury in the event of a seizure. Some recommendations include:

- Ensure that the person never swims alone.
- If the person has a driver's license, he should not drive an automobile for a period of time after a seizure and may even have his license revoked. State governments have rules regarding this recommendation. Although few of our patients drive, it is important to follow the state regulations (see www.epilepsy.com/epilepsy/rights_driving).
- Teach the individual to be cautious with activities that could cause injury from a sudden fall (for example, activities at elevated heights).
- When starting a new medication, observe for possible new side effects that could lead to injury.

♦ Consider changing jobs if the job setting could be dangerous for someone with seizures. For example, if the person cooks French fries and
is near hot oil or works near machinery, consider an alternative job or
different job responsibilities.

♦ Avoid medications that list seizures as a possible side effect. They can
make seizures worse in someone with a seizure disorder.

STROKES

Strokes are rapidly developing injuries to the brain caused by disruption to the
blood supply. The resulting injury to the brain can cause a variety of symptoms including weakness (usually on one side of the body), speech impairment, confusion, and
vision impairment. The symptoms depend on where in the brain the injury occurs.

Strokes caused by atherosclerotic disease seem to be less common in people with
Down syndrome. Atherosclerotic disease (plaques in the arteries, "hardening of the
arteries) is less common in people with Down syndrome (see Chapter 9). However,
several disorders that can result in strokes are more common in Down syndrome;
these are highlighted below.

CAUSES

There are two general types of strokes:
1. **Ischemic strokes:** These occur when the blood vessels that supply
the brain are blocked. The resulting lack of blood causes an infarction
(an area of dead brain tissue).
2. **Hemorrhagic strokes:** These occur when bleeding into the brain tissue causes an injury to the brain.

In people without DS, atherosclerotic disease (narrowing of the arteries) is a common cause of stroke. As noted above, atherosclerotic disease is uncommon in people
with Down syndrome and therefore does not appear to be a common cause of strokes
in adults with DS.

When ischemic strokes do occur in people with DS, the cause is more likely to be:

♦ **Moyamoya disease:** This condition affects the blood vessels of the brain. It is
more common in people with DS (although still not common overall) and can
cause ischemic or hemorrhagic strokes. The disease primarily affects children.
The first symptom is often a stroke or recurrent transient ischemic attacks (or
"mini-strokes") due to blockage in the blood vessels. The symptoms are often
muscular weakness or seizures. Adults with the disorder usually have a hemorrhagic stroke. Moyamoya tends to run in families. Treatment requires surgery to

restore blood flow to the brain by opening narrowed blood vessels or bypassing blocked arteries.

◆ **Microangiopathic disease:** In this disorder, small blood vessels in the brain become occluded (blocked), causing an ischemic stroke. The brain, like other organs, has large and small blood vessels that supply it with blood. Microangiopathic refers to disturbance of the small blood vessels. In people with DS, this disease most often seems to occur when protein builds up in the brain and compresses the small vessels from outside the vessel. The build-up of protein is one of the changes seen in Alzheimer disease (see Chapter 20). It should be noted that sometimes the damage to these small vessels can cause bleeding (hemorrhagic stroke).

◆ **Tic disorders** such as Tourette syndrome cause involuntary movements or vocalizations. Tic disorders are somewhat more common in people with Down syndrome. Sometimes when an individual has tics that involve rapid movement of the head and neck, this can cause compression of the blood vessels (vertebral arteries) in the neck that carry blood into the posterior brain. Infrequently, this compression can cut off the blood supply to the brain and result in a stroke.

◆ **Vertebral Subluxation:** As discussed in Chapter 13, people with DS are at risk of having vertebrae in the neck slip and compress the spinal cord. Sometimes this compression can pinch the arteries that travel from the vertebrae to the brain. If the blood flow is cut off in this manner, an ischemic stroke can result.

◆ **Blood clots:** Blood clots are collections of platelets and clotting factors (proteins). Clots can form in the heart, break loose, and travel to the brain and then cause a stroke. Clots in the heart are more common when there are abnormal valves or other congenital anomalies. Sometimes the clot may include bacteria when an abnormal valve or a patch that was surgically implanted becomes infected with bacteria and then an infected clot breaks loose. Because of this risk of clots, *it is important that anyone who has had a congenital heart defect repaired continue to see a cardiologist in adulthood* (see Chapter 9). As discussed in Chapter 16, blood clots can also be a side effect of birth control pills.

Hemorrhagic strokes can be caused by:
  ◆ Moyamoya syndrome (see above);
  ◆ microangiopathic disease;
  ◆ aneurysms (out-pouchings in an artery that can rupture (aneurysms *do not* appear to be more common in people with DS);
  ◆ hypertension (high blood pressure) (as discussed in Chapter 9, however, hypertension is uncommon in people with DS and, therefore, rarely a cause of strokes in people with DS);
  ◆ unknown causes.

PREVENTION

Because of the variety of risk factors that could result in a person having a stroke, most people are urged to exercise and eat a healthy diet to reduce their chance of a stroke. This approach is less likely to reduce the risk of strokes in people with Down syndrome, given their lower incidence of high blood pressure and atherosclerosis.

We certainly don't want to imply that teens and adults with Down syndrome do not need to exercise and eat right for a variety of other reasons. However, to reduce the risk of strokes in a person with Down syndrome, it is more important to focus on specific risk facts the individual has. For example, regular follow-up with a cardiologist and periodic echocardiograms should be considered if the person had heart surgery earlier in life. Managing tics, assessing for cervical subluxation (see Chapter 13), and assessing for Moyamoya disease (if the person had a previous stroke or TIA) are other beneficial approaches to preventing strokes in people with DS.

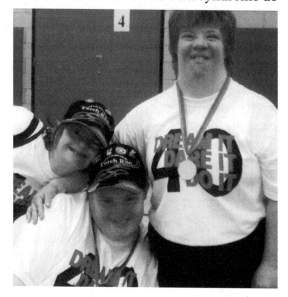

TREATMENT OF STROKES

If a stroke is caused by a sudden blockage of a large blood vessel, urgent (within a few hours) restoration of the blood flow can minimize damage to the brain. This requires rapid evaluation in the Emergency Room and then treatment to remove the blockage. For this reason, it is important to know the warning signs of stroke (see box) and get help immediately if you suspect one is occurring.

Warning Signs of a Stroke

Signs that someone may be experiencing a stroke include:

- ◆ sudden confusion, trouble speaking, or understanding,
- ◆ sudden trouble walking, dizziness, loss of balance or coordination,
- ◆ sudden trouble seeing in one or both eyes,
- ◆ sudden numbness or weakness of the face, arm or leg, especially on one side of the body,
- ◆ sudden, severe headache.

Treatment may include:

- If a blood clot has formed in the heart or the person is at risk for a blood clot, warfarin (Coumadin) (a blood thinner) may be prescribed.
- For obstruction or narrowing of large vessels, a surgical bypass procedure may be performed. Medications may also be prescribed.
- For small vessel disease, an adult or children's aspirin a day may be prescribed. However, studies do not clearly show that this is a beneficial treatment. It may actually cause more problems because hemorrhage can also occur in small vessel disease in people with DS and an aspirin can increase the risk of that occurring.

Anyone who has had a stroke will need ongoing follow-up care. Depending on the cause, circumstances, and other factors, the primary practitioner, a neurologist, a cardiologist, or other specialist may be involved in that care. Some people also need to see a physiatrist (rehabilitation physician). Physical and occupational therapy are recommended to help the individual regain motor skills, skills required to perform activities of daily living, walking ability, and other skills that may be impaired after a stroke. Speech-language therapy may also be helpful if the person's speech or swallowing is impaired. Finally, if the person becomes depressed due to the stroke or associated loss of skills, he may benefit from treatment from his primary physician, a psychiatrist, and/or a counselor.

Chapter 18

Sleep Problems

Marie, age 23, was struggling at her job at the local fast food restaurant. She had always done a wonderful job helping to prepare the food. However, in the last few months, she was making more errors, seemed to be having difficulty concentrating, and was falling asleep on her breaks. Her mom reported that she had never been a "good sleeper," but in the last year or so was snoring more loudly, had become a restless sleeper, and was falling asleep at the movies, while eating dinner, and while talking on the phone. Marie also had less interest in doing activities and keeping in touch with her family and friends, and seemed more irritable.

After an assessment at the Adult Down Syndrome Center, Marie was referred to the Sleep Lab at the hospital and was diagnosed with sleep apnea. After discussion with the sleep specialist, she was advised to lose about 20 pounds and to work on getting at least eight hours of sleep per night, and was prescribed CPAP (continuous positive airway pressure). Over the next few months, Marie's work production returned to its previous level, her mood improved, and she became more interested in socializing with her family and friends again.

Sleep problems are common in people with Down syndrome (DS). Like other people with intellectual disabilities, they often have abnormal sleep patterns. This is likely due, at least in part, to neurological differences in the sleep centers in the brain. A number of studies have shown sleep problems in children with DS. For instance, one group of researchers found that 40 percent of children and adolescents don't sleep through the night (Carter et al., 2009). Sleep apnea, a condition in which breathing stops or is greatly reduced during sleep, is also more common in people with DS. Some of the sleep problems can be improved with good sleep habits (sleep hygiene), while others may require further intervention or medication.

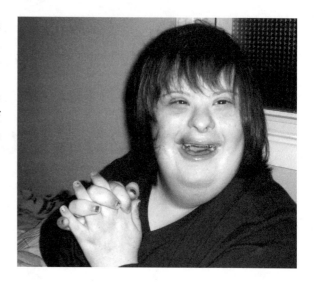

Inadequate or inappropriate sleep may affect people in a wide variety of ways. Some of the changes we have seen include:

- ◆ fatigue,
- ◆ poor work performance,
- ◆ depression and other mood disturbances,
- ◆ anxiety,
- ◆ psychotic behavior,
- ◆ muscle aches and pains,
- ◆ worsening of a variety of health issues, and
- ◆ reduced ability to focus or attend to tasks.

Note that falling asleep in the car is not listed as a problem above. It is characteristic of the great majority of our patients with DS—whether they have sleep problems or not.

SLEEP HYGIENE

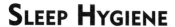

Good sleep starts with good sleep hygiene. While it is important to be aware of potential sleep problems in people with DS, something that it often overlooked (by people with and without DS) are the day-to-day sleeping habits known as "sleep hygiene." Just as good dental hygiene involves a set of planned activities such as brushing and flossing your teeth, the choices and plans you make during the day can also affect how healthily you sleep. Sleep hygiene is addressed in Chapter 2.

TROUBLESHOOTING SLEEP PROBLEMS

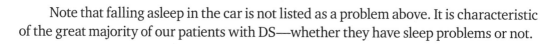

If there is an apparent sleep problem, start by keeping track of bedtimes, wake-up times, and the other issues listed above. Try to make some of the sleep hygiene modifications to fit the individual's particular needs. If the person with DS is living independently and has no supervision at night, it might be a good idea to arrange for someone to spend a night or two with her to monitor what goes on at bedtime. (Refer to the story in the section on "Developmental Age vs. Chronological Age" in Chapter 1 about the women who were staying up late watching TV.)

If those measures don't work and the sleep disturbance is affecting the person, additional treatments can be considered:

- **Melatonin** is a naturally occurring hormone. It has been used to treat jet lag. It seems to help people fall asleep and "reset" their internal clock when traveling across time zones. It is also used for sleep disturbances not associated with travel. We have recommended it for a number of teens and adults with DS and it has helped many of them improve their abnormal sleep. We usually recommend starting with 2 mg before bedtime and increasing to 4 mg in a few weeks if 2 mg doesn't work.

- **Sleeping pills** such as zolpidem (Ambien), zaleplon (Sonata) have been effective for some of our patients with sleep problems. There is a theoretical use of becoming dependent on these medications. Therefore, consider limiting the length of time these medications are used. It may be helpful to use them for a few weeks while implementing measures to improve sleep hygiene and addressing other physical and mental health issues. Sometimes a short course will "reset the clock" and a person will continue to sleep well after the medications are discontinued.

- **Trazadone** (Desyrel) is an antidepressant medication that we have had little success with in treating depression. However, we *have* had success with using it at bedtime to improve sleep. We generally start at a low dose (25-50 mg), usually no more than 100 mg, but occasionally have gone as high as 200 mg. Unlike the sleeping medications in the previous paragraph, it does not have a dependency risk.

- **Antihistamines** such as diphenhydramine (Benadryl) or hydroxyzine are allergy medications that tend to make people drowsy. If taken before bed only, the medication can make some people drowsy enough to use it as a sleep aid. Antihistamines can be useful sleep aids for people with or without allergies.

Sleep Apnea

In order to understand what sleep apnea is, it is important to know what normal sleep is. Normal, uninterrupted sleep consists of a cyclic pattern alternating between rapid eye movement (REM) sleep and non-rapid eye movement (non-REM) sleep. REM sleep is also called dream sleep because this is the stage of sleep when dreams occur. Someone with normal sleep typically has several periods of REM sleep per night.

There are several benefits of REM sleep:

- Certain types of memory are consolidated in REM sleep. This helps in learning new skills the person has been practicing in the daytime.
- REM sleep may have a direct benefit in reducing stress.

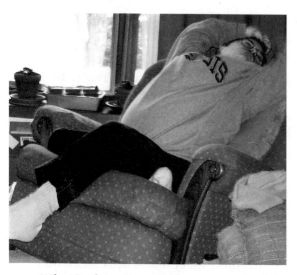

Many physiological changes occur during REM sleep. For instance, there is a decline in chin muscle activity, all the muscles in the body except the diaphragm relax (become atonic), and breathing becomes irregular. Consequently, during normal REM sleep, the pharynx (airway) narrows because of muscle relaxation, causing added resistance to air movement through the airway. During normal sleep, this causes reduced air movement and a slight increase in carbon dioxide in the body.

What is sleep apnea? Sleep apnea is defined as a complete cessation of breathing from any cause during sleep. This results in decreased oxygen in the blood or increased carbon dioxide (a greater increase than would be seen in normal sleep). The pauses in breathing usually last 10 to 20 seconds but can last as long as 120 seconds. In severe cases, the person may experience more than 500 attacks of sleep apnea per night.

Someone who has apnea will wake up enough (often without being aware she is waking) to open her airway. Due to this rapid wake and sleep cycling, sleep is poor, the person has repeated episodes of insufficient oxygen in the blood, and REM sleep is poor.

Sleep apnea is divided into two major types. The most common is **obstructive sleep apnea,** which is caused by obstruction of the airway. The person continues to try to breathe, but the obstruction prevents movement of air into and out of the lungs. This is the most common type in people with DS. The less common type is **non-obstructive (central) sleep apnea.** In this type, there is a problem in the brain or nervous system that controls breathing. The person's airway may be open and the muscles may be fine, but the signal to breathe is not sent or doesn't reach the muscles. There is also a condition related to apnea called **hypopnea,** in which the person gets less oxygen than usual due to obstructions such as enlarged tonsils, but breathing doesn't completely stop.

Sleep apnea is increasingly recognized as a significant cause of health problems and even death. More than 1 percent of the general population is affected, with a dramatic increase in the elderly. Approximately 4 percent of middle-aged men have obstructive sleep apnea, whereas women are much less frequently affected. It is quite common in both men and women with DS, however—and in children and teens, as well. A recent study found that 94 percent (all except one) of the 16 subjects with Down syndrome had sleep apnea (Trois et al., 2009).

Risk Factors for Apnea

Obesity is the major risk factor for obstructive apnea. However, many obese people do not have sleep apnea and some people with sleep apnea are not obese. Typically, conditions that narrow the upper airway increase the risk of apnea. These conditions include enlargement of the soft palate, uvula, tonsils, adenoids, or tongue; deposits of fat near the airway; and structural abnormalities.

People with DS are more likely to develop obstructive sleep apnea due to the following factors:

- ◆ a relatively small midfacial region and relatively large tongue, which contribute to narrowing of the airway;
- ◆ narrower nasal passages and narrowing in the airway below the pharynx (the area behind the nose and mouth, including the throat);
- ◆ chronic inflammation of the nasal passages and enlarged lymph tissue (including the tonsils and adenoids);
- ◆ obesity;
- ◆ reduced muscle tone in the pharynx (maintaining an open airway is dependent on the muscle tone in the pharynx).

The use of sedative medications, and, perhaps, antihistamines may also contribute to decreased muscle tone.

DIAGNOSIS OF APNEA

The most common symptoms of sleep apnea are:

- ◆ a long history of loud snoring, combined with
  - ➤ restless sleep,
  - ➤ excessive daytime drowsiness, and
  - ➤ early morning headaches (although people with DS do not often complain of headaches; see Chapter 17).

Other symptoms may include:

- ◆ difficulties concentrating,
- ◆ depression,
- ◆ irritability,
- ◆ personality changes,
- ◆ heartburn due to increased reflux of stomach contents into the esophagus during obstruction,
- ◆ a persistent cough or aggravation of asthma symptoms if secretions are aspirated into the lungs during obstruction,
- ◆ increased shortness of breath and fatigue over time.

If a person with DS has some of the above symptoms, she should consult with her medical practitioner—whether or not pauses in her breathing while sleeping have been observed. It is worth nothing, however, that a study by Dr. Sally Shott and colleagues (2006) showed that sleep apnea was present a lot more than was suggested by parents' observations and report.

We refer our patients who have symptoms indicative of sleep apnea to a sleep specialist. (Typically, these are neurologists, pulmonologists, or otolaryngologists who have received additional training in sleep medicine.)

The doctor will take a history of the person's symptoms and also do a physical exam. He or she will rule out thyroid disease as a cause of fatigue. If apnea is present, the physical will usually, but not always, reveal obesity and excessive soft tissue in the mouth, pharynx, and neck. With advanced disease, the right side of the heart will be weakened. As a result, the physical may show failure of that part of the heart. (Specifically, the right side of the heart doesn't pump well and pressure builds, which causes retention of fluid in the extremities, the liver, and other tissues.) When someone has sleep apnea, the laboratory tests are usually normal except low levels of oxygen and high carbon dioxide may be found in the blood.

An overnight sleep study is needed to definitely diagnose sleep apnea. During the study, eye movements and muscle tone are recorded, an electroencephalogram (EEG) measures brain waves, and an electrocardiogram (EKG) measures the electrical activity of the heart. The test also records respiratory movements, movement of air in and out of the nose and mouth, and oxygenation of the blood.

A sleep study involves attaching electrodes and other measuring devices to various parts of the person's body. The person is then asked to fall asleep in a bed while the sleep technicians monitor and record data from another room. Most people with DS tolerate the procedure fairly well. A sedative can be given, if necessary, but sedatives can worsen sleep apnea and are generally not recommended. A parent or other familiar person is allowed to stay in the room if necessary for the person's piece of mind. If the person just can't tolerate the sleep study, it may be helpful to make a video of her sleeping at home. This will not provide all the data that a sleep study will, but may provide some helpful information for the professional who is trying to determine whether apnea is present.

The sleep study report indicates the number of pauses (apnea) in breathing and number of decreased (hypopnea) breathing episodes. The Respiratory Distress Index is a measure of the total number of apneas plus hyponeas divided by the total sleep time. This is a measure of the number of events (apneas and hypopneas) per hour. Different sleep specialists may label anything above 5 to 15 as sleep apnea.

The sleep study report will also include data on the person's oxygen saturation levels during sleep. Oxygen saturation is a measure of the amount of oxygen in the blood. In people without sleep apnea, this level normally doesn't go below about 90 percent while sleeping. It may go as low as 40 percent in some people with sleep apnea. Low oxygen can have serious consequences for all the tissues/organs in the body, which is a major reason why treating sleep apnea is crucial.

TREATMENT OF SLEEP APNEA

If obstructive sleep apnea or hypopnea is found, there are several alternatives for treatment:

- ◆ If the patient is overweight, the first consideration is for her to try to lose weight. (See Chapter 2.)

◆ A change in sleeping position may be helpful, since many people have less or no sleep apnea if they don't sleep on their back. Encouraging the person to sleep on her side or on her abdomen can be helpful. Sometimes pinning a sock to the back of the person's pajama top and putting a tennis ball in the sock will keep the person from sleeping on her back.

◆ Eliminating sedatives and alcohol also helps some people.

◆ A mouthpiece may be prescribed by a dentist to help keep the person's airway open while she is asleep. (See box on page 248.)

For many adults with DS and apnea, the strategies above are not sufficient and/or the person is not able to lose enough weight. If so, the doctor will likely recommend supplemental oxygen, CPAP, or surgery to reduce the obstruction. If the person has central, rather than obstructive sleep apnea (less common in DS), she might also be prescribed medications (acetazolamide or theophylline) that stimulate the sleep centers of the brain.

SUPPLEMENTAL OXYGEN AND CPAP

For some people, breathing in supplemental oxygen while sleeping is enough to treat apnea. This treatment involves using a nasal cannula (the two-pronged device commonly used in the hospital to deliver oxygen) attached to a source of oxygen (for example an oxygen tank or an oxygen concentrator) at night to boost the amount of oxygen the person takes in while sleeping.

Generally, however, if the oxygen is to get to the lungs, oxygen alone is not enough. Most people with DS who have apnea need to use CPAP (continuous positive airway pressure) instead. In this procedure, air (and sometimes oxygen) is delivered by a mask that fits over the person's nose or the mouth and nose. It delivers a positive pressure to the airway to keep it open. In a sense, the machine delivers a puff of air under pressure to open the airway. Some adults with DS have trouble tolerating the CPAP mask. Some ways to encourage use of the mask include:

◆ Try the mask during the day while awake.

◆ Wear the mask for only a short period at night and build up the duration over time.

◆ Have someone keep the person company until she falls asleep with the mask on.

◆ Watch the movie *Top Gun* in which Tom Cruise is a fighter pilot who (of course) wears a mask while flying. ("If it is good for Tom Cruise, it is good for me.")

◆ Videotape or take a photograph of the individual wearing the mask to help remind and encourage her to wear the mask.

◆ Develop a reward system for wearing the mask.

◆ Although it is generally advisable to avoid giving sedatives to people with sleep apnea, some doctors may recommend a sedative to help the person fall asleep with the mask on or to allow someone to place the mask on her face after she falls asleep.

Mouthpieces

There are some mouthpieces available that can help patients with sleep apnea. The mouthpiece helps keep the airway open while the person is sleeping. These are often provided by a dentist who has been specially trained in addressing sleep apnea. Mouthpieces are generally recommended for mild to moderate sleep apnea but not for more severe cases.

Just as with CPAP, people with DS may resist using a mouthpiece. We have very limited experience with our patients trying the mouthpieces, nor were we able to find published information about using mouthpieces with people with DS. This is an area for further investigation in treating sleep apnea in people with Down syndrome.

CPAP machines do make some noise and can disturb bed partners or roommates. However, the noise is often less distracting than the loud snoring associated with untreated sleep apnea.

The CPAP machines are portable and should be taken on vacation. Security personnel at airports may closely inspect the CPAP machine, but regulations require that it be allowed as a carry-on piece of luggage. Like all medical devices, it does not count as either a passenger's carry-on or "personal bag." To limit delays at security, bring a letter from the doctor who is treating the sleep apnea or a copy of the Department of Transportation Fact Sheet (available on the American Sleep Apnea Association website—www.sleepapnea.org/news/travel.html).

SURGICAL TREATMENTS

For some people who have apnea, treatment may include surgery to open the airway. Removal of nasal polyps, correction of a deviated septum, or removal of enlarged tonsils and adenoids can sometimes help. However, often there is also obstruction in other parts of the upper airway and a more extensive surgery is required. An otolaryngologist (ENT physician) can examine the upper airway with a laryngoscope (a small scope placed in the mouth to view the upper airway). However, if the exam is done while the person is awake, it will not necessarily show the narrowing that occurs during sleep.

If the ENT determines that tissues in the mouth and throat are constricting the airway, he or she may recommend doing a uvulopalatopharyngoplasty. This is a surgery that removes the uvula, redundant soft palate tissue, tonsils, and adenoids. Recovery from this surgery can be painful, partly because every time the person swallows, it will hurt the raw areas where tissues were removed. We have generally found that this surgery may improve but not eliminate the obstructive sleep apnea. Consequently, the person with DS may still require CPAP after surgery. In other words, the benefits may not be worth the risks and discomfort.

If the decision is made to do surgery involving the airway, it is important to make sure the people doing the surgery are aware of concerns related to smaller airways in individuals with DS. Breathing problems may be more likely during recovery. We strongly advise at least one overnight stay in the hospital for monitoring.

When there is no other available treatment, some patients require a tracheotomy (hole in the neck) to allow them to breathe around the obstructed airway. Tracheotomies are created while the person is under general anesthesia. The ENT surgically creates a hole through the person's neck and into the trachea. A tube is then placed in the hole to keep it from closing. Tracheotomies require regular care, including daily cleaning, and usually need to be suctioned periodically to remove mucous. An adult with DS who lived somewhere that did not provide 24-hour nursing care would likely be required to move to a facility with 24-hour nursing care.

A tracheotomy can affect speech and eating. Additional instruction and therapy as well as additional valves for the tube may be needed. Given the risks and discomfort of surgery, the presence of the tube, the extra nursing care required for tracheotomies, and the possible effects on speech and eating, for most adults with DS and apnea, it makes more sense to try to adapt to CPAP.

Should Everyone with Down Syndrome Be Screened for Apnea?

In light of the high incidence of sleep apnea in people with Down syndrome, how difficult it is for observers to accurately assess whether sleep apnea is present, and the serious complications of sleep apnea, should all people with Down syndrome be screened for sleep apnea? If universal screening is recommended, how often?

At this time, there has not been a recommendation to screen all adolescents and adults with Down syndrome for sleep apnea. However, we are becoming more and more convinced that this is a much larger problem than previously recognized. At the Adult Down Syndrome Clinic, we are more frequently recommending consultations with a sleep physician and sleep studies. We consider these evaluations for patients with mood and behavioral changes, decline in skills, fatigue, obesity, and a report of sleep problems. Unfortunately, the more individuals we recommend for a sleep evaluation, the more individuals we find who cannot cooperate with the sleep study. Additionally, the more people diagnosed with sleep apnea, the more we find that cannot use CPAP.

Over time, we hope there will be improved methods of diagnosing and treating sleep apnea that will be easier for people with Down syndrome to tolerate. Until that time, we continue to work with our sleep lab and sleep specialists to encourage our patients to optimize their sleep treatment.

If sleep apnea is not treated, serious complications can arise. In addition, the chronic sleep deprivation of sleep apnea and the poor oxygenation can lead to significant changes in mood and behavior that can be misinterpreted as purely psychological problems. Unfortunately, if this happens, a medication with sedative effects may be prescribed to help with these changes. The sedation could make the sleep apnea worse, which could then lead to even greater mood and behavior disturbance.

RESTLESS LEGS SYNDROME

Restless legs syndrome is another sleep disorder. This does not appear to be more common in people with DS, but in general occurs more frequently as adults grow older. Restless legs syndrome is characterized by an irresistible urge to move the legs. This can occur during the day, increases with rest, and can be most significant for some people while they sleep.
Treatments include:
- ◆ daily physical exercise,
- ◆ encouraging regular sleep patterns,
- ◆ hot baths and leg massage,
- ◆ keeping the legs warm (e.g., with warm socks),
- ◆ intense mental activity,
- ◆ avoiding caffeine, alcohol, and tobacco late in the day,
- ◆ taking supplements for iron, folate, or magnesium deficiencies,
- ◆ medications.

The drugs of choice are so-called dopamine agonists (medications that mimic the effects of dopamine, a chemical produced by the brain that affects several parts of the body, including parts of the brain). These medications include:
- ◆ ropinirole (Requip), and
- ◆ pramipexole (Mirapex).

These medications do have a number of side effects, including some potentially serious reactions. Be sure to discuss the risks and benefits with the individual's doctor if one of these medications is recommended.

TEETH GRINDING

Teeth grinding (bruxism) while asleep is a fairly common problem for people with DS. Usually there is no clear cause. Sometimes, however, it may be associated with anxiety or other mood changes, so it may be helpful for the person's mental health to be assessed. Teeth grinding can also be associated with misalignment of the teeth.

Generally the focus is on preventing damage to the teeth from grinding. We recommend consulting with a dentist to see if a mouth guard would be helpful in protecting the teeth. Getting a mouth guard may be especially important for adults who have retained their baby teeth into adulthood and do not have permanent teeth to replace them. If the adult with DS resists wearing the mouth guard, you may have to try some of the suggestions above for getting someone to wear a CPAP mask.

Chapter 19

Promoting Healthy

Sexuality and

Abuse Prevention

Staff at the ADSC were asked to help evaluate whether two adults with Down syndrome were able to have a consensual sexual relationship. Both Dave and Mona lived in separate apartments in a complex managed by the agency providing residential service. Agency staff believed that Dave was not sexually active or experienced. There was great concern that he would be forced into something that he did not want or did not fully understand. Mona, on the other hand, had had a former relationship and was thought to be sexually experienced.

A meeting was set up at the ADSC with all relevant parties to sort out the issues. Dave and Mona were invited, as well as longtime staff. Dave's sister was also invited because she was very actively involved in his life and had a very close relationship with him. Mona's family lived out of state, but they stayed in touch with her and staff by phone. Through careful questioning of Dave, Mona, and their family members, we gradually began to understand what each of them expected from a "sexual relationship."

Many of the parents and other caregivers who visit the Adult Down Syndrome Center express concerns for the safety of their family member with DS. Worries that the person "can be taken advantage of by others" are quite common. There are concerns that the individual with DS may be conned out of valuables, or hurt by others, but the primary concern is often with sexual abuse. This chapter will therefore discuss ways to promote education about sexuality and the person's body as a means of preserving the person's physical and emotional well-being, as well as ways to help victims of abuse heal.

WHY DO ADULTS WITH DS NEED SEX EDUCATION?

We have heard some families express concerns as to whether sex education is truly necessary for their sons and daughters with DS. They may be concerned that they "are opening the door and stimulating an interest that wasn't there through sex education." This in an argument used by people who are not in favor of sex education in general. There is little support for this argument. Research has consistently shown that teens educated in sexual matters are far more likely to abstain from sex, and far less likely to have unwanted pregnancies and venereal diseases such as HIV (D. Kirby, 2008; 2007).

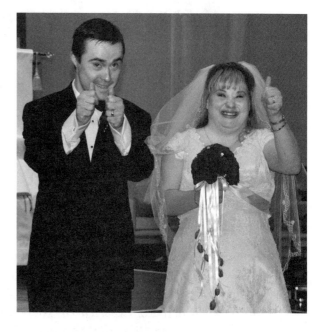

In other words, people who receive sex education are more, not less, responsible with their sexual behavior. In our experience, this is also the case for teens and adults with DS. In close to 20 years of practice at the Adult Down Syndrome Center, we have seen no evidence that sex education increases inappropriate sexual activity—or any sexual activity, for that matter. Perhaps more importantly, we also agree with educators such as Terri Couwenhoven and David Hingsburger that sex education reduces the possibility of victimization by sexual predators. Why is this important? Studies suggest that people with DS and other disabilities are at far greater risk of being victims of sexual violence (Furey, 1994; Sullivan and Knutson, 2000). One study suggests that almost half of people with an intellectual disability will experience ten incidents of sexual violence in their lifetimes (D. Valenti-Hein and L. Schwartz, 1995).

OBJECTIONS TO SEX EDUCATION FOR PEOPLE WITH DS

Despite the availability of very good educational material (see Resources section below), and despite the risk for sexual violence, some parents and caregivers still believe that sex education does not apply to their family member with DS. They may state that their family member with DS "has not shown much interest in sexuality." Other families believe that the person with DS has an interest in stars like Hannah Montana or the Jonas brothers but no real interest in sexuality with people in their day-to-day lives. This may be true. For many, sexuality and sexual intimacy may not have a strong appeal. Instead, they may prefer to hug and be close to others without the complication of sexual intimacy. Still, we believe there are a number of very compelling reasons to carefully consider sex education regardless of the degree of interest or level of sexual activity observed by caregivers.

First, consider that the person's interest in sexuality may not be something he will show or tell a parent, even if he can. Many people with DS value their privacy—particularly related to their bodies and sexuality issues.

Second, consider that people with DS may be exposed to sexuality whether or not they want to be. This is not just because people may be exposed to some form of sexual assault or abuse. (We discuss this in detail in the later part of this chapter.) More likely, they will be exposed to sexual issues through their normal day-to-day experiences. This is especially the case now as more teens and young adults are included in community work, school, and social settings. How much do they see and how does this affect them? We find that this depends on the person, his age, stage of life, and a host of other factors. We don't, however, believe it is always easy for caregivers to know who is interested in or affected by sexuality.

Additionally, many people with DS want to be like "everyone else." How do you think they experience the hugging, fondling, and kissing going on in the entrances and hallways of their middle or high school or the hormonally charged behavior at the school dances? From what we hear and see at the ADSC, these experiences clearly affect a significant number of people.

Many people with DS are also exposed to sexual issues through TV and movies. But, you may say, you don't allow them to see the "wrong type of TV or movies." Can you monitor every movie, TV show, or visit to every relative's or friend's house? Not likely. Again, you may be right—the individual may not see or respond to this type of exposure, but how do you really know?

Something else to consider is that many people with DS have a delay in maturation. Their interest in sexuality may change as they continue to grow and develop. For example, although interest in sexuality may not be present in middle school and early years of high school, it may fully develop later on. Don't be lulled into believing these issues will never exist because they don't exist in the early years.

Third, some parents are concerned that knowledge about sexuality may harm their child or at least have no benefit. They may ask, "What is wrong with sexual innocence?" The truth is that people with DS are far more likely to be hurt if they are not given sex education. As Terri Couwenhoven states in her book on sex education for children and teens with DS, "Experts concur that information about sexuality—particularly facts about bodies, sexual feelings, and rights to choose or not choose sexual partners—is an essential element of exploitation prevention programs for individuals with cognitive disabilities." In others words, ignorance is the perpetrator's friend. Sexual predators are far more likely to target people who have no training in sexual matters. Those ignorant of sexuality and their bodies are far less likely to know what constitutes inappropriate sexual behavior and far less likely to know how to get help when a sexual attack occurs.

Fourth, some families believe that their family member with DS is unlikely to be exposed to a predator. In fact, they are far more likely to come into contact with a predator because most are dependent on a small army of staff in schools, worksites, group homes, and transport services. It is important to consider, too, that the vast majority of perpetrators are known by the victim (Baladerian,1991). It may be the very caregivers who are a part of the person's daily life—those they most trust and depend on—who offer the most risk. It may also be difficult for the person with DS to tell on someone that they depend upon for daily care, food, or privileges.

Some people with DS may avoid victimization by caregivers if they have good intuition for people. They may instinctively know who to avoid. On the other hand, they often have little choice in who is hired to care for them.

Fifth, some parents may be concerned that sex education material will be beyond their son's or daughter's understanding if they have limited reading abilities or other academic limitations. However, knowledgeable sexual educators use concrete visual cues and illustrations, which are the most effective learning strategies for many people with DS. Additionally, there are materials designed to meet the needs of individuals at any age, development stage, or level of adaptive skill.

Still, many parents worry that sex education will go right over their son's or daughter's head. How can this help to protect someone from a sexual predator if they truly don't understand about boundaries and sexuality? We believe that even if people do not fully comprehend the concepts, they still take in the key ideas visually. Once this material is in memory, they are far more likely to use this information to protect themselves if they are confronted by a predator.

In our previous book (*Mental Wellness in Adults with Down Syndrome*), we described behavioral characteristics that many people with DS have, including a superb visual memory. When shown visual images by sexual educators (such as about appropriate boundaries), they take in these images and store them. They may not have an occasion to use this information for some time. It may go "over their head" metaphorically, but it still goes "in their head" literally in terms of stored images. If or when they are confronted by possible sexual violence (such as someone making inappropriate comments, or threatening to touch them inappropriately), this triggers the stored memory, which then can offer guidance and avoidance behaviors at the very time they need it.

There is one more thing to consider related to visual memory abilities and development. As mentioned previously, sexual development is often delayed in people with DS. We have seen many people in their late twenties or even early thirties who were developmentally in the thick of their "teen years"—and for many, this also means having an healthy interest in the opposite sex. Again, even if they are not ready to "understand" information at the time they are taught it, this information is there for them in their memory bank when they are developmentally ready to use it.

Finally, and perhaps most importantly, we have consistently seen that being educated about sexual issues may play a critical role in reducing the severity of a sexual trauma. In our experience, people who have no exposure to sex education are far more likely to be shocked and overwhelmed because they have no warning or basis to make sense out of the experience. Those with exposure to sex education programs are far more likely to recognize what is going on. This can greatly help to moderate the shock and devastation of the experience. We give a number of examples of this when we discuss sexual trauma, in the last section of this chapter.

There is no question that the language limitations of people with DS may limit their ability to communicate sexual violence. Still, the best available sex education materials are in a visual and concrete format that is easy for people to see, store in memory, and then use when needed. This material not only helps people to manage when confronted by a sexual predator, but may give them the tools to communicate what happened to significant others. For example, they may point to pictures in the sex education manual or even pantomime sexual acts because they have seen these scenes before in sex education courses.

In short, what we have consistently seen is that people with DS who are exposed to sex education classes are better able to understand and manage the shock if they are exposed to abuse and to communicate what has happend to others. This, in turn, greatly increases their ability to manage and recover from the experience.

SEX EDUCATION FOR TEENS AND ADULTS

In our practice at the Adult Down Syndrome Center we have found that quite a few people with DS either engage in some type of sexual activity or have ambitions to do so. In these instances, it is important for caregivers to promote a healthy attitude about sexuality. Otherwise, the urge may be expressed in the wrong place and at the wrong time, such as at school or work, much to the horror and embarrassment of the family.

There are healthy ways to approach this issue. For example, many families encourage (or at least, don't discourage) masturbation, as long as it is behind closed doors in one's bedroom or bathroom. (Note that sex educators caution that public and private bathrooms need to be carefully differentiated, so that the individual learns that public bathrooms are not appropriate places for masturbation.)

In our own practice, many families find practical ways of dealing with masturbation. For example, a number of families have found that "do not disturb" cards (similar to those used at hotels) are useful. They give these cards to the family member with DS, with a few instructions for use. When the person wants to express an urge, he simply puts the card outside his door, and others know to respect his privacy. When done, he removes the card from the doorknob and life goes on.

RESOURCES FOR EDUCATING ADULTS WITH DS ABOUT SEXUALITY

There is a growing body of literature on sexuality written specifically for people with Down syndrome and other intellectual disabilities. Terri Couwenhoven, M.S., has written a book entitled *Teaching Children with Down about their Bodies, Boundaries, and Sexuality* which we highly recommend. Couwenhoven's work is designed to inform and educate parents and caregivers but also includes illustrated teach-

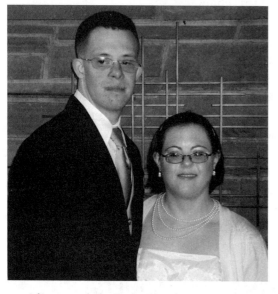

ing materials for people with DS to use in learning about the boundaries that protect and guide them responsibly in relationships and social situations. The book covers a wide range of topics, from basic concerns about hygiene, privacy, masturbation, social skills, and essential safety issues in the community, to more advanced subjects such as sexual intimacy, dating, and marriage. Families can find something for sons and daughters at every level of skill and every stage of development.

Another author whose books we highly recommend is David Hingsburger. Of particular interest is his book on avoiding exploitation, *Just Say Know: Understanding and Reducing the Risk of Sexual Victimization of People with Developmental Disabilities.* Hingsburger has also written helpful works on such topics as masturbation for both men and women and intimacy between consenting adults, which augments Couwenhoven's material.

Both Couwenhoven and Hingsburger's work are well received by teens and adults because they deal with real relationship issues in a respectful and intelligent manner with clear, concrete illustrations that are helpful for people with DS. Equally important, they also offer practical suggestions to caregivers such as for setting up a private space at home or for dealing with problems such as masturbation in public settings.

Additionally, we also recommend a video program for schools and residential and other service providers: *Circles I: Intimacy and Relationships,* by Leslie Walker-Hirsch. This program also uses visual cues very effectively to show appropriate social distance of family, friends, and others as well as how to deal with social and intimate relationships. Other programs specifically designed to help protect and guide people with disabilities in the community include the *Safe Life* program (www.safelifeproject.org) and *Safety Awareness for Empowerment* (SAFE) (www. waisman.wisc.edu/hrtw/Publications.html).

We cannot stress enough how important this material is for the safety and education of people with DS. No matter the person's age or level of skill or function, these issues will affect him. For some people, the effect will be quite profound, particularly during the teen and adult years.

Interest in Sexual Relationships

As discussed previously, we have found that many adults with DS have no real interest in sexual intimacy. These relationships may be too complex or demanding, or it may be difficult to find a sensitive partner. We also know many adults who *are* sexually active with their partners or who have an interest in sexual intimacy with a partner.

Sometimes it can be difficult to determine exactly how much intimacy a given adult with DS truly wants. For example, one important concern is with the person's real level of knowledge and understanding about sexuality. What exactly does he mean when he says he wants a sexual relationship? Does he mean sexual intercourse or some other type of sexual activity between partners, or does he have a whole different idea about what "sex" means? And does the prospective partner have a realistic understanding of what sexual activity entails? Equally important when looking at sexuality between "consenting adults," is the sexuality truly consensual or is it imposed or forced by one of the partners?

The case story about Mona and Dave that began the chapter and continues in the section below illustrates the confusion that can arise when two adults have an imperfect understanding of sexual intimacy.

Mona and Dave

As described above, staff from the agency serving Mona and Dave wondered whether these two adults were both really looking for a consensual sexual relationship. The ADSC agreed to try to find out. We first met with Mona and one trusted staff member. We asked her if she would mind telling us if she had had a sexual relationship with a former boyfriend. She had no problem answering this question. She stated that her former boyfriend had "put his penis in my vagina." From her statements and other corroborative information, we were fairly certain that she had been sexually active. She also stated that she did want to have sexual intercourse with Dave.

When we talked to Dave, we found that he believed "sex" involved "hugging, kissing, and holding hands," but he made absolutely no mention or reference to other types of sexual intimacy. According to Dave's sister, she had a very close relationship with him that allowed an open discussion of any topic. We asked her to take him aside and ask him more directly about his interest in sex, which she agreed to do. What Dave told her confirmed her suspicions about his lack of understanding and interest in sexual intimacy. At the end of her discussion with him she gently asked whether he would take his clothes off when having "sex" with Mona, and he answered somewhat indignantly "of course not." When his sister pushed the issue by asking for any details that would indicate that he either had or wanted to experience sexual intercourse, he clearly indicated no. A trusted male staff person asked Dave the same questions, and he gave this staff person the same answer.

Dave had many strengths and skills. He was very independent, had wonderful social skills, and a solid work record, and he had a collection of movies and music that would be the envy of any collector, and yet he had no interest in engaging in any form of consensual sex. He wanted a female companion to hug, and to share walks, affection, and other good and important things with, but had no desire for sexual intimacy.

The next step was to discuss Dave's lack of interest with Mona. A trusted staff person who was very close to Mona told her that Dave was not interested. What she had not told us when we talked to her earlier was that she had already figured this out. Apparently, on several occasions she had tried to touch "his privates" as a form of foreplay and he had staunchly refused. (She may have been a little embarrassed to tell us this when we first talked to her.) Given Mona's understanding of the situation, we then gave her the choice of either finding someone else who might have more interest in sexual intercourse or staying with Dave. She decided to stay with him and they have shared a close and mutually beneficial relationship for many years without sexual intercourse.

SUPPORTING PERSONAL PREFERENCES

Through our work at the Adult Down Syndrome Clinic, we have encountered a number of adults who have had consensual and mutually beneficial sexual relationships with a partner, and who regarded their sexual intimacy as just one aspect of a rewarding relationship. We have also encountered many individuals, both male and female, who have chosen to have sexual relations and intimacy with members of the same sex. Again, as long as it is apparent that the relationship is truly

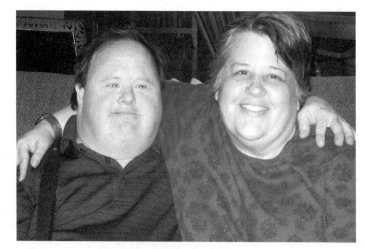

consensual, not based on force or intimidation, and not harmful to either partner, we would not recommend trying to block or interfere with the relationship.

We will not deal with these issues in more depth here because of the availability of the excellent resources mentioned above. We heartily recommend a review of these publications to help guide adults with DS to healthy sexual relationships.

THE POTENTIAL FOR SEXUAL VIOLENCE AND ABUSE

As mentioned previously, research shows that women and men with DS are at greater risk of being victims of sexual violence and abuse. Sexual educators, professionals, and advocates in the field have pushed for better screened and trained staff and for sex education classes to better educate people with DS about how to protect themselves. Fortunately, there is more acceptance and understanding of the problem than in the past. In many communities, there are special clinics or health professionals in emergency rooms who are trained to deal sensitively with victims. Law enforcement and legal professionals are quite often a part of these teams to help to bring the perpetrator to justice. Terri Couwenhoven reports that some of these programs have adapted to meet the needs of persons with DS, but many others are reluctant due to a lack of experience working with people with DS.

Understanding the Terminology

There are several different forms of inappropriate sexual behavior which are all sometimes placed under the umbrella of "sexual violence." The Centers for Disease Control and Prevention (CDC) defines four categories of unwanted sexual behavior forced on a person unwillingly:

♦ Sexual harassment—Unwanted sexual talk, use of sexual language, or comments. Unwanted exposure to materials that is sexual in nature.

♦ Voyeurism—Staring at a person who is undressing or doing private things without their knowledge or permission.

♦ Exhibitionism—Unwanted exposure to a person's private parts.

♦ Sexual assault—Forced attempts to touch or fondle genital/private body parts. Attempted or forced acts of sexual intercourse (oral, anal, or vaginal).

SIGNS OF POSSIBLE ABUSE

Often, people with DS who have been sexually assaulted are unable to tell others directly what has occurred. There are a number of reasons they can have trouble confiding in other people, even trusted family members. First, people with DS tend to have difficulties with expressive language. Second, they may not have received sex education, which would help them to recognize and to find words or nonverbal means to communicate what happened. Many times too the severity of the trauma may limit the person's ability to communicate.

Given these problems, how do caregivers know that sexual abuse may have occurred? Sometimes, there is no definitive way to know, but quite often there are major changes in mood and behavior that may offer clues that the person has been exposed to an intense trauma. Sometimes these changes occur very quickly and dramatically and sometimes they develop over time.

People severely traumatized by sexual violence may show some or all of the following behavioral changes:

- ◆ They may become moody and irritable.
- ◆ They often show symptoms of depression, such as losing interest in things they previously enjoyed (e.g., music or crafts).
- ◆ Many withdraw and refuse to go out to social events or even to socialize with family.
- ◆ Many people who have beneficial "grooves" that help them organize and manage their daily lives and activities will develop less productive compulsive behaviors. (See Chapter 1 for more on this.)
- ◆ Many either use self-talk for the first time or increase their self-talk, and may do it in public areas even if self-talk was previously confined to private spaces. Often self-talk will be negative and include comments such as "no" or "stop."
- ◆ They may express foul language or comments that are uncharacteristic of them.
- ◆ They may make self-critical comments such as "I'm stupid" or "I'm bad."
- ◆ Many people regress in skills and become more dependent on others.

Perhaps most disturbing is the development of a state of self-absorption that takes more and more of the person's attention and focus. Typically this will include self-talk, described previously. Even if the person does not talk out loud, he may act like he is communicating with some invisible person or entity. In this state, people appear to be out of touch with the world and reality and can look very much as if they have a form of psychosis. It is often difficult to pull someone back from this self-absorbed state.

One other very telling indication that someone has experienced a sexual trauma is that the victim will vehemently refuse to do something that had been a normal and enjoyable part of his daily routine. This often indicates the place or source of the trauma. In the case stories that follow, this was a ride service for one victim, and a job site for another. Many others also have general anxiety and fearfulness, or are afraid to leave the home or go to public places or places where there are strangers. They may also become more clingy and afraid to be alone or apart from significant others.

When Victimized by Sexual Violence or Abuse

No matter how careful you are, there is no way to protect a person with DS all the time, and as the expression goes "sometimes bad things happen to good people." There is no question that being the victim of sexual abuse is a catastrophic occurrence. Mental health practitioners working with the general population report that sexual abuse is a major cause of mental and emotional problems. Physical abuse, which involves forcing one's will on another person through intimidation, physical harm, or threats of physical harm, is extremely destructive to the human psyche. Sexual violence through rape, molestation, or any other form of sexual intimidation or assault takes this a step farther. Sexual violence is an act of aggression as well as a violation of the victim's most intimate physical and emotional boundaries and sense of integrity.

Most victims of sexual violence require a great deal of support and counseling to put their lives back together. Treatment will often start with a physical exam to document any evidence of the abuse and to treat any physical damage or trauma caused by the assault. Treatment for the emotional trauma emphasizes steps toward reducing self-blame and shoring up the person's sense of control, trust, and confidence.

First Steps in Diagnosis and Treatment

If you know or suspect that an individual with DS has been the victim of a sexual assault, he should be seen by his primary physician or a physician in an emergency room for a physical exam within 72 hours of the assault, if possible. The exam needs to be thorough, yet gentle and respectful.

There are three purposes for this exam:
- to help identify medical evidence to prosecute the offender(s),
- to screen for injuries and medical conditions and begin medical treatment, and
- to reassure the victim and family members about the person's physical well-being.

We often refer the individual to the emergency room for the initial physical exam after an assault. Emergency rooms are usually equipped to perform the appropriate exam, collect the necessary testing and documentation for future forensics, and make referrals as needed for additional services. After this initial exam, we then treat the patient for ongoing medical and mental health problems related to the abuse.

During the exam, pictures and other documentation may need to be taken. Blood tests and cultures may be done to assess for sexually transmitted diseases or pregnancy. If the exam is done within several days of the assault, medications to prevent pregnancy will also be discussed. Afterwards, the individual and his family should be referred to a healthcare provider who can help coordinate ongoing care and provide for therapeutic services.

If abuse is documented, the health care provider will report the abuse to the appropriate officials, and involve the police, as needed. Reporting varies with the age of the individual (child vs. adult) and where the person lives (family home, type of residential facility). For example, in Illinois, it might be the Office of Inspector General, the Department of Public Health, the local police department, or others.

Effects of Sexual Abuse on People with DS

How are people affected by sexual violence and abuse? As with any human experience, there is a wide range of responses, depending on a number of factors. These include:

- personal factors such as the victim's age, development, maturity, level of sex education, and network of support
- the severity and duration of the sexual violence, as well as how the person personally experiences violence in general
- whether or not the perpetrator is a stranger (Often, those who are known pose a more serious threat. If the individual knows his assailant, it will often undermine his most basic sense of trust and make it difficult to blow the whistle on the perpetrator.)
- the person's ability to verbalize the assault to others
- the availability of trained and sensitive professionals
- other issues that cannot always be predicted or anticipated.

In our experience at the ADSC, all victims of sexual assault are traumatized to a greater or lesser degree. The case stories below provide an overview of the range of emotional responses we have seen.

Example of a Less Severe Trauma

Jean was molested by a substitute driver for a ride service when riding home from her worksite in the early evening. She was the last of four riders to be let off. The driver pulled over and parked the van, then proceeded to sexually molest Jean by touching her breasts. At first she was shocked and surprised and did not respond. However, when the driver tried to unbutton her pants and exposed his penis, this was too much, and Jean voiced the loudest "No" she could muster. Then she screamed.

Jean had taken a number of sex education classes which included exploitation training. As a result, she knew what was going on and had some idea how to respond. Fortunately, although the driver had parked some distance from the nearest houses, he may have been afraid they were close enough for Jean's scream to be heard. This made him stop. He got back in the driver seat and drove Jean the short distance home. Then he made her promise not to tell anyone "or else."

When Jean went into her house, her mother noticed her distressed expression. When she asked what happened, Jean burst into tears. Her mother comforted her and gently, patiently questioned her about what happened, asking a series of yes or no questions. For example, "Did something happen to you today—yes or no? Did it happen in the morning—yes or no? Afternoon—yes or no? Did this happen at your job site; in the van, etc.?" When it became clear that some type of sexual assault had occurred in the van, her mother called the ADSC phone line and was directed to bring Jean to the ADSC clinic immediately.

Dr. Chicoine met with Jean and her mother to do a history and to conduct a physical exam. Dr. McGuire also discussed the situation with Jean, in the presence of her mother, to help to assess the level of trauma and to give supportive counseling. Following the appointment, Jean and her mother went to the police station in their community to report the incident. The perpetrator was arrested that evening by the police. He was found to have a record of abuse in another country which had not been uncovered when he took the job at the transport company.

Jean continued to come for weekly supportive counseling at the ADSC. She seemed to gain more and more strength as the weeks passed. With support from her family and counseling, she was able to tolerate a court experience, and the perpetrator was eventually prosecuted and sent to jail for a lengthy sentence. Following her court appearance, Jean continued to regain her sense of security and confidence in herself. One of the ways that she was supported was to make certain that wherever she went, there was a trusted person she could check with at each step in her day. She was understandably fearful of being alone.

One key area of concern that remained for Jean was transportation to and from work. The ride service was suspended for her because it reminded her of the traumatic experience. Instead, her mother, who had a flexible work schedule, drove Jean to work. People with DS often have exceptional visual memories which may make them at risk for re-experiencing traumatic events through flashbacks. (This issue is discussed in more detail in the next case example below.)

Although Jean was able to discuss the sexual assault with her mother and with medical, police, and legal professionals, she did not dwell on the incidents in counseling. For Jean, as for other victims of sexual violence discussed below, the memories of the event may have been too traumatic to recall without experiencing some of the pain and anxiety of the original event. Still, she continued to make progress in counseling and after approximately one and a half years, she and her family described her as back to normal.

Despite the severity of the sexual abuse Jean experienced, several factors made the trauma less severe and led to a fairly speedy recovery. First, the sexual violence occurred one time and not over a period of time. Second, she had no real relationship with the perpetrator, which made it easier turn him in. Third, the assault was identified almost immediately by her mother, and her treatment and recovery started without delay. Jean did not feel like a passive victim in the experience, which greatly helped with her recovery. Perhaps most importantly, she had been exposed to good sex education courses.

It is our belief that the sex education made all the difference for Jean. She was able to recognize the assault for what it was and to takes steps to fend it off. She was also able to communicate the details of the assault to her mother and a host of other professionals, which also greatly facilitated the recovery process. She had an excellent network of support in place to guide and protect her through her period of recovery.

EXAMPLE OF MORE SEVERE TRAUMA

Although Jean was able to verbalize details about the sexual assault to her mother and others, we more often find that people with DS who have been victimized are unable to tell others what happened. This can delay diagnosis of the problem and lead to delays in treatment that prolong the person's recovery process.

This occurred with Rebecca, age 24, a very well-adjusted woman who lived with her supportive family in an Illinois suburb. Rebecca worked in the mail room of an insurance company and was also busy and involved in a wide variety of social and recreational programs and had many friends.

One day Rebecca's family became very alarmed when she showed a dramatic change in mood and behavior. She was brought by her family to the ADSC for an evaluation. A physical exam was conducted. There were some minor medical issues, but none that suggested an assault or shed light on such a dramatic change in Rebecca.

She did show symptoms of intense anxiety, depression, and withdrawal. What most concerned her family was that she seemed "totally out of it." She could barely respond to family members, and was scarcely able to do even the most basic daily living tasks because she was so distracted and occupied with her own thoughts and self-talk. Although Rebecca had a history of self-talk, she had generally used it to conduct a positive review of her day, and only in her room. This new self-talk was constant, and went on in community settings where she had never talked to herself before. Her family also noted that her self-talk involved self-critical comments such as "I'm bad," and statements like "shut up" which she had never made before. While she was making these comments, she often grimaced and made odd hand gestures as if she was "batting at bugs" or pushing someone away.

One telling indication of Rebecca's trauma was that she refused to return to her job. This was very unusual because she loved her job and would always be punctual for her van ride to work. Every morning since the change in behavior, her family had to help her get dressed (something they had not had to do for 20 years). Once Rebecca was dressed, though, she absolutely refused to leave her house to go to work. Her refusal was also notable because this was the one time when she was very direct and communicative with her family. She was able to state very loudly and clearly "NO" when her family tried to push her out the door. Most of the time her ability to focus and respond to even normal requests and statements were very limited.

To try to get to the bottom of Rebecca's behavioral changes, staff of the ADSC and members of her family met with supervisory staff at the job. The supervisory staff at her job were equally concerned and surprised. Rebecca had been a model employee who was very well regarded by the other employees, both with and without intellectual disabilities. For her part, Rebecca was also unable to verbalize any problems or issues that would help to explain her behavior.

Fortunately, an explanation began to emerge several months after Rebecca began refusing to go to her job. The break came when one of the housekeeping workers came forward to tell her supervisor that she had observed a part-time mailroom employee take Rebecca into an empty room and close the door. This housekeeping staff person spoke only Spanish and was very fond of Rebecca. When she heard that Rebecca had experienced what others called a "breakdown," she realized that what she had observed might be of importance, and reported what she'd seen to her boss. After this, several other employees reported that they had observed the mailroom employee talking to Rebecca.

When this information was divulged, a meeting with Rebecca and her family, staff from her jobsite, and ADSC staff was arranged. Her family was very upset but not completely surprised by the possibility that she was the victim of sexual violence. The police were also called immediately after the meeting and an investigation was started. Unfortunately the man in question had quit his job and reportedly moved out of town. Attempts by the police to find this man were unsuccessful.

The police recommended that Rebecca's family contact an agency that specialized in helping children and adults who had been sexually abused. The agency in question had an excellent reputation for working with children and adult victims. Although we were not sure they would adapt their program to work with a young woman with DS, the family met with agency staff and they agreed to work with Rebecca, provided ADSC staff would be available for consultation. During this time, we continued to see Rebecca and her family for ongoing support, while also offering advice to the staff of the special team on a number of key issues. For example, the team professionals noted a particular concern with the negative self-talk, regression in skills, and self-absorption, which appeared to be "psychotic" in nature. We reassured them that this was a more typical response for a person with DS to a violent sexual trauma. Rebecca's family met with the special team staff for approximately one month. They had many questions and concerns about the sexual violence, which the agency was able to address.

Rebecca and family also continued to meet weekly for six months at the ADSC and then monthly for another four years. Even now Rebecca still comes to the Center every six months, although her symptoms are markedly improved. Still we to continue to monitor progress to ensure that she maintains the gains she has made.

WHAT CAUSED REBECCA'S SEVERE SYMPTOMS?

What caused the severity of Rebecca's symptoms, especially the self-absorption that interfered so dramatically in her day-to-day life? In our experience, people with DS are very susceptible to Post Traumatic Stress Disorder (PTSD) (DSM IV-TR). This is a condition in which people who are traumatized re-experience the traumatic event over and over after the original trauma (in what is sometimes called a flashback). People with DS are particularly susceptible to this disorder because they have exceptional visual memories (see Chapter 5 in *Mental Wellness in Adults with Down Syndrome* for more on this). They tend to store the visual images they see in their daily lives in memory, then may replay a stored memory when they see something in their immediate environment that reminds them of the memory. Of importance, when they do recall a stored memory, they tend to replay the experiences as if it is happening all over again, which includes the emotions experienced during the original event.

Many parents and other caregivers are quite amazed to find that the person with DS can replay a memory from five, ten, or twenty years in the past, and recall the details and the feelings from the original event as if he is there all over again. This skill may be good or bad depending on whether the memories are good or bad. For example, the person may replay a past memory of enjoyable activities with family and friends. He may also entertain himself by replaying favorite movies stored in memory. People who have this visualization skill may also be able to use it to remember useful tasks as long as the task involves use of visual illustrations or cues.

Unfortunately, having an exceptional memory may also make the person with DS more susceptible to recalling a bad memory such as a sexual trauma. Additionally, if a severe trauma is involved, it is not dependent on an external reminder to play. When traumatized by a sexual assault, many people with DS cannot shut off the memory from playing over and over. As a result, they spend much of their time trying to fend off the memory. They are so caught up in this process that they tend to lose touch with the here and now and have great difficulty dealing with day-to-day experiences. This is why some people appear to be so out of touch with reality and why it is often so difficult to pull them back from this self-absorbed state. Caregivers are justifiably terrified when this happens because it appears as if they have "lost" their family member.

In a sense they have, but the good news is that the person with DS can recover from this type of trauma. What is required is an enormous sense of patience and determination from the caregivers and the professionals treating the person. We strongly recommend using activities that are interesting and stimulating to the person who has been traumatized. The purpose of this is to begin to get the person "out of his head" and back to a here-and-now focus. Frankly, it may take years to gently coax someone back from the brink of his own private hell. Still, it is all worthwhile when you begin to see the glimmer of hope and interest.

Perhaps the biggest deterrent to this process is the frustration and hopelessness caregivers can experience, particularly if there is little response for a long time from the person with DS. However, patience and effort do pay off and people do come back.

Some may never totally return to the way they were prior to the sexual violence, but at least they can again go about their lives with a sense of purpose and direction.

MANAGING THE TRAUMA IN TREATMENT AND DAILY LIFE

One very important issue is the question of how to manage the trauma. Should the incident or incidents of abuse be brought up by parents, caregivers, or a professional counselor in therapy to help the person "work through the trauma"? In fact, we have not found this to be at all productive and in many cases it can be very harmful. Usually, the best strategy is to help the person block his memory of the incident or incidents of abuse and divert his attention to something positive or stimulating to focus away from the incident.

The reason for this is, again, because of the capacity people with DS have for remembering events in the past as if they were happening right now. Asking someone to replay this experience is like asking him to put salt on a wound. It can shock and overwhelm him all over again, rather than allowing him to control and manage the experience. Even for victims of sexual abuse who don't have DS, discussion of sexual incidents in therapy is often a very gradual and moderated process in order to be truly therapeutic and not traumatizing.

We recommend too that places or people that remind the person of the trauma be avoided so as not to provoke a replay of the traumatic experience.

REBECCA'S TREATMENT

To return to our case example, Rebecca's family was devastated by what they rightly called the "loss" of their daughter. They saw a transformation from a vibrant, loving, social, accomplished, proud, and independent young woman to a woman who could barely respond to them and who had regressed to the degree that she could barely care for her own hygiene.

The most important messages that we could offer Rebecca's family was hope that she could eventually recover based on our experience working with many others who had experienced a severe sexual trauma. Beyond this there are a number of important treatment considerations.

We have found that psychotropic medications may help some people who cannot sleep and who have more severe compulsive behavior changes (see below for Sam). However, these medications rarely change what families describe as the quality of being "out of it" or "in another world" and which we call self-absorption.

The recovery process can be painfully slow, but progress can be made. After the trauma, the person with DS often shuts down to preserve his sense of emotional health. During this period, it may be very difficult to get the individual to do anything. Getting him dressed and ready to go out is a major undertaking. If he does go, he often has great difficulty focusing his attention outside of himself. In this early stage, it may not help to push the person.

At some point, the hunkering down and isolation from other people and activities becomes totally unproductive. The best thing then is to get the person moving and active, in order to help him "get out of his head" and away from the negative thoughts and memories. Anything that interests and stimulates him is useful to break the internal focus and self-absorption. Often what stimulates and interests is not what used to interest and stimulate, so you need to get creative. For example, Rebecca's parents found that she had an interest in reruns of "Happy Days" on TV. This progressed to other shows and other interests that began to keep her mind off the past. She also began to do word search puzzles and to latch hook, neither of which she had done before. Once Rebecca began to come out of herself, her parents started inviting close family and friends to visit. Because Rebecca was at home, she was able to visit them but then go back to the safety and security of her bedroom when she could no longer maintain her focus.

Rebecca, like others who have been traumatized, strongly resisted going out of the house to work, socialize, and participate in recreational activities. We assured her parents that with careful planning, and protective measures, she could begin to return first to recreation activities and then to a work setting. We also told her parents that this opens up a world of people, activities, and other productive things which no family can supply at home. We don't underestimate the fear and difficulty that this may initially generate, but it is very important for the traumatized person to go out into the world to fully recover. Having said this, there are certain places and events that may never bring anything but terrifying memories and flashbacks. In the above example, Jean should probably never go on a ride service to work. Rebecca will never go back to her former job. There is simply no way to make this a safe place for her, no matter who is there to comfort her. Her memories are just too vivid and strong to change the feeling she has for this place.

Rebecca's parents plotted out a plan of first going to social and recreational events with a parent present. Several interesting recreation programs were selected for Rebecca. She balked the first several nights, but still managed to go. Once there, she was fine as long as a parent or trusted staff person was nearby. In time, she felt safe enough for her parents to stop going. Still, she kept a cell phone with her to call her parents or the recreation manager anytime she felt nervous or frightened. She actually used this twice. Once to test that she could contact someone and the second time for help managing a young man who had no bad intentions but who was a little too interested in Rebecca for her comfort. Interestingly, over time Rebecca has become very comfortable with this young man and her interest in him represented a major positive step in her recovery.

Finally, Rebecca braved a return to a new work environment. The setting she went to was a sheltered workshop. Her family looked very carefully at the agency and was reassured that the workshop responsibly cared for the people in their programs. Within several months, Rebecca was able to go every day without fear or trepidation. In time, she was able to go beyond this setting to work on a cleaning crew with participants from her program, three days per week.

After close to four years of recovery, Rebecca is now participating in a wide variety of recreational and social events and she works in job she enjoys and is proud of.

She still continues to have some times when she goes back into her self, but these times are fewer and farther between. Fortunately, she has so many activities and she really has little time to mull over the past.

Comparing Rebecca to Jean, above, we believe there were several factors that made the trauma far more severe and the recovery far more painful and arduous. First, the abuse probably occurred over a period of time, although we are not sure, given Rebecca's inability to communicate what happened. Second, she had some type of relationship with the perpetrator, which may have made it far more difficult to turn him in. Third, the assault was not identified immediately and her treatment and recovery were also delayed. Fourth, she had not taken any sex education courses that could have prepared her to react to the assault.

Rebecca's parents stated that she was "innocent" of sexual issues. They didn't think she would be exposed to a predator, but there were also no sex education classes or programs in her high school that she was able to attend. We believe this contributed greatly to the severity of the trauma. We believe she was not able to recognize what was occurring when assaulted. Without prior warning or knowledge of sexual exploitation, she was rudely and abruptly thrust into an experience that shocked, overwhelmed, and devastated her. In an attempt to deal with this, she was doomed to replay the experience over and over. Only years later with help and assistance of her family, friends, and a host of professionals was she able to gradually and painstakingly free herself from her unpleasant memories.

Male Victims of Sexual Abuse

Although the above examples were of women, we have also seen a number of men who were victims of sexual abuse. One man with DS, Leo, was raped by a male employee at his job. This was understandably a shocking and horrendous experience for him. Like most victims of a violent sexual crime, he was angry, humiliated, and filled with a great sense of shame and self-blame, although he was a passive victim of the experience. Like Rebecca, he was very fearful of going into the community. Also like Rebecca, he had difficulty blocking the experience from replaying in his mind, especially in the evening. Still, Leo did not slip into the state of self-absorption that was so destructive to Rebecca.

What made the difference for him? There appear to be several similarities with Jean's situation (described above) which seemed to help moderate the severity of the experience, and encouraged a more speedy recovery despite the severity of the sexual assault. As with Jean, the assault occurred one time and not over a period of time. Leo had no real relationship with the perpetrator, which made it easier to turn him in. The assault was identified almost immediately by staff in the workplace. Family and the police were also called immediately. As with Jean, perhaps the most important factor may have been the fact that Leo had been exposed to good sex education courses. As a result, he was able to recognize the assault for what it was. Even though he could not stop the rape, he was able to tell his family and a number of professionals.

Leo did continue to have great deal of fear when going out into the community. Like for Rebecca, we helped his family to find safe places and safe people he could turn to during the day. Over the course of several years, he made gradual but definite progress. Although the trauma was very severe and the process of recovery was long and painful, we still believe that the sex education classes increased his ability to manage the experience and to recover more quickly.

A second young man, Sam, was molested at the age of 19 by a long-time male companion who also had an intellectual disability. Sam was a very friendly, easygoing young man who had many strengths and resources. He had a strong network of family support. He was active in sports and recreations programs and was liked and accepted by his peers.

Sam had done well in his first year of a high school transition program. In his second year, however, he began to show symptoms of depression and anxiety that were very uncharacteristic for him. He became more moody, tense, and irritable and he refused to go to many social and recreation activities he had enjoyed. He also had an increase in unproductive compulsive behaviors which were unusual for him. For example, he began to take the garbage out every few hours. He was also far more rigid about his schedule and about the placement of objects in his room and the house.

Of greatest concern to Sam's family were nightly rages that were very peculiar in nature. Sam would repeat negative or teasing comments made by others to him as a form of self-criticism. His excellent memory provided numerous examples of these comments made by others from the past. (Many of these comments were actually made in fun but were now distorted by him into criticism.) Sam used all of these comments to criticize and chide himself. As the night wore on, the self-criticism became increasingly angry and agitated. He rebuffed all attempts by his family to help him to stop or to divert his attention. This would go on for hours until he finally would fall asleep exhausted.

When Sam came to the Center for his first evaluation, we asked the family if they were aware of any changes or stresses that would account for the change in his behavior. They could think of no reasons. One week after this meeting the school called the family and the family called the Center to report the discovery of the molestation. We were not completely surprised by the call. Sam's change in behavior showed a pattern that we have often found to be associated with a trauma in our patients. We just were not sure what type of trauma it was.

The revelation of Sam's molestation brought a small sense of relief to the family, to know what was causing the problem, but also a terrible sense of dread and anger. They learned that Sam's molester was his "friend" of many years. The molestation occurred while he and this peer rode back and forth on the van to high school. One day, an aide who just happened to be riding the bus observed the molestation. When school authorities investigated, they found that another boy was molested on the bus as well. Apparently the perpetrator had also been the victim of molestation by an older student who was not in special education. Following the investigation, the perpetrator was taken off the bus and moved to a special therapeutic program. However, as Sam's parents stated, "the damage was already done" to Sam.

In comparing Sam's situation to those of Jean, Leo, and Rebecca, there were several factors that made the trauma more severe for Sam compared to Jean and Leo but also less severe compared to Rebecca.

First, Jean and Leo were victims of one incident, whereas Rebecca and Sam appear to have had repeated exposures to sexual abuse over the course of several months. Second, Jean and Leo did not know their perpetrator, whereas both Sam and Rebecca had some type of relationship with their perpetrators. In fact, Sam's longtime friend was the perpetrator. Third, Rebecca was the only one who had not had any sex education classes. However, for Leo the fact that the perpetrator was a friend and peer with an intellectual disability may have confused the issue for him. It may have also made it harder for him to communicate the abuse to others. Still, Leo did have knowledge about sexual exploitation through sex education classes. This may have helped to reduce the severity of his response to the trauma compared to Rebecca.

Like Rebecca, Sam did tend to replay the experience over and over, but this usually only occurred in the evening. He did not go into the state of self-absorption that was so devastating to Rebecca. Again, we believe Rebecca was so "out of it" because without sex education she had no warning or means to understand her assault. Rebecca was unable to continue her normal life activities because of her severe withdrawal. In contrast, we believe Sam showed much of his attempts to deal with his trauma through his nightly rages. These rages were disturbing to Sam's family, but, unlike Rebecca, Sam was able to focus his attention on his school and work tasks and was also able to continue to go about his recreation activities once the process of treatment was started. The self-criticism would start at night during quiet time because this was the time when he did not have other activities that engaged his attention.

SAM'S TREATMENT

Sam's family was very concerned with the effect of the sexual abuse on him. After a complete physical to rule out any health issues, Center staff recommended a multimodal approach to treatment with which the family agreed. This included a psychotropic medication, the antidepressant, sertraline (Zoloft), to help reduce symptoms of depression, anxiety, and compulsive behaviors. (Many people with DS have obsessive-compulsive tendencies, or "grooves," that are generally beneficial. Under stress, however, these compulsions can become less productive, as they did with Sam's placement of objects.)

After the initial evaluation, Sam and his family came for bimonthly supportive counseling sessions. The victim's significant others are often devastated by an attack on their family member, and they need a great deal of support to continue to provide strong support to the victim. One very positive message that we were able to give the family was that Sam did not retreat into a self-absorbed state, such as Rebecca, above, did. For the most part, he was still able to go about his daily life and activities until the evening when the trauma would surface in the form of his self-critical rages.

Changing the Channel. We offered Sam a strategy for dealing with his nightly rages that turned out to be very effective. We introduced a simple cognitive behavioral technique (see Chapter 13 in the *Mental Wellness* book for more on this). This involved teaching him to say "change the channel" while making an exaggerated movement of his hand, as if he was turning a TV channel. This is a surprisingly effective technique for helping people manage negative thoughts, especially when used in combination with other treatments such as psychotropic medication.

It is interesting to note too that although Sam had negative thoughts, he did not discuss the incidents of sexual abuse. We took our cues from Sam and focused the "change the channel" technique on the thoughts and feelings that bothered him and no more. For Sam, as for others traumatized by sexual abuse, we did not believe that a focus on the sexual incidents would be productive.

Rebuilding Self-Esteem: We recommended that Sam's family give him a great deal of praise, particularly when he was able to control his angry rages. We thought a major part of his trauma was the wound inflicted on his self-esteem, which seemed to be manifested by the intensity of his self-criticism. It appeared that Sam blamed himself for the molestation. He then used his memories of previous teasing or criticism by others to castigate himself. This is similar to what happens to victims in the general population who feel they somehow were to blame for an assault even when they were passive victims. The fact that Sam's nightly rages were out in the open allowed us to give him tools and encouragement to block his negative thoughts and intense self-criticism. In time, we were able to gradually discontinue the antidepressant as his self-esteem, mood, and temperament improved with his recovery.

WHEN ABUSE IS SUSPECTED BUT NOT PROVEN

In each of the four case examples described above, we were able to verify that these individuals were the victims of sexual abuse even though two of them were not able to communicate this to others. We would be remiss if we did not talk about other individuals we have seen who also may have been sexually exploited. These individuals showed behavior patterns similar to those described above, but there was never any identification of a predator or of an unwanted sexual experience.

Each of these people showed significant self-absorption, depression, and regression—signs that they could have been exposed to severe trauma. Many of these individuals were also fearful of going out to shopping centers or other places where there were crowds of people, or refused to go places or engage in activities they had previously enjoyed. For many of these people, the world will never again be a truly safe or trusted place. So much is lost, and yet they do fight back and regain much of their focus, energy, and passion for life, given much time and support by others who care for them.

Some do's and don'ts when there is strong suspicion of abuse but no proof:
- ◆ Don't force the person to go somewhere he absolutely refuses to go, even if it was a place he once loved and enjoyed.
- ◆ Do try to avoid crowds or noisy places.

- Don't push for answers he cannot give, such as what happened or why.
- Don't ask repeatedly if he was hurt or victimized.
- Don't try to push activities he does not want to do.
- Do allow some time to heal and recover but not so long that the person has excessive idle time to mull over thoughts.
- Do remember that idle time can provide an opportunity to replay negative memories.
- Do look for creative ways and means of keeping the person's mind from his negative thoughts and experiences.
- Do find activities that are interesting or stimulating to the individual, even if not of interest before.
- Don't expect quick changes; the person may need years to recover.
- Do look for small and subtle changes; progress is progress.
- Do find others who will support and nurture you.
- Do remember that the person's mental health and stability depends on your mental health and stability, so take care of yourself.

Summary

◆ ◆ ◆ ◆ ◆ ◆ ◆ ◆ ◆ ◆ ◆ ◆ ◆ ◆ ◆ ◆ ◆ ◆

People with DS need to learn about the boundaries that protect and guide them responsibly in relationships and social situations. Moreover, sex education is an essential deterrent to sexual violence and it may help to reduce the traumatic effects and speed up recovery if it occurs. Fortunately, there are excellent sex education materials available for people with DS, as described above. Books such as *Teaching Children with Down Syndrome about Their Bodies, Boundaries, and Sexuality* should be an essential part of education for all people with DS.

If sexual abuse does occur or is suspected, the person will need a great deal of support to process what has happened, regain his or her self-esteem, and move on to some semblance of normal activities. Parents, caregivers, and professionals may want to refer to the above list of do's and don'ts to ensure that the person is able to heal in his or her own way, without reliving the trauma.

Chapter 20

Alzheimer Disease and

· · · · · · · · · · · · · · · ·

Decline in Skills*

· · · · · · · · · · · · · ·

Carl, age 53, was seen at the Adult Down Syndrome Center for his annual evaluation. He had lost 15 pounds in the last year. He was eating everything served to him, but his family reported that he was less likely to ask for food or to help himself to food between meals. He was exercising regularly, but this was not a change for him. Further evaluation did not reveal any other cause for his weight loss. Although Carl had no reported decline in skills or memory impairment, we advised his family to monitor him for changes in these areas over the next several months.

Three months later, Carl returned to the ADSC. He had lost 2 more pounds. In addition, his family noted that he now sometimes needed more prompting to complete a task. He usually could complete a task with one or two steps but sometimes he would appear confused in the middle of a multistep task. Further evaluation did not reveal a cause for this change.

We discussed the possibility of Alzheimer disease (AD) with Carl and his family. We also discussed possible medications, but the family decided to hold off on medications at that time. We sent Carl for a computed tomography (CT) scan of the brain, which showed mild atrophy.

As requested, Carl returned again to the ADSC in three more months. His family now reported that he was having some memory

---

* This chapter is reprinted with changes from Chapter 23 in *Mental Wellness in Adults with Down Syndrome: A Guide to Emotional and Behavioral Strengths and Challenges* by Dennis McGuire and Brian Chicoine (Woodbine House, 2006).

impairment for recent events. His memory for events in the past remained intact. After further discussion, Carl was started on the medication memantine (Namenda), which is frequently prescribed when Alzheimer disease is diagnosed.

When Carl came back to the Center three months later, his memory had improved but was not back to its original level. He was doing better with his tasks and his weight had stabilized.

Alzheimer disease (AD) is one of the most commonly diagnosed and misdiagnosed mental disorders in adults with Down syndrome. On the one hand, the condition is often blamed for a decline in skills when the real culprit is depression, a treatable medical condition such as thyroid disease, a change in hearing or vision, or any of a number of less serious causes. On the other hand, AD can appear at an earlier age in people with DS. In addition, while the incidence of AD in people with DS is not clearly defined, some data suggest that it is more common and some suggest that the incidence is similar to that in the general population, but beginning at a younger age.

Since Alzheimer disease can greatly complicate the care of any adult, including one with DS, accurate diagnosis is very important. If the cause of mental decline is not AD, there are usually treatments that can enable the person to regain her usual abilities. If the cause is Alzheimer's disease, there are treatments that may help the person function better temporarily.

WHAT IS ALZHEIMER DISEASE?

Alzheimer disease (AD) is a progressively degenerative neurological condition that affects the brain. AD is a form of dementia. There is progressive destruction of brain cells, especially in certain parts of the brain. People with AD experience progressive impairment of memory, cognitive skills, and daily living skills, as well as psychological changes. There is presently no cure for AD, but there are treatments that can, at least temporarily, reduce its effects.

People with AD have physical changes in their brains known as plaques and tangles. The plaques result when amyloid protein builds up between neurons (nerve cells) and forms clumps. (Little is known about the normal func-

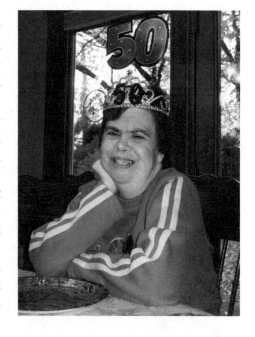

tion of amyloid protein in the brain). The tangles are the remnants of collapsed microtu-bules. The microtubules are a normal part of the nerve cell whose function is to transport nutrients and other substances in the cell. In AD, a protein (tau protein) that is an im-portant part of the structure of the tubule is abnormal, leading to the collapse of the mi-crotubules into tangles. These changes are usually found by examining a piece of brain tissue (generally only done after a person's death) under a microscope. Experimentally, they have also been found with PET scans. In addition, as the disease progresses, com-puterized tomography (CT) or Magnetic Resonance Imaging (MRI) scans of the brain can depict the destruction of many cells because the brain begins to atrophy or shrink.

The cause of AD remains unclear. In a few cases, however, there seems to be a fa-milial link associated with a gene on chromosome 21 for at least some people with AD.

How Common Is Alzheimer Disease?

In the general population, the incidence of AD is increasing as the population ages. The incidence of AD in the general population is listed as 10 percent for people in their 60s, 20 percent for those in their 70s, 40 percent for those in their 80s, and 50 percent or more after age 85.

The incidence among people with DS is not known, although a great deal has been written about AD in DS. A number of years ago, when researchers did autopsies on people with DS who had died from a variety of reasons, they found changes in the brains of all those over age 35 that were similar to those found in the brains of adults with AD. Much discussion and investigation has taken place since then. Some believe that because of these changes in the brain, all people with DS will get AD if they live long enough. Others believe that not all people with DS get clinical AD (decline in cognitive skills and other symptoms outlined later in the chapter).

Our experience suggests that not all people with DS develop the symptoms of AD. We suspect that the incidence of clinical AD might be similar to that in the general population but that it occurs, on average, 20 years earlier than in adults without DS. The youngest person with DS we have seen with symptoms of AD was in his mid-30s. Whether the incidence is the same or higher in people with DS, AD does not seem to be universal when one considers the development of symptoms. There are other causes for a decline in cognitive skills (as discussed later in the chapter), and, therefore, it is important to remember that people with DS deserve an evaluation for these other causes rather than an assumption that any decline is the result of AD.

We have treated many older adults with DS who showed no evidence of mental de-cline. One was a woman believed to be one of the oldest, well-documented people with DS. She died in 1994 at the age of 83, with no evidence of decline (Chicoine & McGuire, 1997). In one study published in 1996, researchers showed a small decline in function with age in adults with DS (Devenny et al., 1996). This decline was comparable to that seen in healthy adults who do not have mental retardation. Other researchers showed a similar lack of decline in function except for those with AD (Burt et al., 1995). So, despite the universal finding of changes in the brain, we do not see the decline in function that would be expected if all adults with DS were getting clinical AD.

DIAGNOSING THE CAUSE OF DECLINING SKILLS

What if we assumed the diagnosis of AD in all adults with DS over the age of 40 whose cognitive skills were declining? Because studies suggest that all people with DS over the age of 35 have microscopic changes in the brain consistent with AD, this conclusion is sometimes made. When we evaluated our patients, however, that is not what we found. In fact, if we had assumed that all of our patients over the age of 40 with declines in function had AD, we would have been wrong 2/3 of the time. Only 1/3 had AD. The other 75 percent are being treated successfully for other conditions. There is no cure for AD at this time, so detection of treatable conditions is a vital element of patient care.

Since many other health problems can cause dementia (loss of cognitive abilities), it is imperative to evaluate for these other conditions before making the diagnosis of AD. Unfortunately, this is not always done for people with DS. One of the concerns expressed by the parents who originally asked us to start a clinic for adults with DS was that their sons or daughters were not being given an appropriate work-up when a decline in skills was noted.

There is no specific test that definitely diagnoses AD. Finding a pattern of decline in neurological and psychological function makes the diagnosis. The medical and behavioral health team must also rule out other illnesses and conditions that cause symptoms that are similar to those seen in AD. This diagnostic process is similar for adults with and without DS.

When a patient comes to us because of a decline in abilities, we provide a thorough medical and psychological evaluation. In our evaluation, we assess for a variety of conditions, particularly those that are more common for adults with DS.

CONDITIONS TO RULE OUT

To rule out causes of decline other than Alzheimer disease, we consider:
- depression and other psychological concerns,
- sleep apnea,
- thyroid disease,
- vitamin B-12 deficiency,
- metabolic diseases such as kidney disease, diabetes, or calcium abnormalities,
- celiac disease,
- loss of hearing or vision,
- atlantoaxial instability or other cervical (neck) problems,

- heart disease,
- seizure disorder,
- normal pressure hydrocephalus,
- medication side effects.

Additional possible causes that we have not seen in our patients:
- syphilis, and
- acquired Immune Deficiency Syndrome (AIDS).

Another possible cause of Alzheimer-like changes may be chronic, undiagnosed pain. Adults with DS can have a global decline in function in response to pain and illnesses that do not directly cause a loss of function. This appears to be an emotional or psychological response to the trauma of pain or illness.

In addition, it is important to remember that people with DS seem to age more rapidly than others. For example, when they are 55, we consider them to be more like someone without DS at 75. It is important to remember that an adult with DS may be experiencing changes due to the aging process at a younger age than in a person without DS. We have seen a number of patients who were slowing down because of age and age-associated health issues. Often these factors were not being considered or addressed and the changes were attributed to behavioral challenges. Addressing them from an aging perspective puts the changes in a whole new light.

Tests for Decline in Function

The tests we recommend for all our adult patients who are experiencing a decline in function include:
- CBC (complete blood count),
- electrolyte panel including serum calcium,
- thyroid blood tests,
- serum Vitamin B12 level,
- vision and hearing testing, and
- 25-OH Vitamin D.

Additional tests that may be helpful based on the findings on the history, physical, and lab tests include:
- lateral cervical spine x-ray in flexion, extension, and neutral positions (to rule out cervical instability),
- liver function tests,
- RPR (for syphilis),
- HIV testing (for AIDS),
- CT scan or MRI of the brain (to assess for tumors and normal pressure hydrocephalus and to look for atrophy),
- blood testing for celiac disease (anti-tissue transglutaminase),

◆ EEG (for seizures),

◆ sleep study.

Neuropsychological testing is part of the evaluation for Alzheimer disease for people who do not have an intellectual disability. However, this testing is more difficult in people with DS and other intellectual disabilities. The underlying intellectual disability makes it difficult for people with DS to perform most of the tests and, therefore, the tests are less accurate. There are, however, a few tests (see below) that, when done sequentially over time, are thought to be more effective. Usually, however, we find that by the time testing shows a cognitive decline, the decline and diagnosis are clear from the person's behavior. In our experience, referring our patients for these tests has not been necessary. We are able to get similar information by asking parents and other caregivers to update us on symptoms, particularly over time.

There are also three tests specifically designed to measure symptoms of Alzheimer disease in people with DS. These include the *Dementia Scale for Down's Syndrome* (Huxley et al., 2000); *The Dementia Scale for Down Syndrome* (Gedye, 2000); and the *Dementia Questionnaire for Mentally Retarded Persons* (Evenhuis et al., 1990).

These tests may be an aid to diagnosis for trained mental health or medical professionals, as they help point out key areas that need to be considered when ruling out other causes. However, results of these tests should not stand alone as the diagnosis of AD. There is still no definitive test to make the diagnosis. The diagnosis is still based on a process of excluding every other possible cause for the person's loss of skills. The three tests mentioned here should only be part of a total assessment involving a thorough physical exam, and extensive information gathered from caregivers regarding skill and memory loss, environmental and developmental stressors, etc.

Symptoms of Alzheimer Disease in Adults with Down Syndrome

Most symptoms (see table) are similar to those seen in people with AD who don't have DS, with the exception of seizures, gait problems, and swallowing difficulties. Seizures tend to occur much more frequently and at an earlier stage in AD in people with DS. Recurrent, uncontrolled seizures can lead to a more rapid decline. People with DS are also more likely to lose the ability to walk earlier on and to have earlier difficulties with swallowing and with aspiration. The aspiration becomes especially problematic if it leads to recurrent pneumonia or decreased eating or drinking.

Especially earlier in the course of the disease, the functioning level of a person with AD often fluctuates. These fluctuations may occur over several days or weeks, from day to day, and even within minutes or moments. A skill may come and go over these periods of time. As the disease progresses, the person's skill level will decline and her periods of better functioning will be shorter and not as functional as before.

Alzheimer Disease Symptoms in Adults with DS

COGNITION
- Slowing down/decreased energy/sluggish
- Decreased ability to follow directions
- Seems to understand less/confusion
- Difficulty organizing things
- Staring into space/"mask face"

MEMORY
- Increased forgetfulness
- Losing things
- Forgetting where going/why went
- Wandering
- Getting lost
- Not recognizing people
- Needs more reminders/prompts

CONCENTRATION
- Decreased concentration/ attention span
- Easily distracted/not focusing

TALKING
- Difficulty finding words
- Decreased speech/articulation/vocabulary

PERSONALITY
- Decreased interest/participation in activities
- Flat mood/apathy
- More withdrawn/less social
- Seems depressed/less smiling
- Less cooperative
- Mood swings
- Crying easily
- Irritability/easily upset
- Temper flares/outbursts
- Yelling/swearing
- Pushing/hitting/kicking/biting
- Excessively fearful/new fears
- Loss of inhibition
- Increased self-talk
- New behaviors/changing old routines
- Doesn't like being alone (new)
- Increase in routines/rituals

SLEEP
- Problems falling asleep at night
- Problems staying asleep at night
- Refusing to get out of bed/sleeping more
- Day-night reversal
- Daytime sleepiness/increased naps

WALKING/POSTURE
- Afraid of uneven surfaces/stairs
- Walking less
- Walking slower
- Decreased step length
- Unsteady when walking/holding for support
- Leaning to one side
- Falling

FOOD-RELATED
- Takes more time to eat a meal
- Decreased appetite
- Weight loss
- Choking/gagging/difficulty swallowing
- Urinary incontinence
- Stool incontinence

MOVEMENT
- Unusual movements/tics
- Myoclonic jerks/jerking movements
- Witnessed seizures

HALLUCINATIONS
- Hearing things that aren't there
- Seeing things that aren't there

284 of Alzheimer Disease and Decline in Skills

TREATMENT OF ALZHEIMER DISEASE

There is no treatment presently available to cure AD. However, treatments are available to temporarily improve memory and daily skills as well as some of the associated symptoms.

Researchers have proven that medications that slow down the breakdown of choline can improve the function of people with AD. Nerve cells communicate with each other via neurotransmitters (chemicals) that pass from cell to cell. One of these transmitters, choline, is the chemical used for communication by many of the brain cells that are destroyed in AD. Medications that slow down the rate of breakdown of choline (cholinesterase inhibitors) prolong the ability of the choline to transmit the message to the next cell. These medications work by blocking cholinesterase, the chemical that breaks down choline. Taking these medications can improve the function of the cells, and thus the function of the person with AD. Unfortunately, this improvement is temporary and the medications' effectiveness decreases as more cells are destroyed and fewer cells are sending and receiving signals via choline.

The cholinesterase inhibiting medications presently available include: donepezil (Aricept), galantamine (Razadyne), rivastigmine (Exelon), and tacrine (Cognex). Tacrine (Cognex) is rarely used now because of liver toxicity side effects and the need for frequent monitoring of blood tests. The others—donepezil (Aricept), galantamine (Razadyne), and rivastigmine (Exelon)—seem similar in their benefits and side effects.

One side effect to watch for with these medications is gastrointestinal upset and/or anorexia (decreased appetite). Many people with AD require assistance and encouragement to consume enough calories and appropriate nutrition any way. If they develop these side effects, it may be even more difficult to maintain good nutrition. In addition, seizures, although not common, can be a side effect as well. If the person is taking one of the medications and develops seizures, the question arises whether the seizures are secondary to the medication or the AD. Unfortunately, there is no way to determine which is the cause. A decision must then be made as to whether the benefit of the medication exceeds the downside that it could be causing seizures.

Memantine (Namenda) is another medication used to treat AD. It works differently than those that slow the breakdown of choline. It may slow calcium influx into cells and slow nerve damage. It does this by binding to N-methyl-D-aspartate receptors (which are involved in memory). (Technically, this makes it an NMDA receptor antagonist.) In our experience, the medication is effective in temporarily stabilizing or even improving function in adults with DS who have AD, and it is generally well tolerated. It is indicated for moderate to severe AD and we usually add it to one of the cholinesterase inhibitors. Memantine can also cause seizures, although this is not a common side effect.

All medications presently prescribed for AD have potential side effects. They can all contribute to increased agitation in some individuals with DS. Some patients have become sedated when one or both categories of medications were used. Also, unfortunately, some individuals actually seem to have a more rapid or greater cognitive decline while taking the medications. We have found no way to determine whether the further decline is secondary to the medication or the disease except to do a trial off the medication.

Unfortunately, neither the cholinesterase inhibitors nor Namenda stop the destructive process of AD. Eventually, too many cells are damaged and the effect of the medication diminishes.

PREVENTING OR DELAYING ALZHEIMER DISEASE

There is great interest in possible ways to prevent Alzheimer disease in people with and without DS. To date, there is limited information available about prevention in people with DS. However, it is reasonable to look at methods that have been studied in people without DS and apply that information to people with DS (unless information becomes available that disproves benefit in people with DS).

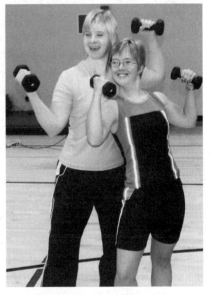

Currently, these are the major strategies recommended for preventing or delaying AD in adults in general:

- **Keep physically active.** Studies have found associations between physical activity and improved cognitive skills or reduced AD risk. As of yet, it has not been shown that the physical activity actually caused the improvement in cognitive skills or reduces the risk of AD. Nor has it been disproved that the people who are more likely to exercise are those with higher cognitive skills and reduced AD risk to begin with. But there is no harm in encouraging adults with DS to exercise, and there are proven benefits to staying physically fit above and beyond preventing AD. Consider at least thirty minutes of exercise at least three times per week.

- **Watch what you eat.** There are data that suggest (but don't prove) that these foods reduce the risk of AD:
  - ➤ Mediterranean diet (many fruits, vegetables, and beans; moderate amounts of fish; low to moderate amounts of dairy foods; small amounts of meat and poultry; regular but moderate amounts of wine; and olive oil),
  - ➤ blueberries, strawberries, and cranberries,
  - ➤ green leafy vegetables,
  - ➤ broccoli.

◆ **Stay involved with friends and family.** Having many friends and acquaintances and participating in many social activities is associated with reduced cognitive decline and decreased risk of dementia.

Until we know further, the best course for everyone is to eat a healthy diet, exercise regularly, and enjoy time with family and friends.

Research into Medications to Prevent AD in People with DS

As discussed above, people with Alzheimer disease develop plaques and tangles in their brains. Since adults with Down syndrome have these plaques and tangles even if they don't have symptoms of AD, many have wondered if the same medications used to treat Alzheimer disease might help people with DS who don't have AD. Several studies have therefore focused on the use of cholinesterase inhibiting medications in people with DS.

Dr. Priya Kishani at Duke University did a small non-blinded study in the late 1990s that suggested donepezil (Aricept) might help cognition in people with DS (Kishnani et al., 2001). ("Non-blinded" means the doctors and participants knew who was receiving the Aricept vs. a placebo.) However, we subsequently did a small double-blind study at the Adult Down Syndrome Center and found no benefit for cognition in young adults with DS who showed no signs of AD (Johnson et al., 2003). ("Double-blind" means that neither the doctors nor the participants knew who was receiving active medication.) Two of the adults in our study who received Aricept did seem to have improved speech. After the study, they continued the Aricept but the effect didn't last and the Aricept was discontinued in both within six months.

More recently, Eisai Pharmaceuticals and Pfizer sponsored a study on the use of Aricept in 6- to10-year-olds with DS. As of this writing, the study is listed on www.clinicaltrials.gov as cancelled due to "sufficient evidence of efficacy not met." A similar study in children with DS aged 11 to 17 was also stopped in the early phases of the study reportedly due to lack of difference in the outcomes in the group taking the Aricept and the group taking placebo. This study was terminated in December 2008.

TREATMENT OF ASSOCIATED SEIZURES

◆ ◆ ◆ ◆ ◆ ◆ ◆ ◆ ◆ ◆ ◆ ◆ ◆ ◆ ◆ ◆ ◆ ◆

As mentioned above, adults with DS are more likely to develop seizures as a complication of Alzheimer disease. The seizures seen in AD may be tonic-clonic (grand mal) or other types. In addition, myoclonic jerks are often seen. Myoclonic jerks are quick, uncontrollable movements of the arms or legs without any loss of consciousness.

Anti-seizure medications can be effective in treating the seizures associated with AD. Those prescribed include: phenytoin (Dilantin), carbamazepine (Tegretol), valproic acid (Depakote), gabapentin (Neurontin), levetiracetam (Keppra), lamotrigine (Lamictal), clonazepam (Klonopin), topiramate (Topamax), and other anti-seizure medications, depending on the type of seizure. These medications can cause drowsiness and increased confusion. We have found this to be particularly true of phenytoin (Dilantin). Carbamezepine (Tegretol) has anti-cholinergic properties (the opposite of cholinesterase inhibitors) and, therefore, could contribute to increased confusion.

We wait until seizures develop before starting anti-seizure medications, in light of the potential side effects and the fact that not all people develop seizures. It is important, however, to bring the seizures under control as soon as possible. Uncontrolled seizures seem to contribute to a more rapid rate of decline.

The one exception to the rule of treating seizures early seems to be the myoclonic jerking. These brief movements are often well tolerated and don't cause significant problems. However, if they become frequent, they can be bothersome and should be treated with medication. In addition, sometimes the jerks can cause a person to fall, especially if she is becoming unsteady on her feet. Treatment is also warranted in this situation. We have found valproic acid (Depakote, Depakene) to be particularly helpful for myoclonic jerking. Other anti-seizure medications can also be beneficial.

TREATMENT OF PSYCHOLOGICAL, PERSONALITY, AND BEHAVIORAL CHANGES

◆ ◆ ◆ ◆ ◆ ◆ ◆ ◆ ◆ ◆ ◆ ◆ ◆ ◆ ◆ ◆ ◆ ◆

Alzheimer disease often causes psychological, personality, and behavioral changes. Changes may include sleep problems, depression, anxiety, agitation, compulsiveness, paranoia, hallucinations, and others. These symptoms can often be reduced through behavioral strategies. Sometimes medications can also help. Further information regarding specific medications for specific symptoms is provided below.

One key issue for treating people with AD is to limit the negative impact of the medication. People with AD are often more susceptible to side effects of medications such as sedation, increased confusion, and further loss of skills such as walking or swallowing. Therefore, it is important to carefully monitor the medications prescribed and their benefits and negative effects. Prescribing smaller doses, less frequently, for a shorter duration may be effective and can help to limit side effects.

OBSESSIVE-COMPULSIVE DISORDER

Some degree of compulsiveness is common in people with DS. That is, they often feel they have to do certain things in certain ways and/or have repeated thoughts about certain things. However, the development of Alzheimer disease may increase this behavior. Some of our patients developed obsessive-compulsive disorder that was, in retrospect, the earliest sign of AD.

We have found that helping someone use compulsive tendencies in a positive manner is likely to be more effective than trying to use behavioral techniques to eliminate this tendency. If the individual has a need to be repetitive, try to redirect her to a healthier behavior than a non-functional or harmful behavior.

For example, if a person is getting stuck on watching the same movies over and over or another unhealthy behavior, work with her to develop picture schedules that include healthy behaviors such as exercise, interacting with others, playing games that are mentally stimulating, etc.

Unfortunately, for some individuals, the obsessions or compulsions are very specific to a certain thing, person, or behavior, and redirection is impossible. If the problem is not responding to behavioral approaches and is affecting the person's ability to participate in daily life, we generally recommend the use of medications. We have found that the medications known as selective serotonin reuptake inhibitors, particularly sertraline (Zoloft) and paroxetine (Paxil), work well.

DEPRESSION

Depression is common in people who have Alzheimer disease. To make matters confusing, depression can occur independent of AD, it can mimic AD (which is why ruling out depression is part of the diagnostic process for AD), and it can be part of the symptoms of AD. Supportive treatment is essential for a person with depression, whether or not she has AD. Offering reassurances, listening to concerns, and encouraging participation in activities are some of the many ways to support a person with depression. Encouraging exercise is recommended because exercise can greatly improve the mood of people with depression.

Medications are also necessary sometimes. We have found the newer antidepressants to be particularly effective. These include: sertraline (Zoloft), paroxetine (Paxil), citalopram (Celexa), escitalopram (Lexapro), and venlafaxine (Effexor). Although any of the antidepressants may cause some agitation, fluoxetine (Prozac) seems to cause it more often in people with DS. Typically, the agitation does not begin immediately, but is delayed until the person has taken the medication for several weeks. In our experience, paroxetine (Paxil) causes agitation less frequently than fluoxetine (Prozac), but when it does cause agitation, it tends to occur sooner— within several days to a few weeks after starting the medication.

Another medication prescribed for depression is bupropion (Wellbutrin), but it has a greater theoretical risk of seizures (which are already a concern in AD). The older antidepressants such as amitriptyline (Elavil), desipramine (Norpramin), and others are probably effective as well. However, we tend not to use these medications because of their greater incidence of anti-cholinergic side effects. People with DS seem to be more sensitive to these side effects even when they do not have Alzheimer disease. There is also the concern that blocking the effect of choline in the brain will result in a greater decline in skills. As discussed above, medications that promote choline activity may reduce the symptoms of AD.

SLEEP DISTURBANCE

Many people with AD have sleep disturbances. Often the typical day-night sleep cycle is disrupted, and they sleep during the day and are awake at night. This may not be harmful if the person can get adequate sleep, just at a different time. If the environment can allow for this pattern, then it is reasonable not to intervene.

There are several reasons to consider intervention, however. Safety is often the most important reason. If care providers sleep at night, the person with Alzheimer disease will not be as well supervised at night. In addition, stimulating activities are often only available during the day. Therefore, even if safety is not a concern at night, if the person has no activities to participate in during her wake time, it can lead to further decline in her abilities, as discussed previously. In addition, the person who is up at night may be very disruptive to those who are trying to sleep at night. Continued sleep deprivation can be very stressful for care givers.

Treatments for sleep changes can include both medicinal and non-medicinal interventions. We have outlined our non-medicinal recommendations in the "Sleep Hygiene" section in Chapter 2. In addition, exposure to sunlight during the day may help "reset the clock." Activities outside, working or sitting near a window, or other sun exposure during the day may help the brain of a person with AD "know" when it is day versus night and then be more awake during the day and restful at night.

If these recommendations don't help, we move on to medicinal measures. Medications are discussed in Chapter 18. An additional issue to consider in people with AD is that the anti-histamines hydroxyzine, diphenhydramine (Benadryl) (discussed in Chapter 18), and many over-the-counter sleep aids that contain diphenhydramine have anti-cholinergic side effects. As was noted above, anti-cholinergic side effects can, particularly in someone with Alzheimer disease, include confusion. Therefore, we tend to stay away from these products.

ANXIETY

Anxiety can sometimes accompany the psychological decline that occurs in AD. Some anxiety may stem from a direct neurological impairment—that is, from changes in the brain. We suspect that some anxiety may also result from the person's fear of not being able to understand what is happening to her as her abilities decline. Often, anxiety seems to occur during earlier stages, which would seem to go along with the latter idea. It can be very disconcerting to sense that you are losing skills but not have the ability to understand why. This seems to be particularly a problem for those who are losing their ability to walk or who feel a sense of imbalance.

Ways to reduce anxiety include:
- ◆ Providing reassurances (gentle verbal reassurance, encouraging and helping the person do the task that she is having difficulty with, etc.);
- ◆ Helping the person find tasks at which she can be successful;

◆ Providing written or picture cues that help the person find her way or do things (we find that pictures work best);
◆ Removing reminders of things that she can no longer do (e.g., if it frustrates her that she can't cook her own meals any more, removing the microwave may reduce anxiety);
◆ Not arguing with her when she is recalling something incorrectly (unless there is a safety issue involved);
◆ Addressing the difficulty with walking (see later in this chapter).

Medications can also be used to treat anxiety. Many of the newer antidepressants, as discussed above, can help with anxiety. A shorter-acting benzodiazepine can also be helpful. We have used alprazolam (Xanax) and lorazepam (Ativan) with good success. We have also had success using the longer-acting medication clonazepam (Klonopin), although anxiety is not an FDA-approved indication. We generally prescribe very small doses and use them less frequently than would generally be recommended. Real care must be taken when giving these medications to someone with Alzheimer disease. Sedation, unsteady gait, depressed mood, and increased confusion are common side effects.

We have generally found that there is a relatively short period of time (weeks to a few months) that an adult with DS and AD requires anxiety medications, although some of our patients experience anxiety for a longer period. We recommend careful observation for side effects and discontinuing the medications if side effects occur. In addition, wean the medication as soon as possible, as anxiety symptoms decrease.

AGITATED BEHAVIOR

Agitated behavior is another problem that can occur in people with Alzheimer disease. This may include shouting at others, getting physically aggressive, or pacing in an agitated manner.

When agitation occurs, careful assessment is important. An evaluation for medical problems and physical sources of pain may find a cause that is not directly related to AD. Because of the person's reduced ability to understand what is happening or to inform others of her discomfort, she may be using behavioral changes to communicate. In addition, depression, increasing obsessive tendencies or compulsivity, anxiety, and sleep disturbance may cause agitated behavior. Treatment for the appropriate condition may reduce or eliminate the agitated behavior. Sometimes, however, no other underlying cause is found.

Sometimes, agitated behavior can endanger the person with AD or others. It may also be associated with hallucinatory behavior or paranoia (irrational fear). If the agitation is disturbing to the person or is a safety issue, medications can be beneficial. We have found the newer antipsychotics helpful. Risperidone (Risperdal), olanzapine (Zyprexa), ziprasidone (Geodon), aripiprazole (Abilify), and quetiapine (Seroquel) have all reduced symptoms of agitation in our patients. But we have also seen increased sedation, increased confusion, unsteadiness, swallowing difficulty, and increased incontinence in patients taking these medications. However, we start with very tiny doses—e.g., risperidone (Risperdal) 0.25 mg at bedtime—and this has reduced the incidence of side effects.

Some recent findings suggest that taking these medications may increase the chance of stroke in people *without* DS who have AD. Vascular disease seems to be less common in general in people with DS, so the risk of stroke would theoretically appear to be less of a concern in people with DS. However, studies have not been done to assess this risk in people with DS, so be sure to discuss the possibility of stroke with the doctor if these medications are prescribed for an adult with DS and AD under your care.

Hallucinatory behavior and paranoia can also occur without agitated behavior. If this is a significant problem for the person, treatment as described above can be beneficial.

DIFFICULTY SWALLOWING

As discussed in Chapter 11, swallowing dysfunction (dysphagia) is more common in people with DS. Unfortunately, as the person's abilities decline due to AD, she will have increased difficulties with swallowing. Some individuals develop a fear of, or a resistance to, eating. They apparently don't like the sensation they experience when their swallowing is impaired.

As swallowing dysfunction gets worse, the adult with AD can aspirate food or drink into the upper airway and lungs. This can cause choking, gagging, coughing, spitting, and even vomiting. These can all be protective mechanisms to keep the solids and liquids out of the lungs. If food does enter the lungs, it can cause aspiration pneumonitis or aspiration pneumonia. Aspiration pneumonitis is an inflammation of the lungs. Aspiration pneumonia is an infection (pneumonia) in the lungs caused by the germs (typically bacteria) in the person's mouth that are aspirated into the lungs.

It isn't necessary to be eating or drinking to develop aspiration pneumonitis or pneumonia. The person can aspirate her own saliva, which contains bacteria. If the person has reflux or vomiting of acid or food from the stomach, these substances can also be aspirated.

Treatment of swallowing dysfunction can consist of:

- ◆ changing the consistency of food or drink (for example, solids may be pureed and liquids may be thickened);
- ◆ changing the rate of eating (slowing it down and having the person chew each bite more thoroughly);
- ◆ swallowing therapy (provided by a speech-language pathologist).

Another option for providing nutrition is to use a nasogastric (NG) tube (a feeding tube inserted through the nose) or gastrostomy tube (G-tube) (a tube inserted through an opening surgically made in the abdomen) to place food into the stomach. When these methods are used, the person with AD does not have to swallow food or liquids. Unfortunately, she still needs to swallow her own saliva, so she can still aspirate on the saliva and develop pneumonia. See Chapter 22 for a discussion related to deciding whether to include information about the placement of a G-tube in an advance directive.

DIFFICULTIES WITH GAIT AND DEPTH PERCEPTION

Many people with DS who have Alzheimer disease develop gait dysfunction (difficulty walking). Early on, the person may express or display fears of walking, before any actual loss of walking skills is noted. Many people seem to have both an impairment in gait and in depth perception. Some people first become fearful in situations where there is more of a need to use depth perception. Situations where this may occur include:
- stairs or escalators; especially those that aren't enclosed or next to a wall;
- changing from one surface to another;
- glass elevators;
- buildings (often shopping malls) with glass railings overlooking an opening down to the next level.

Many people with DS who don't have Alzheimer disease have mild impairments in walking and depth perception. Worsening of these issues can be a sign that the person is developing AD. As difficulties with gait and depth perception worsen, symptoms and signs may include:
- leaning to one side or the other (sometimes even when sitting);
- needing increased assistance to walk;
- walking more slowly;
- falling;
- sitting down when trying to walk longer distances.

Evaluation and treatment may include:
- encouraging the person to keep walking in order to maintain skills as long as possible;
- having someone nearby to prevent falls;
- referring the person for an eye examination to ensure any visual impairments are treated;
- treating other conditions that can contribute to gait problems (e.g., osteoarthritis);
- referring the person for a physical and/or occupational therapy assessment for guidance in optimizing walking skills and to evaluate for and train the person in using assistive devices such as a cane or walker;
- using a wheelchair for longer distances.

INCONTINENCE

As Alzheimer disease progresses, incontinence (urine and/or stool accidents) is common. However, there are many possible reasons that an older person with DS might have problems with incontinence, so it is important to assess for other causes such as celiac disease (see Chapter 11) or a urinary tract infection (see Chapter 12). When incontinence is determined to be due to AD, the cause, at least initially, usually seems to be that the person is having difficulty recognizing her body's signals or has become unable to respond to the signals.

Treatment can consist of:

- ♦ Timed toileting—reminding the individual to use the bathroom every 2 to 3 hours. We generally don't recommend waking the person during the night because this can cause sleep disturbance and increased confusion.
- ♦ Encouraging the person to use the bathroom at times she previously needed to or now is likely to have accidents. For example, encourage the person with AD to sit on the toilet after a meal to take advantage of the gastric-colic reflex. This is a normal reflex that occurs when food enters the stomach that stimulates the colon to defecate.
- ♦ Use of diapers (as a last resort). Initially they may only be needed during the night or at times when the person does not have ready access to a toilet.

DECUBITUS ULCERS

Decubitus ulcers are sores of the skin caused by pressure and other forces on the skin. Most often they occur where there is a bony prominence—for example, at the ankle, the hip, or the sacrum (the lower part of the back just above the buttocks). Ordinarily, people turn or reposition themselves if their weight or another object is putting pressure on their skin. Unfortunately, as Alzheimer disease progresses, the individual becomes less aware of the sensation of pressure or less able to respond. Friction between the skin and an object such as the bed can also contribute to sores. For example, someone may develop ulcers by scooting in bed, in a chair, or even on the floor, of if she habitually rubs an object against her skin.

Ulcers are painful and can become infected. The deeper they become, the more tissue is damaged (muscle, bone). In extreme cases, the infection can turn into sepsis, a life-threatening condition in which the bacteria enters the bloodstream, or an infection of the bone (osteomyelitis).

Prevention of ulcers includes:

- ♦ frequently turning the person in bed or helping her adjust her position in a chair or wheelchair;

◆ applying padding or other protection over bony prominences to reduce pressure;

◆ avoiding scooting, dragging, or other sources of friction through proper lifting techniques, positioning, and attention to the person's movements;

◆ optimizing nutrition to optimize the health of the skin (this includes making sure the person is getting enough calories and protein, as well as vitamin C and zinc). (With excessive weight loss, there is less tissue to pad bony prominences.)

Treatment of decubitus ulcers varies depending on the size, depth, and other associated problems or complications of the wound. There are a variety of dressings, creams, cleansers, and other products to treat ulcers. Surgery is sometimes needed to remove necrotic (dead) tissue or to create a skin flap (moving skin from one area of the body to cover a wound at another site). Sometimes the person may also need to wear gloves or clothes she can't unfasten herself to keep her from picking at the wound or dressing.

WEIGHT CHANGES

Weight loss is common among people with Alzheimer disease. There appear to be multiple causes, including:

◆ loss of appetite;

◆ loss of muscle mass due to inactivity;

◆ inability to prepare, ask for, or obtain food independently;

◆ inability to understand social cues or the usual schedules for eating (for example, if the person no longer recognizes the time around noon as lunch time, she may skip a meal she would have previously eaten even when she wasn't hungry);

◆ reduced rate of eating.

Sometimes, earlier in AD, the person may actually gain weight. This results when an individual is maintaining her appetite and ability to eat but has become less active.

Treatment of weight loss may include:

◆ providing time and encouragement to eat;

◆ assisting the person in food preparation;

◆ eating with the person (as a cue or reminder for the person to eat);

◆ setting up a schedule to remind the person of usual times to eat (picture schedules seem to work best for most individuals with DS and AD);

◆ adjusting the person's diet to include foods that have a higher calorie content;

- offering liquid supplements such as Boost, Ensure, or Carnation Instant Breakfast made with whole milk (and perhaps a scoop of ice cream);
- trying medications such as megestrol (Megace) and cyprohepatadine (Periactin) to stimulate the appetite. (The FDA has not approved these medications for treatment of weight loss in people with AD, but we have found them to be useful for some individuals. We have had more success using Megace.)
- supplementing the person's food intake with a feeding tube (see under "Dysphagia" earlier in this chapter).

If the person is obese when she develops AD, the weight loss may not be all bad. Losing weight may help improve the person's mobility, or at least slow its decline. However, as AD progresses, weight loss can be a significant problem.

SENSITIVITY TO SURGERY AND ANESTHESIA

Some adults with Alzheimer disease have increased difficulty recovering from surgery and/or anesthesia. This may be due to a number of reasons:

- If the person needs to be immobile following surgery, she may subsequently require therapy or assistance to relearn skills not used when immobile. This can be particularly challenging for someone who has difficulties learning or participating in therapy due to progressive cognitive impairment. Skills lost may include ambulation, using the toilet, and others.
- Endotracheal tubes (tubes sometimes placed in the mouth or nose for breathing during, and, in some situations, after surgery) may cause some swelling and temporary swallowing difficulty. For a person who already has swallowing difficulties, these added obstacles to swallowing may cause enough additional impairment that the person never regains the ability to swallow.
- Similarly, if the person needs to spend a period of time without eating due to surgery, she may lose the ability to swallow or not be able to remember how to swallow normally again.
- The effects of anesthesia can cause temporary confusion. Some people with DS and AD may be particularly sensitive to anesthesia.

Some people with DS and AD may be unable to regain skills after surgery even if they do not perform them for a relatively short period of time after anesthesia.

For these reasons, it is important to carefully consider whether surgery is appropriate for people with DS and AD. Certainly, surgery may be the best option if the person has an illness or condition that is life-threatening or will cause serious additional problems if not immediately corrected. However, the same may not be true for procedures that are more elective. For any surgery, the potential complications noted above add an additional layer of concern and should be reviewed when considering surgery.

Further information about surgery for adults with DS is discussed in Chapter 21.

KEEPING ACTIVITIES AT THE RIGHT LEVEL

Another important aspect of caring for a person who has developed AD is to try to keep her functioning as well as she can for as long as she can. We recommend encouraging her to participate in activities that are at the appropriate cognitive level. If you engage the individual in activities that are not too easy and not too difficult, it will help maintain a higher level of functioning for a longer period of time. Tasks that are too difficult will be frustrating and can lead to a more rapid loss of skills, as well as emotional changes, stress-related behaviors, and unhappiness. Similarly, tasks that are too easy will not allow the person to use the skills that she has and will lead to greater erosion of skills.

Assessing the appropriate skill level of tasks can be difficult, particularly if the person's skill level fluctuates. What was appropriate yesterday may not be appropriate today but may again be appropriate tomorrow. This fluctuation in skills can be a challenge for parents and other caregivers, both from an assessment standpoint and from an emotional standpoint. It's easy to "take it personally" when the person with Alzheimer disease can't do a task that she could do just recently. Caregivers may feel that the person with AD is not trying, is being lazy, or is doing it to spite them.

Even if you or another caregiver previously helped the person with DS develop new skills and greater independence, this emphasis on improving skills must be reassessed when AD is diagnosed. The focus must shift to helping the person maintain skills or to limiting the decline in skills, rather than teaching new ones.

THE RIGHT ENVIRONMENT

In our experience, it is usually best for the person with Alzheimer disease to remain in a familiar environment. A change in environment can be confusing, require her to learn new skills, and be emotionally upsetting. Changing the person's environment would be akin to changing the furniture in the house of a person with severe vision impairment. It requires new learning in order to function in the environment. With the declining intellect of a person with Alzheimer disease, this can be difficult.

As the person's skills decline, *the environment* will need to be adjusted. That is, the environment must be adjusted to meet the needs of the person, not the person to meet the needs of the environment.

The flexibility of the environment is crucial to optimizing care for the person with AD. When her skills first begin to decline, she may do well in her customary environment. As her skills further decline, however, her adaptability does too. Often she will be most comfortable (or perhaps only comfortable) in her home.

Going to work may become too stressful, especially as AD progresses. If the person lives somewhere where leaving the building and going to work is a required part of the schedule, this may become a significant problem. Flexibility in the schedule is helpful to the person with AD who is declining. There may be days when it is apparent that she would best be served by staying home. Ideally, the person will be in an environment where the benefits of work versus the stress of work can be assessed. An alternative program at home should be available on days when it would be better for the person to stay home.

Safety issues may also develop. There is a risk of potentially serious accidents as the person becomes less aware of hazards related to appliances, hot water, and the like. In addition, as her walking skills worsen, she may injure herself on stairs and other household obstacles. Wandering is another potential safety issue for people with Alzheimer disease. You may need to install alarms on doors, windows, or the person's bed or have her wear an identification band or bracelet. Assessing the safety of the environment is critical. A "Home Safety Inspection" by an occupational therapist can be of significant benefit.

Besides assessing how the environment affects the person with AD, it is necessary to assess how the person with AD affects the environment. For example, how does she affect the other people who are living with her? For a person of "normal" intelligence, the stress of caring for, or just living with, a person with AD can be substantial. While we have seen people with DS and other intellectual disabilities "rise to the occasion" when someone they live with develops AD, we have also seen it become an overwhelming stress. One group of three women who lived with a woman with DS who developed AD initially "blossomed" with regards to their own caregiver skills. As time went on, however, the situation became too much for them to handle, so a different living situation was arranged for the person with AD.

Whenever possible, we encourage roommates or housemates with intellectual disabilities to try to provide care for the person with Alzheimer disease. Many people with DS or other intellectual disabilities get "done for" their whole lives with little opportunity to "do for." Assisting someone with AD can provide a real boost to self-esteem for the care provider.

However, sometimes even a seemingly minor stress can create problematic tension in the house. This might occur, for example, when the person with AD is no longer expected to participate in life skills classes, go to work, or follow the daily schedule. The sense of "injustice" can lead to emotional or behavioral problems for the others. Stress can also arise if the person with AD often yells or talks loudly, has irregular sleep patterns that disturb others' sleep, or needs changes in the environment that are stressful for the others.

Sometimes the changes in the person with AD just become too great a stress. All these issues may create a situation where reassessing the environment becomes necessary.

A Change in Environment

If the adult with AD is unable to stay home during the day when she needs to, it can be very stressful for her. The continuous expectation to do tasks that are too difficult or too stressful can lead to emotional, behavioral, and cognitive changes. If she feels overwhelmed by expectations, she might give up and seem to have fewer skills than she actually has. Moving the person to an environment that allows for the necessary flexibility can be of significant benefit. This benefit often outweighs the negative impact of the change associated with a move to a new residence.

Moving may also be advisable if safety issues in the person's current residence cannot be resolved. For example, a move to a safer residence might be in order if the person cannot be safeguarded from stairs or potentially dangerous household appliances or cannot be prevented from wandering.

Finally, it is often best for the person with AD to move to another residence if her caregivers or the people she lives with are overwhelmed with the situation and appropriate in-home assistance is not available. This can be necessary both when the person lives at home with her family or when she lives in a residential facility.

We have participated in a number of successful, appropriate moves to different residences for our patients with DS and AD. Nursing homes, particularly if they offer specialized care for people with Alzheimer disease, can be appropriate. Some agencies have residences for "seniors" that are able to provide appropriate care. Moving back home with family (if the person is living in a residential facility) has also worked for some. Generally, however, this requires some additional in-home assistance for the family.

Duration of Alzheimer Disease

The duration of AD in adults with DS is not clear. In the general population, the course of the disease is thought to be approximately ten to twelve years or even longer. Particularly in people with DS who have a higher degree of functioning before they develop Alzheimer disease, an overall course of ten or so years might be expected. However, our experience suggests that the duration is shorter for many, particularly in those who have a lower level of functioning prior to the onset of AD. In a sense, the further the person has to fall cognitively, the longer it generally takes. We have seen people live one year from the time of diagnosis to the time of death. On average, though, the time from the development of symptoms to death is usually in the three- to six-year range.

Theoretically, people with mosaic Down syndrome may be less affected by Alzheimer disease. Little information is available, however, as to whether that is the case. We haven't had enough patients with mosaic Down syndrome to get a sense of any differences.

Again, the development of seizures (particularly if they are difficult to control) seems to accelerate the decline in some people. Losing the ability to walk and swallow and developing complications as a result of losing these skills also seems to increase the rate of decline.

FUTURE CONSIDERATIONS

At present, many researchers are addressing the issue of Alzheimer disease, not only for people with DS, but for those without. People with DS receive particular attention when it comes to AD because studies suggest that all people with DS develop the neuropathologic changes in the brain that are seen in AD. Since these changes in the brain appear to be universal, researchers wonder why all people with DS do not appear to get the symptoms of AD. Is there something else that is coded on the twenty-first chromosome that may be protective against AD for some people with DS? This question has not yet been answered. It should be noted, however, that people with DS rarely develop heart attacks (myocardial infarctions) and coronary artery disease, so there may be something about DS that protects against some diseases that become more common with age.

The findings in people with DS may be important keys in unlocking the mysteries of AD. In addition, there is a great deal of interest in whether what helps AD may help people with DS when they are younger (before AD is apparent). As discussed previously, Aricept was studied but did not improve cognitive function. In addition, there is a great deal of interest and study related to the potential benefit of vitamins and other medications and how they might benefit or prevent AD in people with DS. Similar research is being conducted as to whether vitamins, supplements, and other treatments may also benefit the cognitive, speech, and other skills of people with DS. There appears to be much to learn that may benefit people with Down syndrome, people with Alzheimer disease, and people with both.

SUMMARY

Although all adults with Down syndrome develop changes in the brain that have been linked to Alzheimer disease, a decline in cognitive and other skills does not appear to be inevitable in older adults with DS. When a decline in function is noted, it is important that the person have a thorough evaluation to look for potentially reversible causes. In our experience, declines in mental and physical function are, more often than not, due to a treatable condition other than Alzheimer disease. While there is currently no cure if the diagnosis is AD, there are many ways to temporarily improve a person's level of function and make her more comfortable. Parents and caregivers should ensure that the adult with DS and AD sees practitioners with experience in providing optimal care for people with AD.

Chapter 21

Inpatient Care

• • • • • • • • • • • •

Darlene, age 23, was taken to the emergency room by her family because she wasn't thinking as clearly as usual. She had been fine the day before, but upon waking that morning she appeared confused. She also wasn't walking as well as usual and seemed unsteady. Her family reported that she had been drinking more fluids and urinating more in the last week. She had no fever, no cough, and no complaints of pain.

When Darlene was weighed, her family noted she had lost 15 pounds since being seen at the Adult Down Syndrome Center six weeks before, even though her appetite had increased. Blood work, urinalysis, and CT scan of her head were done in the emergency room. Her blood sugar was very high and her electrolytes (potassium, sodium, chloride, and bicarbonate) were abnormal. Her CT scan was normal.

Darlene was diagnosed with new onset diabetes mellitus and admitted to the hospital. With appropriate care, her blood sugar and electrolytes normalized and her confusion resolved.

As in Darlene's case, some medical conditions may require hospitalization for people with Down syndrome (DS). Hospitalization may be necessary to treat a condition, to monitor the person for progression of an illness, or to manage pain. While the need for hospitalization is certainly not unique to people with DS, there are some problems that may present differently or require a different approach to diagnosis and treatment. In addition, sometimes the care provided for people with DS in the hospital needs to be modified because of difficulties with communication or comprehension, or other characteristics related to Down syndrome. Issues that can complicate hospitalization for adolescents and adults with DS are discussed below.

ELICITING THE MEDICAL HISTORY

Some people with DS have a limited ability to describe what is wrong and how their illness has progressed. This presents an additional challenge to their care. Some people with DS have limited speech. Others may speak well, but have difficulties assessing and relaying their symptoms. Some patients are reluctant to discuss their symptoms because they remember that when they had previous health concerns they ended up having tests or being hospitalized that they found uncomfortable. All of these problems can present additional challenges to the care of people with DS.

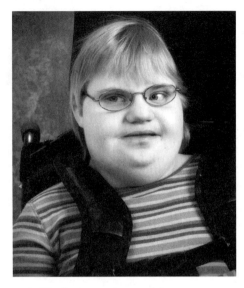

Here are some tips that may help in obtaining the person's history:

- ◆ Speak clearly and use terms the person is likely to understand.
- ◆ If the person doesn't appear to understand the question, ask it again in a different way or use different words.
- ◆ Start with open-ended questions (ones that can't be answered with just a yes or a no).
- ◆ Be careful not to put words into the person's mouth.
- ◆ Consider the use of pictures to help the person explain his symptoms. For example, use the Picture Exchange Communication System (PECS).Use of the picture symbolizing pain and the pictures of different body parts can aid in finding the source of discomfort.
- ◆ Bear in mind that questions involving quantity or time may be particularly challenging (how many, how often, how long). It may be better to try to link the question to something concrete in the person's life. For example, instead of asking "How long have you been feeling this way?" ask "Did your leg hurt during your aerobics class? When you were at the grocery store?" or something of the kind.
- ◆ Family members and other care providers should augment the history, when necessary.
- ◆ Observe—the person's body language may reveal important history both when asked questions and when he is just sitting or lying down.

It is important to try to get at least some of the history from the person with DS. Family members or caregivers may not be aware of some of the symptoms, may under- or over-estimate the significance or severity of a symptom, or may not realize the impact the illness is having on the person with DS.

An important piece of information to obtain is the medication history. Even if a list of medications is available from the doctor's office, the medications should be reviewed. Many adults with DS see more than one health care practitioner. Some see specialists, some go to a local urgent care center or emergency room, and some take additional over-the-counter medications or natural products. Any change in the person's medications may contribute to a change in health in a number of ways. There might be:

- a side effect from a medication or natural product;
- an interaction between a previous medication and new medications that may increase or decrease the effect or increase or decrease side effects;
- worsening of a preexisting medical condition due to a new medication (for example, if an adult who has kidney disease is seen for an ankle sprain by a doctor who doesn't know his full history, he might be prescribed an anti-inflammatory medication that worsens the kidney disease).

It is also essential to find out how the illness is affecting the person's functioning and behavior. The doctors treating the person need to gather information that answer the questions:

- "What is his baseline?"
- "How does he usually act or function?"
- "Is he acting or functioning differently?"

If these questions are not addressed, the correct diagnosis may be missed or the treatment may be inadequate. Particularly if the health care provider is not familiar with the person, he or she may assume that an impairment that is actually part of the illness or disorder is just part of the person's DS.

PREPARING THE PERSON FOR MEDICAL PROCEDURES

Many people—with and without DS—are afraid of what is going to happen to them while hospitalized. Misunderstanding what is going to be done can worsen the situation. For people with DS, it is therefore very important to carefully describe medical procedures in advance. To avoid confusion, we recommend the following strategies:

- Speak slowly and clearly in a room with limited distractions and noise.
- Use simple language and avoid using medical terms that the person may not understand.
- Give the person time to comprehend what is being said.
- Use pictures where appropriate. For example, to explain an x-ray of the ankle, use a picture of a camera, an x-ray machine, and an ankle while explaining what will happen during the x-ray.

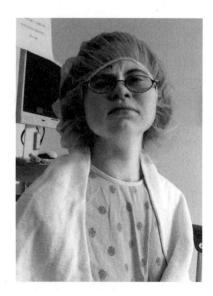

- Use calendars or schedules (especially ones with pictures) to help the person understand when procedures will occur since people with DS often have a limited understanding of time.
- Write a Social Story to let the person know what is going to happen, as well as the sequence of events to expect. Social Stories are a technique developed by Carol Gray that can be used to help the person understand what is going to happen to him and the appropriate way to act in a situation. They can be written with simple, declarative sentences starring the person as the main character and can be illustrated with line drawings or photos. For example: "Eric will get a bracelet at the check-in desk. The bracelet will have Eric's name on it. Then he will go to the surgery center. . . ."
- Try to confirm that the person understands what will happen.
- Enlist the aid of family, care providers, or others who understand the person's communication and comprehension difficulties. These individuals can often help the person with DS understand, or can suggest phrases that are more understandable.
- Avoid terms that may have double meanings (see below).

Connor, age 16, had a fractured leg that required surgery. He was told that he would be "put to sleep." Unfortunately, two weeks prior, his dog had become ill and was "put to sleep." Understandably, Connor was very upset about the idea of being put to sleep until he was given a fuller explanation of anesthesia: He would receive some medication, he would fall asleep, and after the surgery he would wake up.

Other terms with double meanings that may be confusing:
- "going under";
- "a little stick" (in reference to a blood draw or IV);
- you are going to have a "Cat Scan."

ALTERED MENTAL STATUS

Many illnesses or conditions can impair a person's ability to think, cause confusion, make him sedated (groggy or tired), or impair his functioning. As noted above, it is important for family members or care providers to let doctors know whether this is a *change* from the person's usual level of functioning.

If the difficulties do represent a change, there are many possible causes. First, DS itself always causes some degree of cognitive or neurologic impairment. Due to this impairment, the brains of people with DS do seem to be more susceptible to further impairment in response to a variety of health problems. (This is not unique to DS and is seen in many conditions in which there is some cognitive impairment at baseline.)

Infections are a common cause of changes in cognitive abilities. Pneumonia and urinary tract infections are frequently the cause. However, skin infections (for example, cellulitis or abscesses), gastrointestinal infections, central nervous system infections (for example, meningitis), and others can also cause a change in mental status.

There are a number of reasons why infections can cause a change in mental status:

- direct impact on the brain (for example, with meningitis);
- hypotension (low blood pressure), which can make the person feel lightheaded, and if it progresses significantly can cause permanent damage to the brain;
- dehydration, if the person has been drinking less due to the illness (this can result in changes in electrolytes such as sodium and cause confusion);
- fever;
- hypoxemia (decreased oxygen), which can lead to confusion and eventually brain damage;
- anemia (decreased red blood cell count), which can lead to fatigue and low oxygen in the brain;
- toxins produced by bacteria that affect the brain.

Once the infection is treated, the person usually regains his previous level of cognitive function. This may not be possible, however, if the negative effects on the brain continue for too long. For example, there may be permanent brain damage after a prolonged period of low blood pressure or low oxygen.

Neurological problems may also cause changes in mental status. Examples of these problems include:

- stroke,
- trauma (e.g., concussion),
- bleeding in or around the brain (e.g., subdural hematoma),
- tumors.

As in people without DS, these problems can lead to permanent brain damage. People with DS already have impaired cognition and, therefore, these insults to the brain can cause greater impairment or the person may be less able to recover from them. A CT Scan or MRI of the brain can detect these problems and these tests are often part of the work-up done to pinpoint the reason for a change in mental status.

Many metabolic conditions can also cause a change in mental status. (A metabolic problem is one in which one or more of the biochemical systems of the body are affected.) Changes due to a metabolic condition can occur gradually or suddenly. Some metabolic conditions that cause mental status changes are:

- thyroid dysfunction (hypo- and hyperthyroidism),
- uncontrolled diabetes mellitus,
- kidney dysfunction,
- low oxygen to the brain (see infections above; also heart failure),
- liver dysfunction, and
- electrolyte disturbances and dehydration.

As discussed in Chapter 15, thyroid dysfunction and diabetes are more common in people with DS. Inadequate fluid intake and dehydration are also common in people with DS. So, these disorders should always be kept in mind if an adolescent or adult has an unexpected change in mental status.

Psychiatric conditions can also cause a change in mental status. In the hospital, people with DS often experience anxiety or other emotional reactions to their illness or to hospitalization. The stress may cause the person to behave differently or to become confused. A careful assessment for medical/physical causes must be done (see above). Reassurance, support, and the presence of family members, friends, or other familiar people, as well as familiar comfort objects from home, may help calm the person. In addition, if health care providers are aware (or are informed by family members) that these are common reactions, they should take steps to prevent anxiety and watch for early signs of anxiety and agitation. Treatment with anti-anxiety medications in as low a dose as possible is sometimes necessary. Lorazepam (Ativan) and alprazolam (Xanax) are some examples. Occasionally, the anti-psychotic medication haloperidol (Haldol) can be used for a more severe reaction.

Other psychological problems that can result in an altered mental status include:

- acute psychoses or psychotic reaction (such as "ICU psychosis," a recognized complication of being in the intensive care unit—it is related to the severe illness, poor sleep, lack of stimuli that help a person orient to day and time, and other causes);
- post-traumatic stress disorder (see below);
- depression (although this does not usually occur suddenly);
- acute deterioration of many psychological conditions.

Some psychological problems, including anxiety and depression, are fairly common in adolescents and adults with DS. Others, such as psychoses, are relatively rare. More information on symptoms and treatment for mental health problems in people with Down syndrome is available in *Mental Wellness for Adults with Down Syndrome* (McGuire and Chicoine, 2006).

In addition, a sudden or significant change in one of the senses can cause acute changes in a person's mental status. For example, a sudden and severe loss of vision

Post-Traumatic Stress Disorder

Post-traumatic stress disorder (PTSD) is a condition that sometimes occurs in people who have experienced an event that would be extremely distressing to most human beings. This might include a threat to one's life or physical or psychological health. Symptoms of PTSD may include:
- distressing recollections of the event;
- acting or feeling as if the traumatic event is recurring;
- psychological distress in reaction to remembering or reliving the experience (e.g., anxiety);
- psychological symptoms (such as sweating or elevated heart rate);
- efforts to avoid the situation or setting where the event occurred or anything that might remind the person of the situation;
- irritability or outbursts of anger.

For some people with DS, hospitalization can trigger post-traumatic stress disorder. That is, after being discharged from the hospital, the person may experience PTSD symptoms when anything reminds him of his hospitalization. Or, if the person is hospitalized for a repeat visit, she may have PTSD symptoms in the hospital. To minimize that possibility, it is important to reduce the stress of hospitalization. We recommend considering:
- having a family member or friend in the recovery room as the person awakens from anesthesia;
- using an anti-anxiety medication for the trip to the hospital (and/ or prior to the procedure);
- providing good pain control during the hospitalization; and
- having a family member or friend stay with the person during his hospitalization.

(e.g., due to a detached retina) or hearing (e.g., due to a perforation of the tympanic membrane/eardrum) can affect the person's cognition. Pain may also cause the person to become confused.

When a person with DS has experienced a change in mental status, a careful history and physical exam is essential to assess for the conditions just discussed. Lab work and imaging (chest x-ray, CT scan of brain, MRI of the brain) may also be needed. Treatment is based on the findings of the evaluation.

AGITATED BEHAVIOR

Some people with DS get agitated in the hospital. This may occur for a number of reasons. First, their agitation may be a consequence of illness and can be due to any of the causes for changes in mental status addressed above. It is therefore important to consider whether any of these possible underlying medical conditions may be contributing to agitation. Care must be taken not to assume that the person is just upset about being in the hospital and thereby overlook a medical condition.

Second, some people with and without DS find being in the hospital and the procedures that occur there frightening and upsetting. Some of these feelings may be due to fear of the unknown, so explaining what is going to happen can help. Third, pain or the fear of pain may cause agitation. Particularly if the person has had surgery or has a painful condition, pain must be considered. Remember, many people with DS do not complain of pain even when they are experiencing it. Instead, they may react with agitation. Therefore, pain medications are often the first treatment. It is important, of course, to assess for other causes (e.g., low blood pressure, low oxygen) that potentially could be made worse with pain medication.

It may be helpful for the person with DS to be placed on a scheduled course of pain medications, so that they are given every certain number of hours. If the person has breakthrough pain, he may need additional pain medication. The person will either have to ask for additional pain medications or the nursing staff will have to monitor him for signs of pain.

Medical Tests

Some people with DS find it challenging to cooperate with testing—especially if it involves drawing blood. On the other hand, some of our teenaged and adult patients feel as if they have missed part of the care they should have gotten during their appointment if they don't get blood drawn. They are upset if we do not draw blood each appointment.

For those who cannot cooperate with the blood drawing, we consider the use of:

- a topical anesthetic (e.g., EMLA) applied to the skin two hours before the blood draw to numb the area,
- light anti-anxiety medication or sedative,
- combining procedures if the person has to undergo anesthesia (e.g., scheduling blood drawing when a patient is having ear tubes placed).

If significant sedation is required for a procedure, we have it done in a controlled, monitored setting. For example, some patients find MRIs challenging and may require sedation during the procedure. This test involves lying very still inside an enclosed space and enduring repeated loud noises. We have an arrangement with our MRI and anesthesiology departments for an anesthesiologist to be on hand in case sedation is necessary. This ranges from light IV sedation to general anesthesia. Appropriate monitoring is provided by the anesthesiologist.

SEIZURES

· · · · · · · · · · · · · · · · · · ·

As discussed in Chapter 17, seizures are more common in people with DS. When a person with DS who has seizures is hospitalized for any reason, his anti-seizure medications are continued. However, if the person is not able to take his medications by mouth due to a medical condition, this presents another challenge. Some medications commonly taken by mouth (pill, capsule, or liquid) are available in a form that can be given intravenously. These medications include:

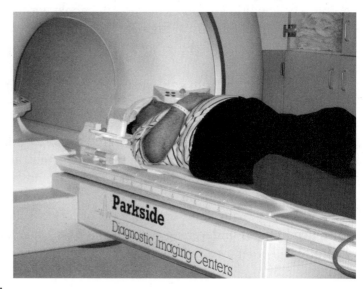

- ◆ phenytoin (Dilantin),
- ◆ valproate (Depacon),
- ◆ levetiracetam (Keppra).

Other medications are not available in a form that can be given intravenously. These medications include:

- ◆ carbamazepime (Tegretol),
- ◆ gabapentin (Neurontin),
- ◆ lamotrigine (Lamictal),
- ◆ topiramate (Topamax).

If the needed medication is not available in an intravenous form, there are a number of options:

- ◆ In some situations, even if the person is not allowed to eat or drink, it may be acceptable to take pills with a small sip of water.
- ◆ A nasogastric tube (NG tube) may be placed through the nose and into the stomach) so medications can be given through the tube.
- ◆ The person may be temporarily switched to one of the medications that is available for intravenous use. In this case, you may want to ask the physician treating the individual in the hospital to consult with the adult's neurologist before prescribing a new medication.

ATLANTOAXIAL SUBLUXATION

Atlantoaxial subluxation is the slippage of the first vertebrae of the neck on the second. The condition is more common in people with DS, and is described in Chapter 13. If the vertebrae slip far enough, the spinal cord will be pinched. This slippage is most common at the first and second vertebrae but can occur at other levels of the cervical (neck) spine.

In the hospital, atlantoaxial subluxation can be of particular concern when someone with DS undergoes general anesthesia. When the head is tilted back to insert the endotracheal (breathing) tube, the vertebrae may slip, pinching the spinal cord.

Everyone with DS should be considered at risk for atlantoaxial subluxation, and a lateral (side) neck x-ray in flexion, extension, and neutral views should be done before any surgery requiring a breathing tube. There are no clear guidelines for how often these x-rays should be done. We consider repeating the x-rays every ten years, but sooner if there are any signs or symptoms of cervical subluxation. If the person with Down syndrome is undergoing surgery and hasn't had a neck x-ray in ten years, we generally will order a set before surgery.

SLEEP APNEA

As discussed in Chapter 18, sleep apnea is more common in people with Down syndrome. Adolescents and adults with DS most often have obstructive sleep apnea. In this type, the person's airway becomes obstructed during sleep and airflow is blocked. Typically, after a period of time, the person arouses enough to open his airway and breathe.

Anesthesia and Sedating Medication

Some people with DS are quite sensitive to sedatives. They may need smaller doses than usual to achieve the desired effect. Conversely, some require very large doses. Some people with DS also waken slowly after general anesthesia and may need more prolonged monitoring.

It is also important to be aware that some reports in the past indicated that people with DS are very sensitive to atropine and can experience an increased heart rate when it is given. (Atropine is sometimes used before surgery to reduce saliva in the mouth.) However, subsequent studies did not support this finding and we have not experienced this as a problem.

If the person with DS has previously had an unusual reaction to sedatives, anesthesia, or atropine, a family member should make sure the anesthesiologist is aware of this.

However, when they are under anesthesia or sedating medications, people with apnea may have a reduced ability to arouse. This may lead to prolonged apnea spells.

If the person with DS has a diagnosis of sleep apnea and uses treatment at home (e.g., CPAP), this should be continued in the hospital. The person may also need to have his oxygen continuously monitored for a period of time after anesthesia or while he is receiving pain medications. This should be discussed with his physician, anesthesiologist, or other health care providers involved in his care at the hospital.

DYSPHAGIA (SWALLOWING DYSFUNCTION)

Swallowing dysfunction is more common in people with Down syndrome, as discussed in Chapter 11. Even if a person with DS does not ordinarily have trouble swallowing when eating and drinking, illness may weaken him, and swallowing dysfunction may occur. In addition, throat surgery, nasogastric tubes, and intubation (placement of a breathing tube) may all contribute to swallowing dysfunction. If the person does experience swallowing difficulties, one possible serious complication is aspirating (breathing in) food or drink.

If there is any doubt that the person is swallowing safely, his eating and drinking should be monitored for any deterioration during the hospitalization. For example, a parent or nurse might observe him while he is eating to see if any choking or gagging occurs. If deterioration is suspected, a speech-language pathologist (SLP) can assess his swallowing abilities. A video swallowing study may also be useful. During a video swallowing study, the patient is given food and drink mixed with barium to consume. The SLP monitors his swallowing and videofluoroscope x-rays are done to trace the progress of the food and note whether any of it gets into the lungs.

BLOOD PRESSURE

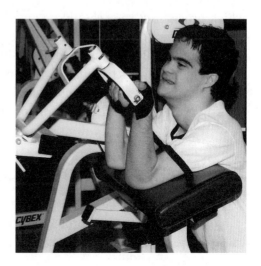

Hospitals often call the Adult Down Syndrome Center with concerns about the blood pressure of patients with DS. As explained in Chapter 9, people with DS tend to have lower blood pressure (BP). The normal BP for most of our patients is 90-110 systolic (the top number) and 50-70 diastolic (the bottom number). BP's that are even lower are not uncommon. These lower readings can cause a great deal of concern in the hospital if the person checking the BP is not aware that many people with DS have a lower BP.

It is important to note the person's previous BP recordings at home or in the office and compare them to the readings in the hospital. If the person has a BP that is similar to his previous recordings and there are no other concerning findings to suggest that the BP is causing problems, then the person checking the BP can be reassured.

CARDIOVASCULAR CONCERNS

Approximately 40 to 60 percent of babies born with DS have congenital heart disease. Most heart defects are now surgically repaired when the person is young, often in infancy. Sometimes, however, the disease has not been corrected. (See Chapter 9.)

Adults who have had heart defects surgically repaired may have structural or rhythm complications later in life. Rhythm problems have been a particular concern with those who have had Tetrology of Fallot repaired. Regular cardiology evaluation is advisable, especially if there are any cardiac complications that are exacerbated by the illness that causes the hospitalization.

For patients whose hearts have not been surgically repaired, cardiology evaluation may be indicated if they are admitted to the hospital for any reason, but especially if heart failure or hypoxemia (low oxygen) are found.

ENDOCARDITIS AND PREVENTIVE ANTIBIOTICS

People who have abnormal heart structures (holes in the heart and abnormal valves), as well as those who have had defects surgically repaired may be at increased risk of endocarditis. Endocarditis is an infection of the heart.

To reduce the risk of endocarditis, antibiotics are given before patients with particular heart problems undergo certain medical or surgical procedures that may increase the risk of infection. As discussed in Chapter 9, the recommendations were changed in 2007 as to who should receive antibiotics before procedures and before which procedures they should be given. In some cases, antibiotics are no longer recommended for people with particular types of defects or repairs when previously they were. Some cardiologists, however, believe that some of their patients should continue to receive antibiotics because of their particular heart problem. We recommend that the patient's cardiologist be consulted in any decisions related to providing or withholding preventive antibiotics while in the hospital.

GASTROINTESTINAL CONCERNS

Two gastrointestinal problems are mentioned here as well as in Chapter 11 because of the need to consider them for people in the hospital.

Gallstones are more common in people with DS and cause abdominal pain. Abdominal pain is one reason someone might be evaluated in the emergency room or in the hospital. However, gallstones may also cause more subtle symptoms such as a loss of appetite or agitated behavior. Therefore, gallstones should be considered in a person with DS who has significant symptoms, especially if they include loss of appetite and/or abdominal pain.

Peptic ulcer disease is another problem that often is evaluated in the hospital emergency room. As with gallstones, symptoms may include abdominal pain, loss of appetite, or a behavioral change. Note, however, that sometimes an ulcer can be "silent" in a person with DS. There may be no symptoms until the person has experienced significant bleeding. This makes it important to consider the possibility of peptic ulcer disease in hospitalized patients with DS.

REHABILITATION AND THERAPIES

When people are hospitalized, others do their daily care for them, they may have foley catheters (to collect and monitor their urine), and they may have limited opportunities to walk and perform other activities for themselves. After hospitalization, they can have difficulty regaining the skills they did not use while in the hospital. For these patients, therapy to address this loss of skills is an important part of their care.

We find this is a need for adults with Down syndrome of all ages. They often need physical and/or occupational therapy in the hospital to help maintain their level of function. This will vary based on the length of the hospitalization, the severity of the illness, and the extent to which they are able or allowed to do things for themselves during the hospitalization.

Unfortunately, some people with DS find it challenging to participate in therapy. Including activities or games the person enjoys may motivate him to participate. People with DS often enjoy listening to music and dancing, so including them in the therapy may be helpful. It is also important to remember that the person with DS might be in pain, even though he isn't saying so. If so, pain medications may help him attempt to make certain movements again.

Getting insurance to pay for physical therapy or other therapies that *children* with DS need to help them make developmental progress can sometimes be challenging. However, the need for the therapies we are discussing here is linked to the hospitalization or illness that caused the hospitalization. Therefore, getting insurance to pay for it is usually not a significant problem. Sometimes the need for therapy can even be anticipated before the hospitalization. If so, it can be helpful for the person with DS to meet with the therapist and see the therapy department before he is hospitalized.

Chapter 22

Preserving Health

and Well-Being over

the Long Term

One of the key issues affecting the health and well-being of teens and adults with Down syndrome (DS) is where and with whom they live.

Some adults with DS continue to live with family members all their lives. Many other adults, however, eventually move out of their family homes. This chapter covers issues related to living arrangements that we have found to have a positive or negative effect on the health of people with DS.

We have limited this discussion to issues that: 1) we have some personal experience and expertise in dealing with, and 2) we feel may be most helpful to people with DS and their caregivers. We first briefly discuss trends in group homes, then the perceptions people may have of group homes, and finally focus on key health and psychosocial issues to consider when look-

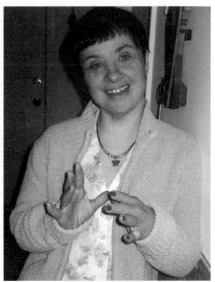

ing at available residential options. We will also look at special issues facing families in which an older adult with DS is still living at home.

To set the stage for these discussions, let's look at a case story that illustrates some of the major concerns for adults with Down syndrome related to life outside of the family home:

Tom lived at home with his family until the age of 25. He then moved into a three-person group home managed by a local residential service provider. Prior to the move, Tom's family had spent a considerable amount of time researching different service providers in their area. They had heard good things about the agency from a variety of sources. They had talked to representatives of a state agency responsible for monitoring residential service providers, and with agencies responsible for processing residential placements. Perhaps most importantly, they had talked to many families who had received some type of service from the agency. All of these people were generally positive about the agency.

When an opening came up in one of the agency's group homes, Tom's family and the agency began the process of moving him into the home. As part of this process, Tom made a series of visits to the home. On several occasions, he visited the house for dinner and for outings to special recreation activities with other house members. He also went for several overnights lasting from one to three nights. Tom seemed very pleased and comfortable in the house. He had a good relationship with the other housemates and with the staff. By the end of his visits, Tom reported to his family that this house was the right one for him and he was ready to move.

Prior to Tom's move, his family was very careful to clarify some key concerns with agency administrators. One of their most pressing concerns involved the provision of health and mental health care for Tom. He had a history of health issues and one mental health issue. Although Tom was generally even tempered, there was one two- to three-month period when he had had uncharacteristic bouts of anger, agitated self-talk, and some symptoms of depression. These changes had occurred about a year before the planned move to the group home.

The staff at the Adult Down Syndrome Center had identified several underlying reasons for Tom's mood and behavior changes. First, he was diagnosed with both hypothyroidism and an uncomfortable acid reflux condition. He was also found to be under intense stress at work, where another participant was teasing and provoking him. Once this situation was identified by his family, the worksite administrators immediately put a stop to the bullying. Tom's reflux and hypothyroid problems were also treated, and within several months he gradually returned to what his family described as his "normal, easygoing self." There were no further incidents of agitation or angry outbursts. Tom did still have a tendency to withdraw and to resist doing activities with friends, but his family worked hard to motivate him to get back into beneficial programs and activities. In time, he was back to a full schedule of social and recreational activities and his enjoyment and enthusiasm had returned.

Although Tom had returned to "normal," his parents were very concerned about how he would weather future stress. More importantly, they wondered how residential service providers would deal with any future changes in Tom's mood and behavior. Would they look for all possible causes, as the family and staff at ADSC had, or would they simply assume this was a mental health or behavioral problem? The answers agency staff gave to the family's questions were reassuring. Agency staff stated that any changes in a resident's mood or behavior would merit a thorough physical exam and a careful look at possible environmental stresses before referral to a mental health practitioner. This was very encouraging. Tom's family were also relieved to find out that the agency would allow Tom to continue to be followed at the Adult Down Syndrome Center, would take him to his appointments there, and would welcome family members if they wanted to come along.

Besides asking questions about health, dental, and mental health care, Tom's family also checked to make sure that the group home scheduled social and recreational activities for all residents. In addition, the family looked at the agency's track record of helping residents locate meaningful and substantial forms of work. They were pleased to find that most people had jobs they enjoyed and that would be considered good jobs by anyone.

Tom's family also wanted to make certain that the agency encouraged family involvement. They were happy to learn that the agency expected regular family visits, as well as get-togethers at the house between all families of the residents.

Despite their positive impression of the agency staff and administration, Tom's family (his parents and his two older siblings) took the step of becoming his legal co-guardians before he moved in. They had heard that sometimes when staff at a group home changes, the new administration may not uphold the promises and expectations between the family and the old administration. They believed that guardianship would give them the legal right to challenge any future decisions that they felt were not in Tom's best interest.

After all the planning and visits, Tom finally moved into the house. His family and staff found the move to be almost anticlimactic. His relationship with staff and other residents was very positive. He enjoyed his new job working at a recycling center, where he did a variety of sorting and cleaning tasks. He also spent several mornings doing assembly work at a workshop that he had attended while still living at home. This gave him an opportunity to stay in touch with his many friends in this workshop and to have some continuity in his daily schedule.

Tom and his new housemates were busy and active, with regularly scheduled sports and recreation activities. He also visited with his family at least once a month, as well as for all holidays and family gatherings. Tom's mother remarked that he had a far better social life than anyone else in his family, including his three older siblings. Overall, Tom was happy and well adjusted. Everyone agreed that the group home was a good move for him.

TRENDS IN RESIDENTIAL FACILITIES

Many teens and young adults with DS see their siblings and peers without disabilities go off to college and establish their own lives and careers, and many view a move out of the family home as a way to establish their own independence.

Usually when adults with DS move from their family home, they go to live in a group home that is managed by an agency and staffed by paid caregivers. There are, of course, many different types of group living arrangements, but the vast majority include some type of shared living arrangement with others who are not blood relatives. Over the past thirty to forty years, the size of group homes has changed. Very large institutions were the norm in the past, but now there are smaller group homes housing one to fifteen individuals. The trend has been for smaller and smaller group homes and for these homes to be scattered in the community. There are still many campus-like settings, but even in these settings, people tend to live in smaller units. This often combines the safety and social benefits of a campus with the benefits of a smaller, family-like residence.

The amount of supervision by staff is also a key issue. Usually, homes are staffed on the basis of how much care the residents theoretically need due to their respective level of adaptive skills. For example, at some homes, staff only provide a few hours of supervision per week at set times; at other homes, staff are present 24 hours a day.

FAMILY PERCEPTIONS OF RESIDENTIAL OPTIONS

One reason families may delay looking at residential facilities, even if their sons or daughters have expressed an interest in moving out, is that they may still have images of large institutional facilities, hidden away from the rest of society. Large facilities do still exist, but they are rare now and usually serve people with very special needs (such as people who have medical issues requiring skilled nursing care).

We often strongly recommend that families contact different agencies to arrange visits to see the group homes in their communities. This may go a long way to dispel any misconceptions or misperceptions they might have. There are other major benefits as well. Families are often good at sizing up different places based on what they believe will work for their sons and daughters.

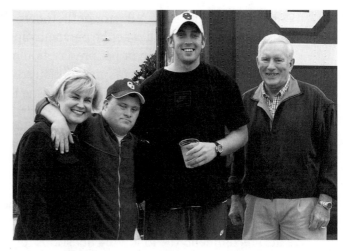

It is just as important to help the person with DS understand about living outside the home. Visiting a host of different residential options may allow her to create a visual image of what her options are and what life would be like outside of her family home. In addition, because many people with DS seem to "read" people and situations, this may help in sizing up which residences "feel" right to them. Visiting a wide variety of houses may also help them to compare and to pick those that may be the best fit for their needs.

Once the individual and her family have identified one or more possible residences, we strongly recommend that the adult with DS pay a series of visits to these settings. Visits to have dinner or to go on outings are a very good way to meet other residents. Staying at the house for a weekend or for overnights is an even better way to experience life in the home. Making these types of advance visits greatly eases the process of adjusting to a new home.

MEDICAL AND DENTAL CARE FOR RESIDENTS

As discussed in the story about Tom, before choosing a home, it is very important to investigate how residents' health care needs are provided for. The administrators should have a clear protocol for dealing with the health care needs of residents. To avoid future conflicts and frustrations, parents or other family members should thoroughly check into this protocol in advance.

Questions we recommend that you ask administrators include:

- ◆ What doctors, dentists, and other health care professions do the staff members rely on to look after the health care needs of residents?
- ◆ What are the health care professionals' qualifications? What is their level of experience in working with people with Down syndrome?
- ◆ Are family members informed each time there is a health issue or problem?
- ◆ Who takes residents to medical and dental appointments?
- ◆ Are families informed of these appointments and are they allowed to accompany staff to the appointments?

- ◆ Can residents go to a doctor of their own choosing and will staff support this choice and take the person to appointments when needed?
- ◆ How are prescription or nonprescription medications managed? Many states have regulations for prescription administration, but many states also allow some individuals to administer their own medications. There may also be some leeway for nonprescription drugs. What are the specific state regulations and agency rules regarding medications?
- ◆ Who pays for medical care that is not paid for by Medicare, Medicaid, or private insurance?
- ◆ Who is allowed access to medical records?
- ◆ How are life-threatening emergencies handled?

We also recommend the following questions related to safety concerns:
- ◆ Are staff trained in CPR (cardiopulmonary resuscitation)?
- ◆ Does the agency have a plan for emergencies? Many states require a plan for fire, including holding periodic fire drills. Does the agency also have a plan for nature disasters such as floods, tornadoes, or hurricanes?

If answers to these questions are vague or not satisfactory, then this may not be the right facility or agency to care for your son or daughter. If there are too many restrictions or negatives, such as refusing to allow parents to accompany staff to appointments or to arrange for their own doctors for medical visits, then this does not bode well for future relations and it could result in less than adequate care for your son or daughter.

One further word of advice: Be sure to find out whether the agency actually follows its stated protocol for health service. You can get this type of information from families of other residents, from state agencies who oversee or regulate group homes in your area, and also from independent or state-mandated case management agencies who help to process applications to group homes.

The vast majority of agencies with residential facilities really do want to do the right thing and they make every effort to care for their residents' needs. Still, our advice is to investigate before you proceed. This can help to reduce a very common area of conflict and dissatisfaction between your family and the staff at your child's group home.

BEHAVIORAL AND MENTAL HEALTH CARE

Agencies should also have a clear protocol for the provision of mental health services, just as for medical and dental care. Again, it is very important to check into this before moving your son or daughter to a residence, even if he or she has no current or past history of mental health problems. Your adult child may be affected by other residents who do have problems, even if she never develops any problems of her own.

As with health issues, there are a number of key questions to ask, but also some unique issues to consider. For example, when it comes to mental health issues, there is often much more at stake in terms of who controls the definition of the problem. This means it is important to understand who makes decisions about the causes and potential treatments of behavioral and mental health problems of residents. How a particular agency makes these decisions may or may not be in the best interest of the person with DS.

If the agency has a considerable say in determining causes and treatments, one key issue to consider is whether it is their policy to get a physical exam for residents when they experience mental health problems. We always recommend this step to rule out any health causes or precipitants to mental health or behavioral problems. Why is this so important? As we have discussed throughout this and our previous book, mental health and health care problems are quite often interwoven and need to be treated as such. This is particularly true for people with DS, who often have conceptual and expressive language limitations that make it difficult to verbalize physical pain or discomfort, as well as to discuss problems or stresses in their lives. Not uncommonly, changes in mood or behavior may be the result of an untreated health problem.

The case example of Tom presented above clearly shows the association between health and mental health problems. Many other examples of this association are provided in other chapters, as well as in our previous book, *Mental Wellness in Adults with Down Syndrome*. From our standpoint, it is critical to ensure that any residential facility you are considering always obtains physical exams for residents when there are changes in mood or behavior.

The next question to ask is who does the agency refer residents to for treating bona fide mental health problems? Do the doctors treating mental health problems have experience working with people with DS? In our experience, many mental health practitioners who are not experienced in working with people with DS use evaluation standards that are not appropriate. (We have written extensively about this in *Mental Wellness for Adults with Down Syndrome.)* For example, these professionals may view self-talk as an indication of psychosis and treat it with potentially harmful medication, when it is usually normal and developmentally appropriate, given the intellectual age of most adults with DS. As a second example, many people with DS have set routines, and caregivers have to be patient in demanding changes in a person's routine. Staff who do not give people time to adjust may create unnecessary stress and resistance, which may be misinterpreted as oppositional behavior (see below discussion on grooves for more on this). This is not to say that mental health problem do not exist and should not be treated—just that understanding the characteristics of people with DS may greatly help to reduce mistreatment.

Another question to ask is how much control families have over the treatment process. Can parents or family members go to psychiatric evaluation and treatment sessions? How much input do they have with the doctor? If the family is not happy with the doctor or the treatment, can they find their own psychiatric or mental health professional? Will the agency support access to a new doctor by taking the family member with DS to appointments and following through on treatment recommendations, even if they have not previously worked with this doctor?

Finally, you should be aware that many states require a behavior plan when psychotropic medications are prescribed. (Psychotropic medications are medications prescribed for mental health problems, including antidepressants, mood stabilizers, and medications for anxiety or for obsessive-compulsive behavior.) Be sure to ask how much input families have for the behavioral evaluation and treatment plan. Also consider asking about the experience and training of the behavior specialists (often called behaviorists) the group home uses. Young and inexperienced behaviorists may be excellent, but sometimes those who have not raised their own children may have unrealistic expectations for "appropriate behavior."

GUARDIANSHIP AND HEALTH CARE ISSUES

Whether or not your adult child is her own guardian will affect how and to what extent you are able to work with residential staff to optimize her health care. If your child is her own guardian, then agency administrators do not have to inform you about any health issues affecting her. By law, they only have to ask your child for her permission to seek treatment. Some agencies may be willing to keep family members informed and involved if the adult with DS informally authorizes sharing of information, but you can't count on this happening. It is very likely that there will be turnover in the agency administrators who oversee your son's or daughter's residence. The people who work with you now may be replaced by staff who are far less interested in working with you or in getting your opinion. We have seen this happen time and time again in our work with families.

The vast majority of agencies work very collaboratively with families. Still, in our opinion, it is worth seriously considering becoming your adult child's guardian if you feel she would benefit from your continued involvement in her health care. Alternately, you might consider obtaining some type of power of attorney, which would give you the ability to make medical, but not other decisions, on your child's behalf.

The same issues that crop up related to guardianship and medical care also occur with mental health problems. Staff may be completely cooperative and open with family with regard to mental health problems, even if the family are not the legal guardians, but why take a chance? Again, there will most likely be turnover in the administrators of the group home. How receptive will these new administrators be to you and your beliefs and wishes for your family member with DS?

Megan's story illustrates some of the possible pitfalls for families when the person with DS is her own guardian and develops mental health problems:

Megan moved from her family home to a four-person group home at
the age of 27. Like Tom's family, discussed above, Megan's family spent time

researching and looking at different group homes managed by different residential providers.

Megan moved into a home that seemed to be a good fit for her needs and wishes. She had a good relationship with the three women sharing the house. All were young and enjoyed being busy and active with social and recreational activities. The house was a very stable and supportive environment. Three staff members had worked at the house for at least five years, and Megan developed a very close, positive relationship with many staff members. Megan's family believed that the workshop she attended could have offered more opportunities for outside work, but at least regular assembly work was available and Megan had many friends at this program. Megan visited with her family regularly and they continued to be an important source of support for her. Of importance, too, Megan's family and staff had developed a good working relationship.

For three years, Megan seemed happy and well adjusted in her residence. In her fourth year, however, her family began to notice some changes in her mood and behavior. At first, these changes appeared to be fairly minor. Although Megan had always had a tendency to chew her nails, she seemed to be chewing them more often and more intensely. She also seemed a little more restless and anxious when she went back to her group home on Sundays after home visits.

Over time, things changed for the worse and her family became increasingly worried. They noticed that Megan was chewing her fingers raw. She also seemed to be tense and irritable most of the time, which was very unusual for her. She didn't seem to sleep well and she was driven for food, which had been a sign in the past that she was experiencing stress. Megan had good speech skills, but like many people with DS, she was not good at articulating what was happening to her.

Megan's family suspected that her mood changes stemmed from something that was happening at her group home, as she seemed to be noticeably more anxious before returning on Sundays after a family visit. Her family began asking questions of group home staff and parents of other residents. What they learned alarmed them. The main agency administrator who had managed residential services had recently retired and was replaced by a man who was rubbing many long-time staff the wrong way. In fact, Megan's longstanding case manager and all of the most caring and experienced staff in Megan's house had left or were leaving and were being replaced by new employees.

Megan's family became even more alarmed when one of the departing staff members reported that Megan was being bullied by a newer resident in the house. This staff person told Megan's family that she was quite concerned about what would happen to Megan when she and the other departing staff were no longer there to protect her. Apparently, this newer resident was very angry (for her own personal reasons). She was targeting Megan because she was the most easy-going resident and the least able to defend herself. As the outgoing staff person predicted, the newer staff did not seem to know what was going on, and this left Megan at the mercy of this angry resident. As the attacks increased, so too did Megan's anxiety. She had difficulty sleeping and was driven to eat more and more. She was self-absorbed at home and on the job, and she was doing a great deal of agitated and self-critical self-talk.

Megan's family asked for an emergency meeting with the new case manager and house staff to discuss the situation. The new residential service director also chose to attend the meeting. The meeting did not go well. The new director seemed to view the family as being on the side of the departing staff, which may have influenced his response to the family. He downplayed Megan's problems with the other housemate while insinuating that Megan had a mental health problem. He gave examples of her agitated self-talk as evidence of mental instability and stated that Megan should go to a psychiatrist he had hired as a consultant to the agency. Megan's parents were stunned by this recommendation. They were good advocates for her but they felt intimidated by the new administrator's demands and their lack of legal right to challenge them.

In fact, Megan was her own legal guardian. Her parents had not seen any good reason to become her legal guardians since they had worked so well with the previous residential director. They felt trapped by the new situation but were also very concerned that Megan could be discharged from the agency if they did not work with this new director.

Things did not improve after the meeting. A new staff member took Megan to the consulting psychiatrist. Unfortunately, this staff member had very little experience with or understanding of Megan. Worse, her family—who knew her better than anyone else did—had little input or say in the diagnosis or treatment. Megan was diagnosed and treated with a medication for psychosis, because of her agitated self-talk. This only aggravated her drive for food while also sedating her. Her anxiety did not improve. Her family believed this was because the real cause of her problems, the bullying by her housemate, was not resolved.

Finally, Megan's family demanded a meeting with the residential director, house staff, case manager, behavior specialist working with Megan, and consulting psychiatrist. They found the psychiatrist to be inexperienced with people with DS, but still very reasonable and responsive to their opinions and requests. In addition, several of the house staff who were present at the meeting had been in the house long enough now to have witnessed the angry housemate's attacks on Megan. Therefore, they corroborated the family's statements. As a result of this new information, *the psychiatrist agreed to gradually discontinue Megan's antipsychotic medication. Equally important, the residential director was far more receptive to the family's opinion about the cause of the problem. He took immediate steps to resolve the problem by moving the woman who was targeting Megan to another, more appropriate house.*

Once the angry resident was moved, Megan's anxiety begin to dissipate. As her anxiety decreased and as the medication was discontinued, she was less lethargic and driven to obtain food. Megan's family was relieved by her improvement, but they also had to admit that there were some hard lessons to be learned form this whole experience. They took a close look at what had happened to Megan and decided to begin the process of obtaining guardianship. They believed that this would enable them to better protect Megan if a similar situation ever occurred again.

Working Collaboratively with Agencies

We do not want to sound overly critical of agencies that run residences for adults with disabilities. We have found that most do their level best to serve the health and mental health needs of people with Down syndrome in their care. Unfortunately, they are often hindered by financial constraints imposed on them by state budgets, Medicaid funding, etc. They may also have a difficult time finding trained and experienced staff or outside medical or mental health practitioners who are able to effectively treat people with DS. Still, they try to treat the people with DS in their care and their families with respect and sensitivity.

We have found that many agencies work very collaboratively with families to solve mental health issues of their family members with DS. Yes, there are sometimes conflicts between families and agencies over who controls the definition and treatment of mental health or behavioral problems. Far more often, however, they are two parties with the same goal—to solve problems as soon as possible. We have found too that many agencies listen to families' concerns and appreciate constructive advice about the choice of treatment or providers. These agencies view the open discussion of facts and ideas by family and staff as an essential part of a good treatment plan. Often family members may also help to locate mental health professionals who can provide a second opinion. We have found that many agencies welcome recommendations from health care practitioners, and they may even begin to use these providers to work with others in their care.

RESIDENCES THAT ARE A GOOD FIT FOR ADULTS WITH DOWN SYNDROME

◆ ◆ ◆ ◆ ◆ ◆ ◆ ◆ ◆ ◆ ◆ ◆ ◆ ◆ ◆ ◆ ◆ ◆

In looking at residential options, it may be helpful to consider how the house will fit the person with DS based on characteristics discussed in this and the previous book (*Mental Wellness in Adults with Down Syndrome*). These issues include the tendency of many adults with DS:

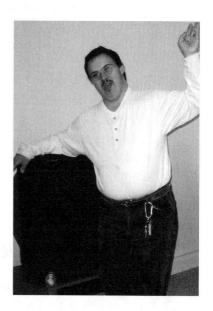

◆ to have grooves,
◆ to be notably sensitive to others,
◆ to have a strong visual memory,
◆ to engage in self-talk, and, sometimes,
◆ to have imaginary friends.

It is also important to consider the need for adequate social and recreational activities. In addition, families will want to consider issues related to providing the appropriate amount of supervision and ensuring that fellow residents are compatible.

GROOVES

As the authors have discussed in previous publications, people with DS tend to follow set patterns and routines that we have called "grooves" (Chapter 9, *Mental Wellness in Adults with Down Syndrome*). In general, grooves are beneficial, giving order and structure to people's lives. Adults with DS tend to be neat and well groomed, to organize and manage their rooms and personal items, to follow through reliably with self-care and work activities, and to have routines that include beneficial activities such as social and recreational programs.

Most families know of these benefits, but many have also experienced some of the drawbacks of grooves. For example, people with DS may be a little too rigid about their routines, and when they are under stress, a groove may become more problematic. Additionally, and perhaps most importantly to this discussion, caregivers need to be patient and accommodating to ensure that grooves are productive.

Not surprisingly, family households or adult residences that are not organized or structured or that are too chaotic may be a poor fit for adults with Down syndrome. Issues such as frequent staff turnover, haphazard changes in schedule and routine, and unkempt or unclean houses can all be especially stressful environments for people with DS. Also, staff who don't know that an adult with DS needs time to process ideas and to shift gears may create enormous stress and unnecessarily precipitate "behavior problems." For example, telling someone with DS to stop what she is doing "NOW" to do some new thing simply doesn't work.

Patience is not only a virtue, but a necessity and it shows respect and understanding for the person with DS. Families know this, after years of living with the person with DS. When looking for an appropriate living situation, it is important to determine whether staff are also aware of the need to allow people with DS to have grooves and routines.

SENSITIVITY TO OTHERS

We have found that many people with DS have excellent "people skills." They are quite often aware of, and sensitive to, other people's feelings. They often reach out to try to help others they sense are in need. On the other hand, this sensitivity may also make people with DS susceptible to the negative feelings and emotions of others in their environment.

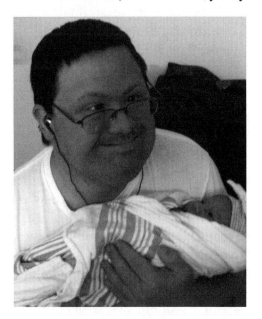

Because of this sensitivity to both positive and negative feelings in the environment, it is important to look for a setting where the adult with DS will be able to feel calm and happy. There are many different types of conflicts in a group residence that may affect someone with DS. There may be conflicts between staff members or between staff and administration, between staff and family members, or conflicts among residents. When looking at a possible residence, it is best to find one with a cheery, less stressful atmosphere, or, at the very least, an environment where there is minimal conflict.

VISUAL MEMORY

Another factor to consider when evaluating the suitability of a group home is whether visual cues are used in organizing the house. Why visual cues? People with DS tend to have strong visual memories. If this strength is capitalized on, it can greatly enhance the person's learning and increase independence. Houses that use visual cues such as writing activities on calendars or posting schedules are more likely to be a good fit for adults with Down syndrome.

On the other hand, most people with DS have difficulties with auditory memory. They tend to have trouble remembering or understanding spoken directions, especially if a long string of instructions is given. Staff who are not aware of this difficulty may believe that a person is oppositional rather than having difficulty understanding or

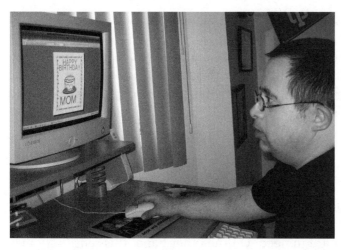

remembering what has been said to her. If staff members primarily give spoken directions, it may increase the likelihood of conflict or tension in the house.

Additionally, visual cues are far more effective at helping people with DS adapt to a change than auditory cues are. Telling people about a change in schedule is simply not as effective as using a visual cue. For example, staff might tell a resident, "We will go shopping before coming home from work tomorrow." When the time comes, however, the person with DS may simply have no idea why she is going shopping rather than going home. This type of misunderstanding often creates a great deal of distress for the person with DS and her caregivers. On the other hand, if we can show the person a calendar or a schedule with a visual representation of the change, she will usually remember this information, and be prepared for the change.

Not surprisingly, calendars and appointment books are very popular among people with DS. They want to be able to predict what will happen to them every day, even if this is the same thing every day. Many staff and families have learned this about people with DS, even though going over the calendar every day may seem redundant, even boring, especially if this means restating the same events every day. Still, when a change is necessary, then the person is far more likely to remember and to deal with this change than if just told that the change will occur.

In sum, a particular residential option is more likely to work for an adult with DS if there is an emphasis on visual learning through the use modeling, observational learning, and supports such as calendars and schedules. If the staff members are not using visual cues but they are willing to learn how to use these types of cues, then this too may bode well for the house.

SELF-TALK AND IMAGINARY FRIENDS

It is fairly common for teens and adults with DS to talk to themselves (self-talk) or have imaginary friends. These habits are often developmentally appropriate, given the intellectual age of people with DS. That is, self-talk and imaginary friends are considered normal in children up until approximately ages five to eight, so these habits are also normal in adults with DS if they have a similar mental age. We do, however, define these behaviors as social skill issues, meaning that self-talk and play with imaginary friends should be conducted in a private space and discouraged in public settings.

Under certain circumstances, self-talk may be an indication of a problem or mental health condition. In particular, self-talk that is predominantly angry or agitated may indicate that the person with DS is experiencing a problem in her day-to-day life. For example, angry or agitated self-talk may occur in adults who are the victims of abuse in a work or residential setting or who have been exposed to tension or conflict in their environment. Agitated or self-critical self-talk may also be a symptom of a mental health problem. If this is the case, there will invariably be other symptoms present as well, such as social withdrawal or a lack of interest in things previously enjoyed.

When considering a possible residence for a family member with DS, consider whether the administrative and direct care staff have experience with, and a normal view of, self-talk and imaginary companions, particularly when there are no indications of agitation, self-criticism, or symptoms of a mental health problem. Even if your adult child with DS does not talk to herself much or at all at this stage, this may change. One reason may be that self-talk is often a means to think out loud and to process new experiences. This may be precisely what an adult with DS needs to do to understand and adapt to a major life change, such as a move from a family home to a group home.

You may be able to avoid a major problem if you determine ahead of time that staff understand when self-talk is normal for an adult with DS. We have actually seen some people who were mistakenly put on medications because staff erroneously believed that self-talk was a sign of mental illness.

OPPORTUNITIES FOR SOCIAL AND RECREATIONAL ACTIVITIES

We cannot overemphasize the need for people with DS to have a regular schedule of social, cultural, and recreational activities. We find that many enjoy going on outings two to four times per week, and at the very least, one time per week. This should

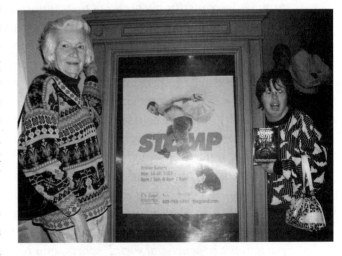

include regular scheduled visits to cultural events, such as concerts, museums, and theaters, as well as to shopping centers and restaurants. Equally important, there should be weekly scheduled participation in sports and recreation programs through a local park or recreation association and/or Special Olympics activities.

Agencies that do not provide these types of programs may simply not care enough about the health and well-being of your son or daughter. Administrators of good group homes will make recreational activities a priority.

APPROPRIATE LEVEL OF SUPERVISION

Agencies that run residences for adults with disabilities have limited budgets. This is often not their fault, but due to state funding issues. Still, it may sometimes be a little too easy for some administrators to under-staff a house as a cost-cutting measure. Many times this may be rationalized as a step that preserves the "rights" of the residents to make their own life decisions. However, for adults with DS and other intellectual disabilities, their chronological age is not the same as their developmental age. They may be thirty years of age but have the reasoning capacity of a nine-year-old.

We have also found that many people with DS have uneven skills. They may be quite mature in certain areas but immature in others. If they are allowed to make choices in areas in which they are immature, this may have a negative effect on their own health and well-being. Here are examples from *Mental Wellness in Adults with Down Syndrome* illustrating how insufficient supervision can lead to health problems for adults with Down syndrome:

Four women with Down syndrome had no supervision after 11:00 at night. They fell into a pattern of staying awake to watch movies and eat junk food until very early in the morning. Despite a high degree of skill in most areas of social and vocational functioning, these women were not able to make a mature decision of when to go to bed. Their behavior led to extreme fatigue in the day time, serious problems on the job, and significant weight gain. Several were showing significant symptoms of depression. The solution was to simply get them the right amount of supervision for their needs. In this situation this meant having a staff member present for 24 hours to ensure that all were going to bed and not staying up late into the morning. With appropriate supervision, all were back on track and doing just fine within three months.

> *Two young men with DS lived in an apartment. Both men and their families were justifiably proud of their ability to manage the household cleaning, shopping, and cooking tasks with only six to eight hours of staff assistance per week (for such tasks as meal planning and money management). Unlike the women mentioned in the above example, these men seemed to be getting adequate sleep and eating healthy meals, and they were very conscientious and reliable in getting to jobs in the community. Over the course of a year, however, both men gained a significant amount of weight.*
>
> *They were both brought to the Adult Down Syndrome Center, and at our suggestion, family and staff took a close look at their daily schedules. They were shocked to find that the two men had almost no activities outside of their apartment. Despite a high degree of independence, they apparently had one major skill deficit. They were not able to schedule and participate in beneficial social, sports, and recreation activities. Instead, they had developed a bad habit of spending all their free time watching TV and movies and playing video games. At our suggestion, family and staff*

actively helped the men arrange a host of activities and transportation to these activities. After they began attending these activities, both began to lose weight and to get back in shape. What is interesting is that both men loved to participate in social and recreation activities. They simply did not have the skill to organize this for themselves despite their other considerable skills.

The key is to support independence at all levels, but to give assistance when needed to allow people to continue to function adaptively and productively in their environments.

Estimating Level of Care Needed for New Residents May Be Difficult

It is not always easy to determine just how much supervision an adult with Down syndrome needs until after she has lived outside the family home for a period of time. One reason is that parents sometimes overestimate just how much care their adult child requires. The person with DS may also underestimate her own abilities.

In a setting where other residents are taking care of their own needs, the adult may rise to the challenge and do what she never knew was possible. In addition, it may be easier for staff to encourage new behavior than for parents or relatives in the family home. This is not just because family members develop expectations of what their children can do, but also because nonrelatives may have more success when teaching someone to do a new task. This is just human nature and is true for anyone, whether or not they have DS. For example, how many parents are surprised to hear from the parents of a friend that their teenage son or daughter is actually able to fry an egg, make their bed, clean up after themselves, etc.? In other words, they can do tasks that they never demonstrated at home. The same may be true for adults with DS who have moved out of the family home.

COMPATIBILITY OF RESIDENTS

One question to consider when looking at a potential residence is who would the adult with DS be living with? Do the other residents seem to be a good fit for the adult with DS? For example, a house with many older adults who are close to retirement may not be a good fit for a young person who has a need for a more active life. The opposite situation can also be problematic, if an older person moves in with young residents who do more than she has the interest, energy, or ability to do.

Despite these generalizations, it is not always easy to predict people's responses to a given situation. For example, some older adults respond to younger residents by becoming more active, which is extremely beneficial for them. Some young people may actually enjoy the slower pace of a house with older individuals. They may enjoy helping others with tasks that require more strength and agility. They may also find that they have more one-on-one time with staff members for outings because other residents are less interested in doing such activities.

It is important not to pigeonhole your son or daughter or micromanage her choice of residences. It may be better to let her try out different living situations rather than to just assume they won't work. Many parents are quite surprised at how flexible and adaptable their adult children are. If an opportunity is not harmful or too limiting, then it may allow the adult to grow and mature by responding flexibly to the new situation.

FAMILY LIVING OPTIONS

We would be remiss if we did not mention that there are viable family living options for adults with Down syndrome. For example:

Laura lived at home with both parents and her younger sister, Molly. Laura's father died when she was in her thirties, but she continued to live with her mother and sister in the house.

When Laura was in her early forties, a number of major life changes affected Laura and her family. First, Laura's mother became ill and physically incapacitated. Molly, who was still living at home, took on the responsibility of caring for both Laura and her mother. During this period, her mother received help with nursing care through a program funded by the state's Department of Aging. Laura did not need any special assistance, and was quite capable of doing her own daily living tasks. She also did some housekeeping chores such as sweeping and cleaning. In addition, she helped care for her mother, especially when the nursing caregivers were not present. Laura was very proud of the help she was able to give to her family. Molly was also very appreciative and pleasantly surprised by her sister's help. Molly was very conscientious about arranging for Laura to continue to go to her work activities and the many recreation and Special Olympics programs she enjoyed. This arrangement seemed to benefit everyone in the household (mother, Molly, and Laura) for many years.

A second major life change for the family occurred when Molly got married. Molly met her fiancé, Bill, while working as a legal assistant in a law firm. Bill was very accepting of Molly's determination to be the caregiver for both her sister and mother. After a big wedding (where there was much dancing and Laura was maid of honor), Bill and Molly moved into a new addition that was built onto Molly's family home. This addition was, in effect, a separate apartment with its own kitchen. Laura and her mother continued to live in the house's original rooms. Then Laura's and Molly's mother passed away. Although this was a painful loss, it did not have a major effect on the living situation in the house. Molly had been Laura's co-guardian, and thus was able to continue in this role after their mother's death.

A third major change in the household occurred when Molly delivered twin girls several years later. This change required some re-thinking because of the new demands on Molly and Bill. Molly and Bill were able to obtain funding for a part-time caregiver for Laura (for approximately twelve hours per week). This caregiver came from an agency serving the needs of adults with disabilities. The caregiver helped Laura with some of the most demanding living tasks (meals and managing her checkbook). But perhaps the greatest assistance was to arrange for Laura to continue to go to her regular recreation and social activities in the evening. This arrangement seemed to work well for Laura and her family, even though there was some turnover in respite staff over time.

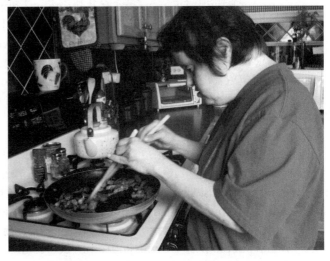

Over the years, Laura and Molly had another important source of support. Their brother and sister, who lived some distance from Laura and Molly's home, also continued to be very actively involved in Molly and Laura's life. These siblings visited several times a year and would stay in the home caring for the twins and visiting with Laura. This enabled Molly and Bill to take care of important business, go out alone, or take vacations without Laura and the twins. Sometimes Laura and Molly visited their brother and sister and stayed in their houses. Laura was also able to visit her brother or sister on her own, which was a real treat for her.

As Molly and Bill's twins grew older, there were new demands on their time and energy, such as attending soccer games, concerts, and school meetings. Still, the arrangement continued to work very well for Laura and Molly. Laura was able to help with childcare and to become very close to her two nieces. With continued opportunities to work and enjoy her community activities, she had a very full life.

LATER LIFE ISSUES FOR ADULTS WHO LIVE AT HOME

As mentioned previously, there are many dimensions to the questions of where and with whom an adult with DS should live. The decisions around these issues become more pressing as parents and the person with DS age. Some adults continue to live with family, but many move on to a group home. Some do so by choice, but others are forced to move to a residence out of necessity.

For people with DS who are still living at home later in life, there is good and bad news. First some of the "bad" news. Adults with Down syndrome age more rapidly than other adults. We find that they often have the health concerns and mental outlook of someone fifteen or twenty years older. Therefore, future planning for people with DS needs to take into consideration an aging process that occurs at a much younger age. (See Chapter 4 in this book and Chapter 10 in *Mental Wellness in Adults with Down Syndrome*.)

Ironically, the fact that people with DS have a premature aging process may give some consolation to families and especially older parents. They may believe that this means they will be more likely to be there for their child with DS throughout the course of their lives. The truth is, however, even with premature aging, we have seen more and more people with DS in their sixties and seventies. And it is not unheard of for people with DS to live into their eighties (Chicoine and McGuire, 1997).

When people with Down syndrome receive the health care they need, they are far more likely to live long, full, and productive lives. This is good news but it also creates a dilemma for many parents and other family members. They have to consider the possibility that their family member with DS may outlive them. This leads to the inevitable question of who will look out for their child when the parent or sibling is gone? This question is not unique to adults with DS. Any time family members or other people are dependent on each other for support and care and these individuals are aging, questions about the continuity of support or care need to be considered very carefully.

A number or studies have shown that there are a large number of people with Down syndrome over the age of 40 who are still living at home with one or both parents (Fujiura, 1998). This is a problem if there is not an adequate plan for the future in place. Without a plan, the adult with DS may face an uncertain future. If an emergency placement has to be found for her after family members pass away, she may end up in a setting that is inappropriate to her needs and also experience great confusion and anguish about the sudden move to a new home. She may also be left with inadequate financial and legal safeguards to ensure the quality of her life. For example, George's parents did not plan adequately for his life without them:

> George lived at home with his parents. His father died when George was in his early thirties, but he and mother continued living together for many years. George had siblings, but they lived far from the family home in another part of the country. They seemed to be very busy with their own lives and did not come to visit often. Like Laura, George had a job and was

initially involved in many sports and recreational activities. Unfortunately, later in life, his mother developed quite a few health problems and was not able to arrange for him to continue to go to his social and recreation programs. George's siblings, unlike Laura's sister, were not willing or able to step in and arrange programs and transportation for him.

When George's mother took a turn for the worse, George even stopped going to work. He was just too worried about his mother and wanted to help her. His mother did begin to receive some in-home nursing care, but these caregivers were only available to help his mother and not George. Gradually, as his mother's condition stabilized, George was able to entertain himself by watching movies and TV and making lists of favorite things, but he never went back to work. This was quite a loss for him because he had had many friends at work and enjoyed doing his job.

Then one day when George was in his late forties, his life changed dramatically. His mother died very abruptly due to complications from a stroke. Although his mother had made some early plans for him to move to a group home, she had not been able to follow through with this process as she became more incapacitated.

After his mother's death, George was moved by the staff of a state agency from his house to an emergency group home. He had great difficulty adjusting to his new residence. Not only was he was dealing with his mother's loss, but he also found the group home to be loud and chaotic. The change from his quiet house to a large and raucous home was just too much for him. George grew very despondent. As time passed, he became more withdrawn and lethargic and he began to refuse to socialize and participate in activities in or outside of the residence.

George was taken to a psychiatrist, who prescribed medication, and he talked to a counselor. He improved somewhat but he was still not very happy or enthusiastic about his life in the emergency group home. Not only was the noise and seeming chaos of the house difficult to deal with, but so was the constant turnover of residents in the house.

After about a year in the emergency placement, George moved to a regular group home that seemed to be far better suited to his needs. This was a stable house with residents who were close to him in age and temperament. This change seemed to give George the boost he needed and he gradually worked his way out of his depression. In time he was back in a workshop, doing his daily living tasks, and he seemed genuinely interested and enthusiastic about his work and social and recreational activities.

If parents are in the position of looking for a group home for an older son or daughter who is still at home, there is some potentially good news for them. Older adults with Down syndrome are often considered a priority by state placement agencies, particularly if the parents are older and/or have their own health issues. This means your child may not have to languish on a waiting list for housing for long. However, many families of older individuals with DS seem to have a negative view of residential options in the community. This is often because they remember the large institutions that used to exist, as well as their negative reputations. It is vitally important that families visit current placements before deciding that a particular option is or is not the right place for an older adult child with Down syndrome.

GETTING INFORMATION OR SUPPORT WHEN CONSIDERING A RESIDENTIAL OPTION

Many families of older individuals may have lost connection with parent associations and other support or advocacy groups in the community. They may have stopped participating in these support group activities once their children entered school and the demands on the family and the child increased. They may also have believed that

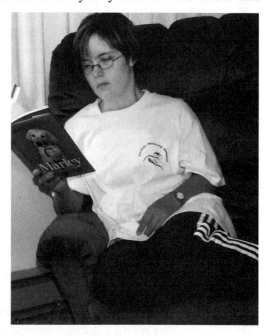

support groups were only relevant to the needs of families with younger children. Unfortunately, without support from a group or from some other helpful source, the process of applying for residential service may seem overwhelming.

There is help available. Often the best step is to reconnect with the local parent association or support group. Families who have strayed from participation, for whatever reason, may be very surprised by the current composition of these groups. Although the majority of participants are still families of younger children, there are also many more families with older sons and daughters. As the population of parents and children with DS has aged and changed, so to has the composition of these groups.

There are enormous benefits for families of older individuals in reconnecting with a group. Members exchange valuable information that is often learned from their own experiences. This may include key information about the best agencies to contact, which professionals are the most helpful, or even which staff are best able to break the process down into manageable steps. This type of information and support from the group may be just what a family needs to proceed with the residential process.

Other potential sources of help and information are the local or national ARC groups, as well as the National Down Syndrome Society and the National Down Syndrome Congress. There are listings of local support groups and some information for families of older individuals on the websites for these associations. Resources are also available through university affiliated programs such as the Rehabilitation Research and

Training Center (RRTC) on Aging with Disabilities. There are a number of these programs in different parts of the country such as the Institute on Disability and Human Development at the University of Illinois at Chicago. You can find this and other programs on the Internet through this link: www.uic.edu/orgs/rrtcamr/clearinghouse.htm.

FUTURE PLANNING FOR OLDER ADULTS WITH DOWN SYNDROME

Previously we discussed how characteristics of teens and young adults with DS may affect their adjustment to a residential setting. Not surprisingly, these same characteristics may also affect the adjustment process for older adults. In our experience, the tendency to follow "grooves" and to be sensitive to others are most likely to complicate the process.

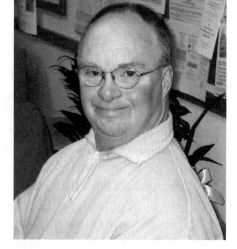

As they grow older, many people—with and without Down syndrome—become more set in their ways. If someone already has groove-like tendencies, this resistance to change can be even more apparent. For older people with DS, it can be extremely difficult to make a major change such as moving out of their home (after 40 or more years) into a group home.

We have definitely seen older adults experience problems in making the transition to a new home. Adjustment can be especially difficult if, like George, the person is forced out of his or her home due to an abrupt change, such as the death of a parent. When the change occurs in a more normal fashion, and not due to an unexpected life event, most people with DS do surprisingly well in adapting. In fact, many older adults with DS seem to become more energized when they move out of the family home. Residential staff often report that they are excited by their new opportunities to be with peers and to go on outings such as to restaurants, movies, shopping centers, dances, social gatherings, and other cultural events. This may be more likely to happen if the person has been living with older, more sedentary parents.

Bianca's story, below, illustrates how an adult with DS who moves to a home with more active residents can get caught up in the excitement and discovery that may have been missing in his or her own family home:

> *As Bianca entered her forties, her parents began to worry about where she would live if either or both of them died or became incapacitated. They started to gather information about local agencies that ran group homes for adults with developmental disabilities. After Bianca's father had a mild*

heart attack, their concern deepened. After his recovery, they moved fairly quickly to contact the right agencies to get the process moving. Fortunately, they received good advice from Margaret, an experienced case manager in a local agency, who assisted them with getting state funding and finding a suitable home. With Margaret's help, they located an opening in a four-person group home.

To prepare her for the move, Bianca had numerous overnight visits to the home. She seemed to be very comfortable with the physical layout and with the other residents. Fortunately, the administrators in this agency were very open to any questions or concerns her parents had for her care, including medical care. They would allow her to continue seeing her primary physician as well as the clinical social worker she had been seeing for help with the anxiety she had experienced after her father's heart attack.

Bianca moved into the group home at the age of 42. Once in her new home, she was delighted to discover how many outside activities were scheduled for members of the house. It had been difficult for her parents to take her to activities recently, especially during her father's recovery. The three other women were various ages, but they all were quite active. They participated weekly in sports and recreational activities through the local special recreation association and a local chapter of Special Olympics. Bianca also began going to a workshop with the other residents. She was happy that there was far more work available and more opportunities for art and craft activities than at her former workshop.

After she moved into the home, Bianca continued to see her family often. Her parents visited her in her new home regularly and she visited her parents in their home at least one weekend a month. Bianca's parents were already her legal guardians, but they added her brother and his wife as co-guardians. Both had a very good relationship with Bianca and they had been very actively involved in her life.

Recently, Bianca's father died and her mother moved into an assisted living setting. Although Bianca was quite sad about her father's death, she continues to visit with her mother at least once a week, which is important to her. She also sees her brother and sister-in-law for monthly visits and holidays, and seems confident that they will continue to be there for her.

As of this writing, Bianca has been in her group home for five years. She had a very smooth transition with just a few minor bumps in the road. For now, she seems very comfortable with her residence and her family support There is no reason to believe this will not continue into the future.

WHEN FAMILY MEMBERS HAVE TROUBLE LETTING GO OF EACH OTHER

• • • • • • • • • • • • • • • • • •

Sometimes when an older adult moves out of her family home, it is far more difficult for the parents and other family members to adapt to change than it is for the person with DS. There are many reasons for this. Perhaps the parent has benefitted from her child's companionship or from her help or assistance. Some parents may find it hard to imagine life without their child in their day-to-day lives.

We find, however, that once family members see that their son or daughter (or brother or sister) is happy, they are more at peace with their decision. It is interesting to note, too, that many staff report that adults with Down syndrome who have recently moved into a group home reserve their sad looks and words of discontent for times when their parents are visiting.

This bring us to another important issue, related to the fact that many people with DS have an exceptional sensitivity to other human beings, especially family and friends. If there is any concern that a parent is in pain, discomfort, or ill health, or is lonely or feeling some type of emotional pain, then it may be very difficult for the person with DS to move out of the family home. We have seen this issue resolved in a variety of ways. Some adults with DS were able to move on when they were convinced that their parent had the care he or she needed—such as from a live-in caregiver or from staff in an assisted living home. In other cases, we have seen parents simply convince their adult child that they were perfectly fine and that it was time for the child to move on. When the adult with DS is reluctant to move out because of concerns about parents, it usually helps to ensure that the person with DS will continue to see her parents regularly.

ADVICE FOR PARENTS ON LETTING GO

What advice can we give to parents who are having trouble letting their children go? First, know that you are not alone in this. So many families struggle with these issues, and you may be able to gain support and encouragement, and to learn strategies for dealing with these issues, from other parents. No on knows what you feel or are experiencing quite like someone who has been in the same situation.

To find parents who have been there, we recommend reconnecting with your local parent organization (ARC chapter or Down syndrome support group). Sometimes these groups have support groups specifically dealing with these issues. If not, you may be able to start such a group. There will be plenty of parents who are interested.

It may also be possible to meet with other families who have family members living in the same group home or with the same agency as your son or daughter. This can happen through gatherings arranged by parents or staff at the group home. For example, many group homes regularly schedule cookouts or holiday parties which include parents and other family members. You may also meet other families by joining fundraiser groups or advisory boards for the agency. By joining such groups you may help to oversee the agency's policies or help to promote its financial solvency while also meeting with others who have similar issues as you and your family member with DS.

Some parents who are having trouble letting go may also benefit from counseling with a psychologist, social worker, or other trained counselor. You may want to look for a counselor who has experience working with people with DS and their families, but it may not be necessary. There are many counselors who are trained to deal with such issues as loss, separation, and leaving home, because these issues are universal, whether or not the family member who is leaving has DS. These counselors may not know about the specific process and procedures needed to obtain residential service or about available group homes. This information may still need to be obtained from agencies and other knowledgeable sources, but these counselors will often know how to help with the emotional issues related to change and loss. Additionally, many counselors deal with issues related to aging—of parents and their adult children alike.

Finally, national and local conferences are often a good place to meet other families facing similar issues as you. Not surprisingly, these parents will often attend workshops that address teen, adult, or aging issues. You may need to speak up and ask those attending if they share your concerns and issues. Trust us on this—there are plenty of parents who will want to talk about these issues. At the very least, you can exchange names and numbers to contact one another by email or phone until the next meeting or conference.

PASSING THE TORCH TO AN APPROPRIATE ADVOCATE

◆ ◆ ◆ ◆ ◆ ◆ ◆ ◆ ◆ ◆ ◆ ◆ ◆ ◆ ◆ ◆ ◆

Even if the person with DS is very good at advocating for herself, it is still very important to have others who are supporting her and looking out for her well-being. This is true for all of us, not just for people with Down syndrome—particularly as

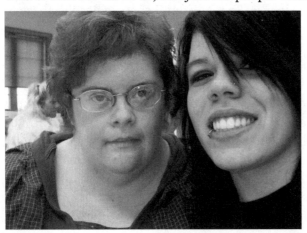

we age. There is, after all, no way to predict how we or our friends and family who support us will fare as we get older.

To help the adult with DS to prepare for the possible loss of key family caregivers, we feel it is important to arrange for at least one and preferably two people to be able to step in as advocates for the person with DS. This will ensure that support continues even if the parents or other family members are gone or unable to serve in this role. Having two advocates increases the chances that at least one person will be available at any given time.

Who to Pick as Advocates?

The people you ask to serve as advocates should truly know the person with DS and have her best interests at heart. This may be a sibling, cousin, another relative, or even a long-time family friend. This person also has to have the right set of circumstances to be able to manage the task. This is a little tricky because you do not want to enlist people for a task that may be difficult for them for whatever reason. This would not be good for the person drafted into the role of advocate and it would certainly not be good for the person with DS. Remember that people with DS tend to be very sensitive to the people in their lives and they may sense that this person is stressed, encumbered, or resentful of this role.

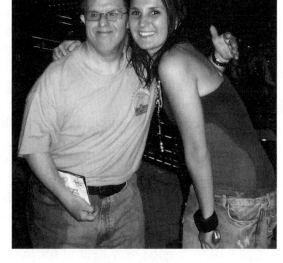

One key issue here is to give the right type of responsibility to the right type of person. This means you need to narrow down what types of support the adult with DS may need. Will she just need an advocate? Or will caretaking responsibility be involved as well?

The distinction between an advocate and a caregiver is very important. Caregivers usually live with the person with DS under the same roof and they are responsible for the person's care. Of course, the level of care varies greatly, depending on the person's needs and level of skills. Still, there are significant responsibilities even when the adult with DS is able to manage many of her own living, vocational, and transportation tasks.

We have seen many siblings, cousins, and close family friends act as the primary caregivers for the person with DS, and for the most part they do this task extremely well. The story of Laura and her sister Molly offers a good example of a family member who chose to be a caregiver and succeeded admirably. The key reason for the success of Molly and other caregivers is that they have freely chosen to do this task and it fits their particular needs, skills, and personality. Most people who are caregivers are also quite adept as advocates. After all, who knows the person's needs, strengths, and limitations better than a caregiver?

Still, this caregiver role is by no means for everyone or even a necessity. In fact, a large percentage of adults with DS live in group home settings, and thus even their parents do not have primary caretaking responsibilities for them. If the role of caretaker is taken over by staff in a residential facility, then the role of advocate is still extremely important to the well-being of the adult with Down syndrome.

THE ADVOCATE'S ROLE

What is the advocate's role? Parents state that the advocate should be like a parent in terms of his or her devotion to and interest in the person with DS. Therefore, it may be helpful to describe what we see from parents who are good advocates, since these would be the same attributes to look for in the ideal advocate.

First and foremost, an advocate needs to care deeply about the person with DS. This often translates into time spent with her. If the person with DS lives in a community residence, the person may make regular scheduled overnight visits and attend holiday celebrations and other family or relevant gatherings.

Second, the advocate must be knowledgeable about the skills, resources, and deficits of the adult with Down syndrome. In other words, he or she should be well aware of the person's strengths and weaknesses. Moreover, she needs to be well informed about the person's history—to include her education, job training and experience, health care history, and any behavioral problems or medical and mental health issues. Some parents educate the advocate and prepare her for the job by putting together a book with all relevant historical and current information on education, vocational, health, and social history. It may also be advantageous to make a book for the person with DS herself about her own care needs. We have used such books at the Adult Down Syndrome Center and find that they are very helpful in having people take an active role in their own health care.

Third, it may be very helpful for the advocate to be informed about the latest research and clinical findings about people with DS. She should be very interested in obtaining new or useful information that can help her advocate for the person with DS. Parents and other family members can also help to meet this need. They may be able to acquaint the advocate with major DS organizations, such as the National Down Syndrome Congress, the National Down Syndrome Society, or the National Association for Down Syndrome, where they can obtain up-to-date information and also meet other advocates online or through conferences offered by these groups. Local DS and ARC organizations can also provide information on important local resources and agencies serving people with DS and other types of disabilities. Many local organizations have meetings and conferences and these conferences can be very informative and a good way to meet other advocates. You can find contact information for many useful local and national groups at www.ds-health.com.

Fourth, this person needs to be available to advocate for the needs and rights of the adult with DS at all relevant meetings at her home or worksite. Again, having two advocates may enable your chosen advocates to manage this task more effectively.

Finally, it is essential to consider whether the advocate should obtain legal guardianship. If, in fact, she is truly going to advocate in the best interest of the person with DS, then this should definitely be a part of the advocate's role—provided the person's family has determined that she needs a guardian. We have found that many people who are planning to assume the role of advocate share legal guardianship with parents or other family members so that there is a clear transition to the advocate in case something unexpected happens to the parents.

CONCLUSION

In summary, how and when an adult with Down syndrome approaches the process of leaving home can have an effect on physical and emotional health. When the process is begun earlier, the adult with DS and her family may have far more time to adjust to a change in living situation. Just as importantly, they may have far more choices of residential settings and a much greater chance of a positive outcome than if the transition is left to nonfamily members to manage.

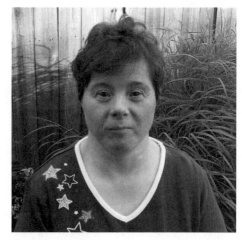

On the other hand, we don't want to discourage families of older individuals who are still living at home. It is never too late to begin the process of helping an adult with DS transition out of the family home, especially if you still want to have some influence on this process. Also, as mentioned above, there may be some advantages to starting late. Placement agencies may waste less time in finding a home for older individuals, especially if parents are elderly. Parents may also be able to get more help for their own needs through the agencies serving the needs of aging individuals. In general, however, even if there is no pressing need for the adult with DS to move from the family home any time soon, it is best to at least contact appropriate agencies and make some type of plan for helping the adult with DS make the transition to a new home.

Chapter 23

Advance Directives

· · · · · · · · · · · ·

"Put him in an institution. Go home and never look back. Tell your family and friends he died at birth." This was the advice that Sean's parents had been given when Sean was born. His sister, Lisa, had heard this story from Sean's parents when they were still living.

Lisa was now Sean's legal guardian. Sean was dying from advanced Alzheimer disease. He had developed severe swallowing problems, had been hospitalized several times in recent months, and was presently again in the hospital on intravenous antibiotics for pneumonia.

Sean was not responding well to treatment this time. Another swallowing evaluation demonstrated that he had now lost his ability to swallow. He was aspirating almost everything he ate or drank, as well as his own saliva, into his lungs. These swallowing problems were the cause of his pneumonia.

Lisa met with Sean's physician to discuss her brother's condition. The physician explained Sean's recurrent pneumonia and swallowing problem. He explained that a feeding tube (gastrostomy tube) could be surgically placed in Sean's stomach through his abdominal wall. Sean would then receive all this nutrition through the feeding tube. Unfortunately, Sean would likely continue to aspirate and develop pneumonia despite the feeding tube. This was because he would continue to aspirate his own saliva, which contained bacteria.

Lisa was saddened by her brother's decline. He no longer recognized her, had lost his ability to speak, and was no longer able to walk. Each hospitalization was uncomfortable for Sean. The blood tests, catheters, and even just the transportation to and from the hospital were challenging for him.

Sean's physician discussed advance directives with Lisa and asked her what the goals of treatment were for her brother. She understood that Sean's condition was incurable and that he would continue to require regular and frequent treatment for pneumonia. The month before, Sean had had a very severe episode of pneumonia and had required intubation (a breathing tube) and a ventilator to help him breathe. "We almost lost him that time," Lisa said while silently wondering if perhaps it would have been a blessing for Sean to have died so he would no longer have to endure the discomfort associated with treatment. On the other hand, she kept thinking about what her parents had been told when Sean was born. Her parents had felt completely abandoned by the medical community. They had felt a real sense that Sean's life was judged to be less important and that he didn't deserve to live; that his living was just a burden.

Lisa clearly remembered what Sean had been like before he had declined so badly from his Alzheimer disease. She said to Sean's physician, "He is such a gift. Are you only offering comfort measures because his life is judged to be less valuable—just like it was so many years ago?" The doctor said no.

Lisa's question helped clarify the discussion regarding Sean's terminal condition. The doctor explained that medical care simply could not prevent Sean's continued decline and recurrent hospitalization and that comfort care did not mean there would be no care and compassion for Sean. Although the focus would no longer be on trying to prevent his inevitable death, efforts would be made to optimize Sean's comfort.

After discussions with her family, with the ethics team at the hospital, and with her parish priest, Lisa decided that she wanted to sign DNR (do not resuscitate) paperwork for Sean. In the event his heart stopped, she requested that it not be restarted (by electrical shock) and that he not receive CPR (chest compressions and assisted breathing). If his respiratory (breathing) status declined again, she requested that he not be placed on a ventilator. She also requested that Sean not receive cardioversion (shocking his heart) or medications if his heart rhythm were to become abnormal, or medication to raise his blood pressure if it dropped. She also decided against having a feeding tube inserted, and, after this hospitalization, she requested that Sean no longer be given antibiotics or be hospitalized, but that he remain at home receiving comfort care. The local hospice agency was consulted and they met with Lisa and helped her obtain support at home to keep her brother comfortable. Lisa's friends, family, and members of her church also supported her and Sean.

Sean completed the treatment for his pneumonia and then returned home. His condition continued to decline, and two weeks later, he developed pneumonia again. A few days later, with Lisa and other family and friends at his side, Sean died comfortably in his home.

ADVANCE DIRECTIVES

Advance directives are guidelines for the ongoing and future care of an individual. Most commonly this information guides treatment decisions in the event of a terminal illness. Generally, it is recommended that everyone think about how they would like to be treated if they become ill. Sharing those desires with others is important so that if the person becomes too ill to make his wishes known, someone else can provide this information. Formalizing these decisions by putting them on paper is recommended.

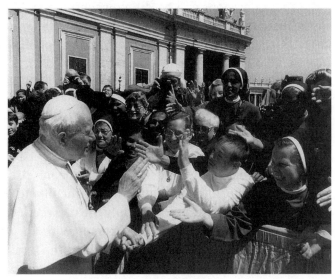

To help in making these decisions about future medical treatment, there is a great deal of information available from physicians, hospitals, health departments, and websites. Often it is the families who are left to make these decisions about the future care of their adult children with Down syndrome (DS). Although many adults with DS can certainly contribute to the discussion about their own future care, the majority will not know how to initiate writing, or realize the importance of having, an advance directive. (See "Including the Person with DS in the Decision," below.)

Advance directive decisions can cover many aspects of care:

- ◆ use of certain medications (including antibiotics),
- ◆ use of feeding tubes,
- ◆ use of intravenous fluids and intravenous medications,
- ◆ hospitalization, and
- ◆ resuscitation in the event of a cardiac or respiratory arrest.

The decision may be fluid over time. A decision to include a treatment in the advance directive may be changed at a later time if the person's health improves or deteriorates.

Laws about advance directives vary from state to state. The specific paperwork that needs to be completed, therefore, varies from state to state. In some states, like Illinois, health care providers such as paramedics, physicians, or nurses cannot follow a "Do Not Resuscitate" order unless it is written on a specific form with appropriate signatures and the signatures of witnesses. Sometimes there are also specific rules regarding decisions when the person himself is not able to make the decision.

Advance directives can be an important aspect of health care. As in Sean's case, in certain situations and at certain times in an illness, limiting certain types of care and focusing on other aspects of care (e.g., comfort measures) may be appropriate. There are medical considerations as well considerations based on personal preferences. It is important to discuss these issues with the health care providers. Generally, it is helpful to consider these decisions before they really need to be acted upon. It can be stressful to consider these decisions for the first time in an emergency room when a quick decision is needed.

These decisions can be difficult for anyone. Many factors are considered in the decision: personal beliefs, religious tradition, previous experiences, and issues related to the particular illness that the person has. For a person with DS, there may be some additional considerations:

- ◆ The person may not be able to participate in the decision process.
- ◆ The person may have a legal guardian.
- ◆ There may be a heightened sense of responsibility in making the decision for someone else. It can be very challenging to make these life or death decisions for oneself, but may be even more challenging if you are making the decision for someone else. Judging someone else's suffering and his goals can be difficult and there may be nagging doubts as to whether it was truly the correct decision.
- ◆ When the parents of a person with DS die, a strong sense of responsibility is usually transferred to the family member or friend who as-

The "Out-of-Towner" Situation

When an individual is making a decision about advance directives for someone else, we generally recommend that he discuss the decision with other family members. This provides the decision-maker with support for his decision, shares the sense of responsibility of making this important decision, and helps avoid conflict later if all the family members don't agree with the course taken. Even if the person making the decision is the legal guardian, and technically does not have to consult the rest of the family, it's often a good idea to discuss the decision, or at least inform family members of the decision.

Involving family members in this way can help avoid what we call the "Out-of-Towner" situation. In this situation, the person making the decision is generally the primary caregiver and is often the legal guardian. The scenario is usually that the adult with DS has developed a terminal disease and the primary caregiver has decided that the goal of care will shift from striving to prolong the person's life or cure the illness to providing comfort care. At that time, someone else, usually another family member, may get involved and disagree with the decision or place a heavy emotional burden on the decision-maker.

We call this the "Out-of-Towner" situation because the person who swoops in at this time is often from out of town. This is not to say that all out-of-town family members behave this way, or that it can't occur with a family member

sumes care or guardianship responsibilities. Sometimes specific instructions are also passed along, although they often don't cover all possible future scenarios. For example, in Sean's situation above, if his parents had specifically stated that Lisa should never allow the medical community to abandon her brother, she may have never been able to see comfort measures as anything other than abandonment.

◆ Sometimes a sibling is taking care of aging parents while also taking care of his or her sibling with DS. Because of the early aging issues of people with DS, at times a person with DS may develop medical conditions (associated with advancing age) at the same time as his parents. If the parents' health declines to the point that they are no longer able to care for their own needs, let alone the needs of the person with DS, the sibling of the person with DS may find himself caring for all of them. Caring for multiple people can overwhelm a caregiver and make it harder to make a decision regarding advance directives. Caregivers in this situation may require additional support to cope with the stress. As in Sean's case, support can come from the patient's physician, family and friends, the ethics team at the hospital, a priest, rabbi, minister, imam, or other religious person, or a hospice.

who lives locally. However, the person who disagrees with the decision has usually had little participation in caring for the person with DS and often has not been around to experience his pain and suffering.

Sometimes the person disagrees with the decision because he lacks information or experience with the illness that the adult with DS has. Usually, including the out-of-towner in the discussion or explaining the condition will improve the situation. Other times, this person may feel guilty because he was not involved in caring for the adult with DS and this is his last chance to demonstrate his concern, even if it may not be appropriate in this situation. This issue may be more difficult to address, particularly because the motivation is often not overtly admitted or addressed. However, discussion and education about the health and prognosis of the adult with DS will usually help the family to come to an agreement.

Sometimes the person who enters the decision-making process relatively late may actually provide insights that were not previously known or considered by the decision-maker. For example, a personal philosophy, religious tradition, or another reason may persuade family members to forge ahead, hoping for a cure, even in the face of an illness for which there is no medical solution. Or the person who comes into the picture at a later time may know more about the parents' desires than the decision-maker does.

INCLUDING THE PERSON WITH DOWN SYNDROME IN THE DECISION

◆ ◆ ◆ ◆ ◆ ◆ ◆ ◆ ◆ ◆ ◆ ◆ ◆ ◆ ◆ ◆ ◆

Everyone has the right to participate in decisions about his own life, including his own health care. In the United States, except for a few exceptions, this legal right is attained when the person reaches the legal age of adulthood, age 18 years. At this time, the exceptions are: Alabama and Nebraska (age 19) and Mississippi (age 21). This

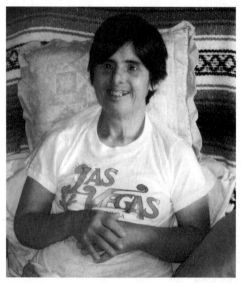

right can be removed if a person is declared legally incompetent and a legal guardian is appointed. This process requires a court appearance before a judge.

Many parents assume that because their son or daughter has DS, they are the legal guardians for him or her even after he or she reaches the age of majority set by their state. This is not true. No matter what the person's condition, his parents are no longer his legal guardians when he reaches the age of majority unless the judge/court system makes the declaration of incompetence and appoints the parent(s) as legal guardian. (In a few states, a person is not considered to have reached the age of majority until he

graduates from high school, whether or not he has reached the usual age of majority.)

An adult with DS who is his own legal guardian generally has the legal right to make the decision regarding advance directives. In some cases, however, a surrogate can be used (see box). Someone who has medical power of attorney over the person with DS can also make decisions about advance directives and other health care issues. If the person with DS has a guardian or has given medical power of attorney to someone else, it is respectful to include him in the decision even if there is no legal obligation to do so.

Including an adult with DS in the decision-making process can be challenging. Although concrete thinking serves people with DS well in daily life, most people have some limitations in their ability to think in the abstract. Death and dying are concepts humankind has tried to understand for centuries. They can be very challenging for people of all levels of intelligence.

In addition, many people with DS have trouble understanding the concept of time. They can get confused when discussing their eventual death as a future event. They can become quite anxious, thinking that their death is imminent. Particularly if a person has Alzheimer disease, he will no longer be able to understand the concepts involved in this decision or be able participate in the decision.

Sometimes it can be beneficial to take advantage of the person's concrete thinking. For example, parents might begin a matter-of-fact discussion about the fact that everyone in the family is going to do an advance directive and ask whether the adult with DS would like to do one, too.

What Happens When There Is No Advance Directive?

What happens if you are very ill, cannot make health decisions for yourself, and do not have an advance directive?

The law varies from state to state. In some states, a health care "surrogate" may be chosen for you if you cannot make health care decisions for yourself and do not have an advance directive. For example, in Illinois, the health care surrogate appointed will be one of the following individuals (in order of priority): guardian of the person, spouse, any adult child(ren), either parent, any adult brother or sister, any adult grandchild(ren), a close friend, or guardian of the estate. The surrogate can make health care decisions for you. In Illinois, a health care surrogate cannot tell your doctor to withdraw or withhold life-sustaining treatment unless you have a "qualifying condition." These conditions are:

◆ a terminal condition,
◆ permanent unconsciousness, or
◆ an incurable or irreversible condition.

If your place of residence doesn't have a health care surrogate law, it is probably safest just to have an advance directive/living will drawn up. You may also wish to consult with an attorney to review the local law.

TALKING TO THE PERSON WITH DOWN SYNDROME ABOUT DEATH

* * * * * * * * * * * * * * * * *

Zeke, a 34-year-old man with DS, struggled with the concept of death. His difficulties began when his parents met with their attorney to modify their will. At the same time, they decided to purchase their own cemetery plots. They also bought a plot for Zeke so that he could be buried next to them. When Zeke heard about this, he became very depressed. He was absolutely convinced that he had a serious illness that his parents and doctor were not telling him about. Despite reassurances from his parents and physician that he was in excellent health, Zeke could not shake his concern that he was going to die in the near future. He was treated with an antidepressant, and, over several months, was able to move on with his life to some degree. It was clear, however, that he still worried about dying because he periodically mentioned his concern.

Sylvia, a 37-year-old woman with DS, had severe cyanotic congenital heart disease. She was born before heart surgery was available for people with Down syndrome and she was now in the end stages of her disease. As her health declined, Sylvia became depressed, anxious, and less and less interested in doing any activities. She began to see someone who was not there, which was very frightening to her. Initially, it appeared she was becoming psychotic. However, over time she was able to talk more about her anxiety and the person she was seeing. It became clear that she had personified death. Her parents suspected that she may have developed this concept from watching a TV program. This person was imaginary, but in contrast to the more usual imaginary friend (see Chapter 1), this was more of an imaginary enemy.

Seeing death as a person was Sylvia's way to try to understand her ill health and her impending death. These images were so frightening and paralyzing for her that risperdone (Risperdal), an anti-psychotic medication, was used to help reduce the impact on her. She was never able to verbally express her concerns about dying, but she did seem more psychologically comfortable on the medication. She subsequently succumbed to her cardiac condition.

The two examples above illustrate some of the pitfalls that can be encountered when helping a person with DS understand death. When discussing death, it usually helps to use simple terms. In addition, we recommend avoiding ambiguous terms like "falling asleep." This can cause confusion and fear of life's daily events.

Many people with DS will perseverate about things they find stressful or anxiety-provoking. Perseveration can cause significant impairment and prevent the person from thinking about or participating in the activities of his life. To reduce the anxiety and stress, we suggest:

- ◆ respectfully acknowledging the person's concerns,
- ◆ expressing empathy and compassion, and
- ◆ gently redirecting him to a different topic.

Religious tradition, personal and family philosophy, or other beliefs may help a person with DS come to grips with death. Particularly if he has known others who have died and has a positive sense of that experience, these views of death can be comforting. Joe told us, "I was with my Aunt Jenny when she died and I know that she is in heaven. When I die, I will be in heaven with her and I know that Mom and Dad will join me some day."

If a person with DS is able to understand and talk about his own death, like Joe, this can be very comforting. He and his family can support each other, allay previously unspoken fears, and develop a better understanding of what death means to them.

In helping the person better understand the concept of death, care must be taken to avoid removing hope and enjoyment of life. People who understand they are going to die often state that this knowledge gives them the freedom to "enjoy the time I have left." However, sometimes knowledge of impending death prevents the person from enjoying his remaining days. Telling someone about his own imminent death may actually be harmful if the person is unable to understand death, or if he would become obsessed with the knowledge to the point where he was unable to participate in other activities, or if he would become overwhelmed with fear or anxiety. In these situations, the knowledge may crush the individual's hopeful enjoyment of his remaining days.

If the person knows he is dying and understands what that means, it should be helpful to help him get his affairs in order. For example, help him to decide who will get his belongings, to see or communicate with people he cares about, and to talk through issues in an advance directive.

It can be a problem when people around the person won't talk to him about his impending death because they want to protect him or think he can't deal with the truth when in reality he truly needs to talk and ask questions about what is happening. Sometimes parents or others even deny that the person is dying if he asks whether he is. Refusing to address the truth can be just as problematic as giving someone too much information or letting him obsess about his impending death.

It can be challenging to predict how someone will respond to discussions about death. You can probably get a sense of his likely response by considering:

◆ his previous response(s) to very stressful situations;
◆ his previous comments about death;
◆ his previous experiences with the death of others;
◆ his present health condition and how he is managing the stress of the illness and other stresses in his life.

As is true for everyone, regular exposure to death as a natural part of life can help an adult with DS deal with these issues. You can help the person develop an understanding of death over time by having him attend wakes and funerals, sharing your feelings and encouraging him to share his, and discussing your own and others' beliefs about death.

Another factor that must be weighed when deciding whether to tell a person with DS about his impending death is the wishes of the guardian or parents. If the adult with DS is his own guardian, he should have been informed of his health condition from the start. He also has the right to decide who should be told about his condition. He can give permission to his physician and family or care provider to participate in the decision-making processes. As his illness progresses, he may become unable to participate in the decision-making process. The family will then be consulted to help make decisions for the person with DS. If the person with DS has a legal guardian, the physician will work with the guardian to determine what information is provided to the person with DS.

For some people with DS, their guardian is the state. In Illinois, for example, the Office of State Guardian (OSG) provides this service for people who need a guardian and do not have family or friends who are willing and able to provide guardianship.

Working with OSG is similar to working with a family member or friend who is guardian. However, the information must be written on specific forms. An OSG attorney reviews the information as part of a more formal review process.

GETTING HELP WITH THE DECISION ABOUT ADVANCE DIRECTIVES

In addition to reading written information about advance directives, you may find it very beneficial to consult with a counselor from the hospital Ethics department. While some families feel they have enough information to decide whether to develop an advance directive and what measures to include in it after discussions with the health care provider and the person with DS, the Ethics counselor can provide additional insight. He or she can help the family and/or person with DS define their goals of treatment and figure out whether the decision is appropriate.

The decision about advance directives is not an easy one. The implications are clearly potentially life-altering for the person who is ill. However, the implications will often extend far beyond the death of the person. Family and guardians may sometimes revisit their decision and have second thoughts about its appropriateness. Carefully reviewing goals, values, and the implications and prognosis of the condition are paramount not only for making the decision but also when survivors reflect back on their decision. Often people second-guess themselves and ask whether they did the right thing. Taking the time to carefully reflect upon all issues can help to reassure you that your decision was appropriate.

HOSPICE CARE

Hospice care is end-of-life care provided by health professionals and volunteers. These hospice workers provide medical, psychological, and spiritual support when someone has been diagnosed with a terminal illness. Under hospice care, the primary goal becomes making the person as comfortable as possible, rather than prolonging his life.

Hospice care can be provided in a variety of settings:
   ◆ at home,
   ◆ at a hospice center,
   ◆ in a hospital, or
   ◆ in a skilled nursing facility (e.g., a nursing home).

Hospice care is usually covered by Medicare, Medicaid, and most private insurances. To qualify for hospice care under Medicare, the life expectancy of the person has to be six months or less.

We have had wonderful success with our hospice providers in caring for our patients with DS. The physical, psychological, and spiritual assistance of the hospice care providers can give the individual with DS a great deal of comfort. This comforting care is extended to the family through psychological and spiritual support. This support for family members and care providers can continue after the death of the patient.

If the adult with DS has an advance directive, it can spell out the circumstances under which he would like to receive hospice care. For example, an advance directive might specify that the person will begin hospice care if he is diagnosed with a terminal condition. Even if a family has not decided on advance directives or hospice care, a hospice consult can be of benefit. The hospice staff can explain their philosophy regarding hospice care, their services, and assist the patient and family in the decision-making process.

Addendum 1: Drinking More Fluids

Name: _____ Date:_____

We recommend you drink more fluids. We recommend you drink at least 6 to 8 cups (cup = 8 ounces or 240 ml) of fluid per day. You will need to keep track of everything you drink to make sure you are getting this amount.

All drinks (beverages) are considered fluids. These include the following:

Common Beverages (Fluids)

Water	Coffee
Tea	Fruit drinks
Carbonated beverages Coke, 7-Up, etc.	Soups
Milk	Fruit juices

There are also some fluids that are not drinks. Any food that begins as a liquid is counted as a fluid. These include the following:

Foods That Count As Fluids

Ice	Ice cream
Ice milk	Sherbet
Popsicles	Gelatin
Italian ice	

It is best to drink or eat fluids that don't have any calories—especially water. This will help you avoid gaining weight.

Measuring Fluids

Every day you need to drink at least 48 to 64 ounces (or about 2 liters) of fluid. This is the same as 6 to 8 cups of fluid.

There are three ways to make sure you are drinking enough fluids:

- ◆ **Method #1:** Add up how many *ounces (oz.)* of fluids you drink or eat every day. If the total is 64 oz. or more, you are drinking enough.

- ◆ **Method #2:** Add up how many *milliliters (ml)* of fluids you drink or eat every day. If the total is 2000 ml (2 liters) or more, you are drinking enough.

◆ **Method #3:** Add up how many *cups* of fluid you drink or eat every day. If the total number is 8 cups or more, you are drinking enough. (This method is the hardest because it involves measuring and adding fractions of cups (1/4, 1/3, ½). We will not discuss it here, but if you are a fraction whiz, feel free to try it.)

Instructions for Method #1 (Adding Ounces of Fluid):

1. First, find out how many ounces your cups and glasses hold. Here's how:
    ◆ Fill a glass with water.
    ◆ Now pour the water into a measuring cup.
    ◆ Write down how many ounces of water are in the measuring cup. This is how many ounces your glass can hold. (You will probably remember this without your notes soon.)
    ◆ If you use several different types of cups and glasses in your home, figure out how much each type holds. (Some might hold 6 ounces. Some might hold 8 or more.) Follow the steps above and write down how many ounces each type holds.

2. Every time you drink something from a cup or glass, write down how many ounces you drank.

3. If you drink something from a bottle or can, look at the label to see how many ounces are in that container. Write down that amount if you finish the whole bottle or can. If you just drink half, divide the number of ounces in the bottle by 2. For example, the bottle holds 20 ounces and you drank half the bottle: 20 divided by 2 equals 10.

4. For the foods listed on the chart above (soup, popsicles, etc.), look at the container or package. It should tell you how many ounces there are in one serving. If you eat one serving, write down the number of ounces for one serving. If you eat 2 or 3 servings, multiply the ounces in one serving by 2 or 3. For example, there might be 8 ounces of soup in one serving. You ate 2 servings. So, 8 x 2 equals 16.

5. Sometimes the serving size for a liquid food is given in cups, not ounces. If this happens, you should know that 1 cup is the same as 8 ounces. (Also, ½ cup is the same as 4 ounces and ¾ cup is the same as 6 ounces.)

6. If you have a drink in a restaurant, there are two ways to tell how many ounces you drank:
    ◆ Ask your server or the person at the counter how many ounces are in the drink.
    ◆ Estimate the ounces by looking at the chart on Estimating Fluids below.

7. At the end of the day, add up how many ounces of fluid you drank or ate. (You can use a calculator!) If the total is 64 oz. or more, you are drinking enough.

Instructions for Method #2 (Adding ML of Fluid):

1. First, find out how many milliliters (ml) your cups and glasses hold. Here's how:
    - ◆ Fill a glass with water.
    - ◆ Now pour the water into a measuring cup.
    - ◆ Write down how many ml of water are in the measuring cup. This is how many ounces your glass can hold. (You will probably remember this without your notes soon.)
    - ◆ If you use several different types of cups and glasses in your home, figure out how much each type holds. (Some might hold 180 ml. Some might hold 240 or more.) Follow the steps above and write down how many ml each type holds.

2. Every time you drink something from a cup or glass, write down how many ml you drank.

3. If you drink something from a bottle or can, look at the label to see how many milliliters are in that container. Write down that amount if you finish the whole bottle or can. If you just drink half, divide the number of ml in the bottle by 2. For example, the bottle holds 500 ml and you drank half the bottle: 500 divided by 2 equals 250.

4. For the foods listed on the chart above (soup, popsicles, etc.), look at the container or package. It should tell you how many milliliters there are in one serving. If you eat one serving, write down the number of ounces for one serving. If you eat 2 or 3 servings, multiply the ml in one serving by 2 or 3. For example, there might be 240 ounces of soup in one serving. You ate 2 servings. So, 2 x 240 equals 480.

5. If you have a drink in a restaurant, there are two ways to tell how many ml you drank:
    - ◆ Ask your server or the person at the counter how many ml are in the drink.
    - ◆ Estimate the ounces by looking at the chart on Estimating Fluids below.

6. At the end of the day, add up how many milliliters of fluid you drank or ate. (You can use a calculator!) If the total is 2000 ml (2 liters) or more, you are drinking enough.

Estimating Fluids

Sometimes you might not be sure how much you drank. No problem! You can use this chart if:

- ◆ Someone serves you a drink and you don't know what size cup it's in.
- ◆ You forget to look at a label to see how many ounces/ml are in a serving.

Type of Beverage	Typical Serving (in ounces or ml)	Typical Serving (in cups)
Carbonated beverages (Soda)	12 oz (360 ml) (small soda in restaurant)	1 ½ cup
Clear broth	6 oz (180 ml)	¾ cup
Coffee/tea	8 oz (240 ml) (large mug)	1 cup
	6 oz (180 ml) (regular-size cup)	¾ cup
	4 oz (120 ml) (small cup)	½ cup
Gelatin, fruited	2 oz (60 ml)	½ cup
Gelatin, plain	4 oz (120 ml)	½ cup
Ice cream	2 oz (60 ml) (about one scoop)	½ cup
Italian ice	2 ½ oz (75 ml) (one scoop or small cup)	½ cup
Juice	4 oz (120 ml) (small juice glass) 8 oz (240 ml) (large juice glass)	½ cup 1 cup
Milk	8 oz (240 ml)	1 cup
	4 oz (120 ml) (in juice glass or on cereal)	½ cup
Popsicle	2 ½ oz or 75 ml	1 whole
Sherbet	2 oz or 60 ml (about one scoop)	½ cup
Cream soup	6 oz (175 ml)	¾ cup
Soup with noodles, rice	6 oz (120 ml)	½ cup
Water	8 oz (240 ml) (regular glass)	1 cup
	6 oz (180 ml)	¾ cup
	4 oz (120 ml) (juice glass)	½ cup
	2 oz (60 ml) (enough to swallow a pill)	¼ cup
Water bottle (from vending machine or store)	about 16 oz (500 ml)	½ liter or 2.1 cups

Replacing Fluids Lost through Exercise

When you exercise, your body loses water through sweat. It is important to replace this water by drinking extra fluids. One way to calculate your needs is to weigh yourself before and after an exercise session. For example, say you walk 2 miles and lose 1 pound. (That weight loss is primarily from water loss.) One pound is equal to 0.45 liters (about 2 cups) of water. Therefore, before, during, or after that walk, you should drink about 2 more cups of fluids (16 oz or 480 ml). This is in addition to the 8 cups (64 oz or 2000 ml) you are already drinking that day.

You can estimate your fluid needs for different amounts of exercise. Keep in mind that hot days will require even more fluids.

Addendum 2: Health Screening Recommendations for Adults with Down Syndrome *(as practiced at the Adult Down Syndrome Center)*

USPSTF: United States Preventive Services Task Force
CTFPHE: Canadian Task Force on the Periodic Health Examination

Condition	Recommendation	Other Special Circumstances	Discussion
Blood pressure (BP)	Annually	Particular attention if: ◆ African-American ◆ Moderate or extreme obesity ◆ First degree relative with hypertension ◆ Previous history of hypertension	USPSTF recommends that BP should be measured "periodically" with the interval left to clinical discretion.
Blood sugar	There is insufficient data to recommend universal screening for diabetes. Consider screening in people who are at high risk.		Due to the higher rate of obesity in adults with DS, we consider checking blood sugar every 1-2 years.
Body measurement ◆ Height and Weight ◆ Calculate Body mass index (BMI) ◆ BMI = (weight kg)/(height m)^2	Annually		USPSTF recommends that body measurements should be measured "periodically" with the interval left to clinical discretion. BMI: Overweight: 25-29.9 Obese: >30

Breast examination	Annually on women (and men) greater than 40 years of age	There are different recommendations from several different organizations. While breast cancer is less common in women with DS, because this is an exam without complications, this recommendation is reasonable. We actually start the breast exams around age 18 - 20 to help the patients get used to the exam and to examine for other potential abnormalities.
Complete blood count (CBC)	Consider annually if person has large red blood cells (common in people with DS)	Screening for the development of anemia
Celiac testing	Once in a lifetime and additionally as indicated by symptoms. Consider every 3-5 years.	The Down Syndrome Medical Interest Group recommends one blood test between ages 2-3. However, celiac disease can occur at any age and is probably more common in middle age. There are no data to direct screening. Therefore, because it can occur at any age, we consider checking every 3-5 years.
Cholesterol	Possibly not indicated	The incidence of coronary artery disease is low in people with DS so this screening may not be indicated. Make the decision for each individual based on risk factors.

Dental	Regularly as recommended by dentist	Consider every 6 months because of the higher incidence of gum disease.
DEXA scans (bone densitometry)	At menopause and every 2 years (if the initial one is normal). In men on high-risk medications. Also for those with celiac disease.	
Digital Rectal Exam of prostate and colon	Not indicated/consider if tolerated.	The USPSTF has indicated that there is insufficient evidence for prostate exams. However, other agencies including the American Cancer Society recommend the exams. For those with DS, based on the life expectancy and the lower incidence of prostate cancer, the exam is not indicated by USPSTF guidelines. However, since there is debate, we consider performing the exam if the person can tolerate it. (See fecal occult blood and/or colonoscopy for discussion on colon cancer.)
Echocardiogram (and/or Cardiology consult)	We recommend these evaluations at least every 5 years in our patients who have had previous surgery. More frequently for those with ongoing heart conditions.	

Fecal occult blood and/or colonoscopy	Not indicated	The incidence of colon cancer is lower in people with DS. There is increased potential for complications due to the greater need for anesthesia for follow-up tests. Therefore, we don't recommend routine screening. (However, at this time, there is limited data.).
Hearing	Every 2 years	Based on studies done on people with intellectual disabilities. (Consider annually in those with recurrent ear infections, fluid in the ears, or hearing aids).
Lateral cervical spine x-rays	There are no data on which to base this recommendation. We recommend every 10 years.	Screening for cervical subluxation
Mammography	Annually after age 40: if woman has a first degree relative with breast cancer (mother, sister), some agencies recommend starting 10 years younger than that relative developed breast cancer (e.g., if mother developed breast cancer at age 45, daughter should get first mammogram at age 35).	There is still much debate, discussion, and study with regards to appropriate screening with mammograms. Recommend counseling between physician and patient with regards to risks of breast cancer and benefits of mammography.

Pap Smears	For women who are not sexually active and not having symptoms: every 3 years (starting at age 21). For those who are sexually active: annually for 2 years, then every 3 years.	We find that many of our patients do not tolerate the speculum exam that is usually performed to obtain the sample. Therefore, we often do the Pap smear blindly (introducing the swab into the vagina without using a speculum to visualize the cervix). We have a very high success rate of obtaining the appropriate cells even without the speculum exam. Therefore, we perform the Pap smear even if we cannot perform a speculum exam.	Pap smears are not indicated for women who have had a hysterectomy for reasons other than cancer. Since the risk of having cervical cancer is negligible in women who are not sexually active and there are risks with anesthesia, we do not recommend sedation/anesthesia for a pap smear if the woman is not sexually active, not having symptoms, and not able to tolerate the exam in the office.
Pelvic exam for ovarian cancer	Regularly with the pap smear		Routine pelvic exam for ovarian cancer is not recommended by USPSTF or CTFPHE. However, CTFPHE states it is reasonable if pelvic done for another reason (pap smear).
Prostate specific antigen	Not indicated. Based on the life expectancy of a man with DS and the lower incidence of prostate cancer.		USPSTF does not recommend PSA testing for any males.
Sexually transmitted diseases	Screen women at risk for Chlamydia and gonorrhea. Offer HIV testing to people (men and women) with another sexually transmitted disease and those in high risk categories.		

Testicular exam	Annual exam	Although there is disagreement on the need for this exam, we recommend it in our patients because: ◆ higher incidence of testicular cancer in men with DS ◆ reduced ability to self-report abnormality ◆ high cure rate of the disease
Thyroid	Annually (TSH and possibly T4)	High prevalence of hypothyroidism in people with DS and likelihood that symptoms will be overlooked.
Tuberculosis	Screen high risk individuals	High risk individuals: Close contacts of someone with TB; people infected with HIV; people who inject illicit drugs; people with medical risk factors known to increase the risk of TB if infection occurs; residents of high-risk congregate settings; people who currently live in a country with high incidence of TB or lived in one within the last 5 years (does not include U.S. or Canada)
Urinalysis	Not indicated for people without symptoms	
Vision screening	Every 2 years—consider more often if the person wears glasses or has a history of eye conditions such as keratoconus or cataracts	Based on a large study done on people with intellectual disabilities. Important to include glaucoma screening.

Immunizations

Condition	Recommendation	Other Special Circumstances	Discussion
Gardasil (human papillomavirus)	We recommend discussing giving the 3-shot series between the ages of 18-26. It is now recommended to offer it to women and men.		In women it prevents cervical, vulvar, and vaginal cancer and genital warts. In men, it prevents genital warts. The second shot follows the first by 2 months and the third follows the second by 4 months.
Hepatitis B	All individuals who live in a residential facility or work in a "workshop" setting.		If no history of hepatitis B or hepatitis B vaccine: draw serological markers (HBsAb, HBsAg, HBcAb). If negative, give 3-shot series; draw HBsAb 4-6 weeks after the third immunization to check for immunity (that the vaccine worked) and consider additional vaccination if vaccine did not work.
Influenza	Annually for all individuals. Particularly those older than 50 years of age, those living in residential facilities, those with chronic health conditions (e.g. diabetes, heart disease, etc), pregnant women who will be beyond their first trimester of pregnancy during the influenza season.		Early aging issues in people with DS led to recommendation of lower age.
Pneumococcus	Those over age 50 and those under 50 with chronic health conditions (heart disease, lung disease, diabetes, etc).		Give one injection at age 50. (Early aging issues in people with DS led to recommendations of lower age.) In higher risk individuals who received their first shot at a younger age, repeat at age 50.

Shingles	A single dose is recommended at age 60 or after	It might be considered at a younger age (e.g., age 50) for people with Down syndrome due to early aging issues, but lack of Medicare reimbursement for people less than 60 years of age has limited its use.
Tetanus-diphtheria-pertussis (dTaP) or diphtheria-tetanus (dT)	Every 10 years	When due for next dT, if haven't received the dTaP since childhood, give dTaP, and in 10 years resume dT every 10 years.
Varicella (chicken pox)	If there is not a history of chicken pox or chicken pox vaccine, give vaccination. It is a 2-shot vaccination given 1-2 months apart	If there is no known history of chicken pox or chicken pox vaccine, we recommend checking a varicella IgG titer to check for immunity. Even without a known history, many people have previously had chicken pox.

Counseling

Condition	Recommendation	Other Special Circumstances	Discussion
Cigarette smoking	For those who smoke, regular counseling regarding smoking cessation.		
Nutrition	Regular nutrition guidance based on BMI calculation and dietary assessment.		
Physical Activity	Regular assessment of physical activity and counseling regarding regular physical activity.		

Resources

Adult Congenital Heart Disease Association
6757 Greene St., Ste. 335
Philadelphia, PA 19119
888-921-ACHA;
www.achaheart.org

Adult Down Syndrome Center
1999 Dempster St.
Park Ridge, IL 60068
847-318-2377
http://www.advocatehealth.com/adultdown
Facebook: adultdownsyndromeclinic
     The ADSC of Lutheran General Hospital is a multidisciplinary clinic that serves adolescents and adults with Down syndrome from Illinois. Although the clinic does not have the resources to serve patients from other states, it maintains a website with information that may be helpful to families and professionals from around the world.

Alzheimer's Association
225 N. Michigan Ave.
Chicago, IL 60601
800-272-3900; 312-335-8700
www.alz.org

American Diabetes Association
1701 N. Beauregard St.
Alexandria, VA 22311
800-DIABETES (800-342-2383)
www.diabetes.org

American Sleep Apnea Association
6856 Eastern Ave., NW, Ste. 203
Washington, DC 20012
202-293-3650
www.sleepapnea.org

American Thyroid Association
800-THYROID (800-849-7643)
www.thyroid.org

The Arc of the United States
1010 Wayne Ave., Ste. 650
Silver Spring, MD 20910
301-565-3842; 800-433-5255
www.thearc.org

Arthritis Foundation
P.O. Box 7669
Atlanta, GA 30357-7669
800-283-7800
www.arthritis.org

Best Buddies
100 SE Second St., Ste. 2200
Miami, FL 33131
800-89-BUDDY (892-8339)
www.bestbuddies.org

Best Buddies Canada
907-1243 Islington Ave.
Toronto, Ontario M8X 1Y9
Canada
888-779-0061
www.bestbuddies.ca

Canadian Down Syndrome Society
5005 Dalhousie Dr., NW, #283
Calgary, Alberta T3A 5RB
Canada
www.cdss.ca

Caring Connections
State Advance Directives Downloads
1731 King St., Ste. 100
Alexandria, VA 22314
800-658-8898
www.caringinfo.org/stateaddownload

Celiac Disease Foundation
13251 Ventura Blvd., Ste. 1
Studio City, CA 91604
818-990-2354
www.celiac.org

Centers for Medicare and Medicaid Services
7500 Security Blvd.
Baltimore, MD 21244
877-267-2323
www.cms.hhs.gov

Disability.Gov
"Connecting the Disability Community to Information and Opportunities"
www.disability.gov

Down Syndrome: Health Issues
www.ds-health.com

Epilepsy Canada
2255B Queen St., Ste. 336
Toronto, Ontario M4E 1G3
Canada
877-734-0873
www.epilepsy.ca

Epilepsy Foundation of America
8301 Professional Place
Landover, MD 20785
800-332-1000
www.efa.org

Eyecare America
The Foundation of the American Academy of Ophthalmology
P.O. Box 429098
San Francisco, CA 94142-9098
877-887-6327
www.eyecareamerica.com

GovBenefits.gov
800-333-4636
www.govbenefits.gov

Moyamoya Disease Information Page
National Institute of Neurological Disorders and Stroke
www.ninds.nih.gov

National Alopecia Areata Foundation
14 Mitchell Blvd.
San Rafael, CA 94903
415-472-3780
www.naaf.org

National Association for Continence
P.O. Box 1019
Charleston, SC 29402-1019
800-BLADDER; 843-377-0900
www.nafc.org

National Association for Down Syndrome
P.O. Box 206
Wilmette, IL 60091
630-325-9112
www.nads.org

National Down Syndrome Congress
1370 Center Dr., Ste. 102
Atlanta, GA 30338
800-232-6372; 770-604-9898 (fax)
www.ndsccenter.org

National Down Syndrome Society
666 Broadway
8th Floor
New York, NY 10012
800-221-4602
www.ndss.org

National Eye Institute
Information Office
National Institutes of Health
31 Center Dr.
Bethesda, MD 20892
301-496-5248
www.nei.nih.gov

National Institute on Deafness and Other Communication Disorders
National Institutes of Health
31 Center Dr., MSC 2320
Bethesda, MD 20892-2320
800-241-1044; 800-241-1055 (TTY)
www.nidcd.nih.gov

Person Centered Planning Education Site
Cornell University
Employment and Disability Institute
Ithaca, NY 14853
607-255-7727
www.ilr.cornell.edu/edi/pcp/index.html

Social Security Administration
Office of Public Inquiries
6401 Security Blvd.
Baltimore, MD 21235
800-772-1213
www.socialsecurity.gov

Special Olympics
113319th St., NW
Washington, DC 20036
202-628-3630; 800-700-8585
www.specialolympics.org

Special Olympics Canada
60 St. Clair Avenue East, Suite 700
Toronto, Ontario M4T 1N5
Canada
416-927-9050
www.specialolympics.ca

State Coverage Initiatives
Robert Wood Johnson Foundation
www.statecoverage.net
  This website gives state-specific information on who qualifies for Medicaid based on how their earnings compare to the federal poverty level (FPL). For example, in Maryland, working adults with disabilities can earn 300% of FPL and still qualify; nonworking adults with disabilities can only earn 74% of FPL.

References

American Psychiatric Association. (2000). *Diagnostic and Statistical Manual of Mental Disorders,* Fourth Edition, Text Revision. Washington, DC: American Psychiatric Association.

Baladerian, N. (1991). Sexual abuse of people with developmental disabilities. *Sexuality and Disability, 9(4),* 323-35.

Bandura, A. (1977). *Social Learning Theory.* New York, NY: General Learning Press.

Barger, E., Wacker, J., Macy, R., Parish, S. (2009). Sexual assault prevention for women with intellectual disabilities: A critical review of the evidence. *Intellectual and Developmental Disabilities 47 (4),* 249-62.

Beck, A., (1995). *Cognitive Therapy: Basics and Beyond.* New York: Guilford Press.

Carter, M., McCaughey, E., Annaz, D., Hill, C. M. (2009). Sleep problems in a Down syndrome population. *Archives of Disease in Childhood 94*(4):308-10.

Cassano, P., and Fava, M. (2002). Depression and public health: An overview. *Journal of Psychosomatic Research 53:* 849-57.

Chicoine, B., and McGuire, D. (1997). Longevity of a woman with Down syndrome: A case study. *Mental Retardation 35:* 477-79

Colombo, M.L., et al. (1989). Ascorbic acid in children with Down's syndrome. *Minerva Pediatrica 41(4):*189-92.

Couwenhoven, T. (2007). *Teaching Children with Down Syndrome about Their Bodies, Boundaries, and Sexuality: A Guide for Parents and Professionals.* Bethesda, MD: Woodbine House.

Devenny D., Silverman, W.P., Hill, A.L., Jenkins, E., Sersen, E.A., Wisniewski, K.E (1996). Normal ageing in adults with Down's syndrome: A longitudinal study. *Journal of Intellectual Disability Research 40:*208–221

Epilepsy Ontario. Epilepsy/seizures in Down syndrome. www.epilepsyontario.org. *Epocrates Essentials.* Version 1.00 (2008). Epocrates , Inc.

Franceshi, C., Chiricolo, I.M., Licastro F., Zannotti, M., Masi, M., Mocchegiani, E., Fabris, N. (1988). Oral zinc supplementation in Down's syndrome: Restoration of thymic endocrine activity and of some immune defects. *Journal of Intellectual Disability Research 32(3):*169-81.

Fujiura, G.T. (1998). Demography of family households. *American Journal of Mental Retardation 103:* 225-235.

Furey, E. (1994). Sexual abuse of adults with mental retardation: Who and where. *Mental Retardation 32 (3):* 173-80.

Heller, T. (1982). Social disruption and residential relocation of mentally retarded children. *American Journal of Mental Deficiency* 87: 48-55.

Hingsburger, D. (1995). *Just Say Know: Understanding and Reducing the Risk of Sexual Victimization of People with Developmental Disabilities.* Richmond Hill, Ontario: Diverse City Press.

Hirsch, L. W. *CIRCLES I: Intimacy & Relationships.* Santa Barbara, CA: James Stanfield Publishing Company (www.stanfield.com).

Johnson, N., Fahey, C., Chicoine, B., Chong, G., Gitelman, D. (2003). Effects of donepezil on cognitive functioning in Down syndrome. *American Journal on Mental Retardation 108 (6):* 367-72

Kanis, J.A., Delmas, P., Burckhardt, P., et al. (1997). Position paper: Guidelines for diagnosis and management of osteoporosis. *Osteoporosis International 7*: 390-406. Kaplan, H.I. and Sadock, B.J., eds. (1995). *Psychiatry: Comprehensive Textbook of Psychiatry.* Baltimore: Williams and Wilkins.

Katon, W., and Ciechanowski, P. (2002). Impact of major depression on chronic medical illness. *Journal of Psychosomatic Research 53:* 859-63.

Kirby, D. (2008). The impact of abstinence and comprehensive sex and STD/HIV education programs on adolescent sexual behavior. *Sexuality Research and Social Policy 5*(3):6-17.

Kirby, D. (2007). *Emerging Answers 2007: Research Finding on Programs to Reduce Teen Pregnancy and Sexually Transmitted Diseases.* Washington, DC: The National Campaign to Prevent Teen and Unplanned Pregnancy.

Kishnani, P.S., Spriidigliozzi, G.A., Heller, J.H., Sullivan, J.A., Doraiswamy, P.M., Krisnan, K.R.R. (2001). Donepezil for Down's syndrome. *American Journal of Psychiatry 158:*143.

Leshin, L. Down syndrome and epilepsy. www.ds-health.com/epilepsy.htm.

Luke, A., Rozien, N.J., Sutton, M., Schoeller, D.A. (1994). Energy expenditure in children with Down syndrome: Correcting metabolic rate for movement. *Journal of Pediatrics, 125(5):* 829-38.

Martinez-Cue, C., Baamonde, C., Lumbreras, M.A., Vallina, I.F., Dierssen, M., Florez, J. (1999). A murine model for Down syndrome shows reduced responsiveness to pain. *Neuroreport 10*(5):1119-22.

Mayo Foundation for Medical Education and Research website. www.MayoClinic.com.

McGuire, D., and Chicoine, B. (2006). *Mental Wellness in Adults with Down Syndrome: A Guide to Emotional and Behavioral Strengths and Challenges.* Bethesda, MD: Woodbine House.

Minuchin, S., and Fishman, H.C. (1981). *Family Therapy Techniques.* Cambridge, MA: Harvard University Press.

Miyoshi, Y., Tajiri, H., Okaniwa, M., Terasawa, S., Fujisawa, T., Iizuka, T., and Ozono, K. (2008). Hepatitis C virus infection and interferon therapy in patients with Down syndrome. *Pediatrics International 50(1):*7-11.

National Institute of Neurological Disorders and Stroke. Moyamoya disease information page. www.ninds.nih.gov/disorders/moyamoya/moyamoya.htm.

National Institute on Aging. Can Alzheimer's disease be prevented? www.nia.nih.gov/Alzheimers/Publications/ADPrevented.

Quint, E.H., and Elkins, T.E. (1997). Cervical cytology in women with mental retardation. *Obstetrics and Gynecology 89(1):*123-6.

Rosenberg, M. (1965). *Society and Adolescent Self-image.* Princeton, NJ: Princeton University Press.

Rubin, S.S., Rimmer, J.H., Chicoine, B., Braddock, D., and McGuire, D.E. (1998). Overweight prevalence in persons with Down syndrome. *Mental Retardation* 36: 175-81.

Scott, J. (1996). Cognitive therapy of affective disorders: A review. *Journal of Affective Disorders 37*:1-11.

Seligman, M. E. P. (1975). *Helplessness: On Depression, Development and Death.* San Francisco: W H. Freeman.

Shott, S., Amin, R., Chini, B., Heubi, C., Hotze, S., Akers, R. (2006). "Obstructive sleep apnea: Should all children with Down syndrome be tested?" *Archives of Otolaryngology—Head & Neck Surgery 132 (4):* 432-6.

Sullivan P., M., & Knutson, J.F. (2000). Maltreatment and disabilities: A population based study. *Child Abuse and Neglect 24 (10):* 1257-73.

Sussan, T.E.,Yang, A., Li, F., Ostrowski, M.C., and Reeves, R.H. (2008). Trisomy represses Apc^{Min}-mediated tumours in mouse models of Down's syndrome. *Nature 451:* 73-75

Trois, M.S., Capone, G.T., Lutz, J.A., Melendres, M.C., Schwartz, A.R., Collop, N.A., and Marcus, C.L. (August 15, 2009). Obstructive sleep apnea in adults with Down syndrome. *Journal of Clinical Sleep Medicine 5 (4):* 317-323.

U.S. National Institutes of Health. Evaluating the efficacy and safety of donepezil hydrochloride (Aricept) in the treatment of the cognitive dysfunction exhibited by children with Down syndrome, aged 6-10. www.clinicaltrials.gov.

U.S. National Institutes of Health. Evaluating the efficacy and safety of donepezil hydrochloride (Aricept) in the treatment of the cognitive dysfunction exhibited by children with Down syndrome, aged 11-17. www.clinicaltrials.gov.

Valenti-Hein, D. & Schwartz, L. (1995). *The Sexual Abuse Interview for Those with Developmental Disabilities.* Santa Barbara, CA: James Stanfield.

Walsh, W., Cross, T., Jones, L., Simone, M., and Kolko, D. (2007). Which sexual abuse victims receive a forensic medical examination? The impact of Children's Advocacy Centers. *Child Abuse and Neglect 31:* 1053-1068

Yokoyama,T., Tamura, H., Tsukamoto, H., Yamane, K., and Mishima, H.K. (2006). Prevalence of glaucoma in adults with Down's syndrome. *Japanese Journal of Ophthalmology 50:*274–76.

Index

About the Authors:

♦ ♦ ♦ ♦ ♦ ♦ ♦ ♦ ♦ ♦ ♦ ♦ ♦ ♦ ♦ ♦ ♦ ♦

Brian Chicoine, M.D., is the medical director of the Adult Down Syndrome Center of Lutheran General Hospital in suburban Chicago. **Dennis McGuire, Ph.D.,** is the Director of Psychosocial Services for the Adult Down Syndrome Center. Together they founded The Center in 1992 and have served over 4500 teens and adults with Down syndrome since its inception. Both authors make regular presentations to parent and professional audiences about their work at the Center.

Brian Chicoine received his medical degree from Loyola University in Chicago from the Stritch School of Medicine. He did his residency at the Lutheran General Hospital Department of Family Medicine in Park Ridge, Illinois, where he currently works. Dr. Chicoine has spent over 30 years working with people with intellectual disabilities in a variety of capacities. The father of three, he lives with his family in Arlington Heights, Illinois.

Dennis McGuire received his Masters degree from the University of Chicago and his doctorate from the University of Illinois at Chicago. He has worked for more than 30 years in the fields of mental health and developmental disabilities. He lives in Oak Park, Illinois, with his wife and son.